CARDIAC
COMPLICATIONS
OF CANCER THERAPY

Edited by
Anecita P. Fadol, PhD, RN, FNP-BC, FAANP

Oncology Nursing Society
Pittsburgh, Pennsylvania

ONS Publications Department
Executive Director, Professional Practice and Programs: Elizabeth M. Wertz Evans, RN, MPM, CPHQ, CPHIMS, FACMPE
Publisher and Director of Publications: Barbara Sigler, RN, MNEd
Managing Editor: Lisa M. George, BA
Technical Content Editor: Angela D. Klimaszewski, RN, MSN
Staff Editor II: Amy Nicoletti, BA
Copy Editor: Laura Pinchot, BA
Graphic Designer: Dany Sjoen

Library of Congress Cataloging-in-Publication Data

Cardiac complications of cancer therapy / edited by Anecita P. Fadol.
    p. ; cm.
 Includes bibliographical references and index.
 ISBN 978-1-935864-24-0 (alk. paper)
 I. Fadol, Anecita P. II. Oncology Nursing Society.
 [DNLM: 1. Neoplasms--therapy. 2. Antineoplastic Agents--adverse effects. 3. Cardiovascular Diseases--etiology. 4. Neoplasms--complications. QZ 266]

 616.1'2071--dc23

                                                                                    2012038603

Publisher's Note

Printed in the United States of America

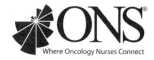

Oncology Nursing Society
Integrity • Innovation • Stewardship • Advocacy • Excellence • Inclusiveness

Contributors

Editor

Anecita P. Fadol, PhD, RN, FNP-BC, FAANP
Assistant Professor, Departments of Nursing and Cardiology
University of Texas MD Anderson Cancer Center
Houston, Texas
Chapter 7. Hypertension in Patients With Cancer; Chapter 10. Heart Failure in Patients With Cancer

Authors

Sarah Anderson, MSN, APRN, ANP-BC
Research Nurse Specialist
Vanderbilt University Medical Center
Nashville, Tennessee
*Chapter 2. Anthracyclines, Trastuzumab, and
   Cardiomyopathy*

Virginia Beggs, MSc, FNP-C, APRN
Nurse Practitioner
Cardiomyopathy and Heart Failure Program
Dartmouth-Hitchcock Heart and Vascular Center
Lebanon, New Hampshire
Chapter 4. Radiation Therapy and the Heart

Courtney L. Bickford, PharmD, BCPS
Clinical Pharmacy Specialist, Cardiology
University of Texas MD Anderson Cancer Center
Houston, Texas
Chapter 3. Targeted Therapies and Cardiomyopathy

Sue Buzzurro, RN, MS, FNP-BC
Nurse Practitioner
Division of Hematology/Oncology
Robert H. Lurie Comprehensive Cancer Center
Northwestern Medical Faculty Foundation
Chicago, Illinois
*Chapter 14. Cardiovascular Evaluation of Patients
   With Cancer Prior to Chemotherapy and Surgery*

Jessica S. Coviello, DNP, APRN, ANP-BC
Associate Professor
Yale University School of Nursing
New Haven, Connecticut
*Chapter 15. Screening and Management of Cardio-
   vascular Risk Factors in Cancer Survivors*

Allison E. Fee, MSN, RN, ANP
Cardiology Nurse Practitioner
University of Texas MD Anderson Cancer Center
Houston, Texas
*Chapter 5. Acute Coronary Syndromes in Patients
   With Cancer*

Cezar Iliescu, MD
Assistant Professor of Cardiology
University of Texas MD Anderson Cancer Center
Houston, Texas
*Chapter 5. Acute Coronary Syndromes in Patients
   With Cancer*

M. Tish Knobf, PhD, RN, FAAN, AOCN®
Professor
Yale University School of Nursing
New Haven, Connecticut
*Chapter 15. Screening and Management of Cardio-
   vascular Risk Factors in Cancer Survivors*

Darla Labasse, RN, BSN, BBA
Cardiac Device Nurse
University of Texas Medical School and MD Anderson Cancer Center
Houston, Texas
Chapter 13. Ventricular Dysrhythmias and Cardiac Implantable Electronic Devices

Tara Lech, PharmD, BCPS
Clinical Pharmacy Specialist, Cardiology
University of Texas MD Anderson Cancer Center
Houston, Texas
Chapter 7. Hypertension in Patients With Cancer; Chapter 12. QT Prolongation and Antineoplastic Agents

Monika J. Leja, MD
Assistant Professor, Department of Cardiology
University of Michigan Hospitals
Ann Arbor, Michigan
Chapter 1. Cardiovascular Anatomy and Cardiac Malignancy

Sheryl W. Murphy, RN, BSN, MSN, FNP
Advanced Practice Nurse, Cardiology
University of Texas MD Anderson Cancer Center
Houston, Texas
Chapter 11. Atrial Dysrhythmias and Atrioventricular Blocks; Chapter 13. Ventricular Dysrhythmias and Cardiac Implantable Electronic Devices

Claire Pace, MSN, FNP-C, ACHPN
Nurse Practitioner, Radiation Oncology
Dartmouth-Hitchcock Medical Center
Lebanon, New Hampshire
Chapter 4. Radiation Therapy and the Heart

Tara Reilly-Donovan, RN, MSN, ACNP-BC
Cardiology Nurse Practitioner
Memorial Sloan-Kettering Cancer Center
New York, New York
Chapter 9. Stem Cell Transplantation and Cardiovascular Adverse Events

Edgar C. Salire, RN, MSN, NP-C
Advanced Practice Nurse, Cardiology
University of Texas MD Anderson Cancer Center
Houston, Texas
Chapter 8. Venous Thromboembolism; Chapter 11. Atrial Dysrhythmias and Atrioventricular Blocks

Brenda Wimberly White, RN, BSN
Research Nurse Specialist
Vanderbilt University Medical Center
Nashville, Tennessee
Chapter 2. Anthracyclines, Trastuzumab, and Cardiomyopathy

Myrshia L. Woods, MHS, PA-C
Physician Assistant, Department of Cardiology
University of Texas MD Anderson Cancer Center
Houston, Texas
Chapter 6. Cardiac Inflammatory Conditions and Cardiac Tamponade in Patients With Cancer; Chapter 7. Hypertension in Patients With Cancer

Disclosure

Editors and authors of books and guidelines provided by the Oncology Nursing Society are expected to disclose to the readers any significant financial interest or other relationships with the manufacturer(s) of any commercial products.

A vested interest may be considered to exist if a contributor is affiliated with or has a financial interest in commercial organizations that may have a direct or indirect interest in the subject matter. A "financial interest" may include, but is not limited to, being a shareholder in the organization; being an employee of the commercial organization; serving on an organization's speakers bureau; or receiving research from the organization. An "affiliation" may be holding a position on an advisory board or some other role of benefit to the commercial organization. Vested interest statements appear in the front matter for each publication.

Contributors are expected to disclose any unlabeled or investigational use of products discussed in their content. This information is acknowledged solely for the information of the readers.

The contributors provided the following disclosure and vested interest information:

The authors have no relevant information to disclose.

Contents

Preface ix

Foreword xi

Chapter 1. Cardiovascular Anatomy and Cardiac Malignancy 1
    Overview 1
    Left Atrial Structures and Masses 1
    Left Ventricular Structures and Masses.. 6
    Right Atrial Structures and Masses 6
    Right Ventricular Structures and Masses 8
    Pericardium.. 9
    Metastatic Tumors to the Heart 9
    Diagnosis of Cardiac Tumors.. 9
    Conclusion 10
    References 10

Chapter 2. Anthracyclines, Trastuzumab, and Cardiomyopathy 13
    Introduction.. 13
    Pathophysiology... 14
    Risk Factors for the Development of Cardiotoxicity.. 14
    Clinical Presentation of Cardiomyopathy in Patients With Cancer 16
    Laboratory and Diagnostic Tests 19
    Management of Cardiomyopathy in Patients With Cancer.................................. 22
    Medical Management 24
    Conclusion 26
    References 27

Chapter 3. Targeted Therapies and Cardiomyopathy... 31
    Introduction.. 31
    Incidence of Left Ventricular Dysfunction Associated With Targeted Anticancer Therapy.................. 32
    Mechanism of Action of Targeted Therapies.. 32
    Monitoring of Left Ventricular Dysfunction With Targeted Therapy 36
    Treatment 37
    Conclusion 37
    References 37

Chapter 4. Radiation Therapy and the Heart 39
    Introduction.. 39

Epidemiology..40
Radiation Oncology Basics 40
Pathophysiology...42
Late Cardiovascular Effects in Patients With Cancer 43
Nursing Implications 47
Conclusion 50
References 51

Chapter 5. Acute Coronary Syndromes in Patients With Cancer **55**
Introduction...55
Pathophysiology and Mechanisms of Coronary Artery Disease 55
Risk Factors and Precipitating Factors 56
Signs and Symptoms of Acute Coronary Syndrome 58
Diagnostic Criteria and Testing...58
Classification of Acute Coronary Syndromes 65
Pharmacologic Therapy 67
Nursing Management..70
Prevention 71
Conclusion 73
References 73

Chapter 6. Cardiac Inflammatory Conditions and Cardiac Tamponade in Patients With Cancer **77**
Introduction...77
Pericarditis 78
Myocarditis 82
Endocarditis 85
Cardiac Tamponade 86
Conclusion 92
References 92

Chapter 7. Hypertension in Patients With Cancer **95**
Introduction...95
Definition...96
Pathophysiology 97
Risk Factors 99
Diagnostic Workup..100
Management of Hypertension 101
Nursing Implications 105
Conclusion 105
References 106

Chapter 8. Venous Thromboembolism **109**
Introduction...109
Pathogenesis..110
Signs and Symptoms 110
Differential Diagnosis 112
Diagnostic Tests 113
Treatment 117
Management of Venous Thromboembolism Recurrence in Patients With Cancer............122
Preventive Measures 123
Nursing Implications 125
Conclusion 126
References 126

Chapter 9. Stem Cell Transplantation and Cardiovascular Adverse Events............................ **131**
Introduction...131
Diseases Treated With Hematopoietic Stem Cell Transplantation 131
Types of Hematopoietic Stem Cell Transplantation...132
Methods of Harvesting Cells 133
Patient Selection..133
Pretransplant Cardiac Evaluation...136
Pretransplant Conditioning...137
Engraftment and Cardiac Complications During Engraftment...139
Cardiac Complications With Stem Cell Transplantation 141
Transplant in Patients With Known Cardiac Disease...151
Long-Term Cardiac Effects 151
Conclusion 153
References 154

Chapter 10. Heart Failure in Patients With Cancer **159**
Introduction...159
What Is Heart Failure?...160
Classification of Heart Failure 163
Initial Evaluation for Possible Heart Failure Diagnosis in Patients With Cancer.......................167
Diagnostic Tests for Chronic Heart Failure in Patients With Cancer......................................170
Management of Heart Failure in Patients With Cancer...173
Symptom Management in Patients With Cancer and Heart Failure 185
Conclusion 185
References 188

Chapter 11. Atrial Dysrhythmias and Atrioventricular Blocks.. **195**
Introduction...195
Basic Electrocardiogram Interpretation 195
Atrial Fibrillation 197
Atrial Flutter..205
Supraventricular Tachycardia 207
Sick Sinus Syndrome 209
Atrioventricular Blocks 210
Conclusion 213
References 213

Chapter 12. QT Prolongation and Antineoplastic Agents **217**
Introduction...217
Incidence...217
Diagnosis 218
Pathophysiology...220
Medications That Cause QT Prolongation...220
Torsades de Pointes 223
Conclusion 224
References 225

Chapter 13. Ventricular Dysrhythmias and Cardiac Implantable Electronic Devices **227**
Introduction...227
Premature Ventricular Contractions 227
Ventricular Tachycardia 230
Torsades de Pointe 232
Ventricular Fibrillation 234
Cardiovascular Implantable Electronic Devices 235

Conclusion 243
References 247

Chapter 14. Cardiovascular Evaluation of Patients With Cancer Prior to Chemotherapy and Surgery.. 251
Introduction..251
Epidemiology..251
Prechemotherapy Evaluation...252
Preoperative Cardiac Evaluation for Noncardiac Surgery 252
Preoperative Management of Anticoagulation 257
Anticoagulation in Special Situations 259
Coronary Stents and Perioperative Major Adverse Cardiac Events...........................261
Conclusion 262
References 263

Chapter 15. Screening and Management of Cardiovascular Risk Factors in Cancer Survivors 267
Introduction..267
Cardiovascular Risk Factors and Cardiovascular Disease in the General Population 268
Cardiovascular Disease Risk in the Diagnosis and Treatment of Women With Breast Cancer 271
Cardiovascular Risk in Men...276
Cardiovascular Risk Identification and Management in Survivorship 277
Screening and Surveillance for Cardiac Risk 277
Management 284
Conclusion 287
References 287

Index 297

Preface

The cardiac complications of anticancer therapy represent an emerging clinical issue not only for established chemotherapeutics but also for the novel molecular targeted therapies used in the treatment of several forms of cancer. Moreover, the burden of cardiac complications in cancer survivors is increasing because the population is aging and because of the potential long-term adverse effects of cancer therapy. Patients undergoing cancer treatment and cancer survivors are depending on us as care providers to be vigilant in evaluating for acute and chronic or late physical effects of cancer therapy—some of which are life threatening and may occur years after therapy.

An abundance of literature on the management of cardiac problems is available, with several comprehensive textbooks and countless journals published on the management of cardiac issues. However, the complexity of cardiac problems in conjunction with a cancer diagnosis in an individual requires the clinician to sort through enormous repositories of information, and finding answers to questions encountered in caring for this patient population can be challenging. The efficient utilization of time is key to finding the appropriate resource to guide clinicians in optimizing care delivery.

This book was developed to provide the essentials of clinical management in a readable and understandable format for busy clinicians. It provides complete yet concise and easily accessible information on the management of the most common cardiac complications of cancer therapy. The contributing authors from well-recognized cancer centers around the country have simplified key concepts from clinical guidelines and integrated clinical experience to help clinicians on a daily basis as they care for patients with cardiac problems in the setting of cancer. The book is organized in a systematic fashion to facilitate easy referencing. It begins with an overview of the cardiovascular anatomy, physiology, and malignancy, followed by the cancer treatments that have potential cardiotoxic side effects. The succeeding chapters cover the various cardiovascular problems that may result from cancer therapy, with a brief discussion of pathophysiologic mechanisms, risk factors, signs and symptoms, diagnostic evaluation, and medical and nursing management. The final chapter explores issues related to cancer survivors, with emphasis on the screening, monitoring, and management of cardiovascular risk factors and long-term cardiac complications of cancer therapy. I hope that this book will help clinicians as they encounter the complexity of the management of the cardiac complications of cancer therapy in patients with cancer and cancer survivors.

Anecita P. Fadol, PhD, RN, FNP-BC, FAANP

Foreword

As increasing numbers of individuals diagnosed with cancer are now achieving long-term survivorship, cardiac complications resulting from cancer therapy are emerging, often many years after completing treatment. These cardiac effects can profoundly challenge the quality and quantity of life for cancer survivors. The challenges are magnified because of the many and varied potential cardiovascular complications associated with cancer therapy. Nursing professionals must become aware of these potential complications and have readily accessible resources to assist in managing their patients.

This is the first clinical reference book on the cardiac complications of cancer therapy written for nurses and mid-level providers. The book takes an integrated approach to the unique issues of cardiac disease within the context of cancer care. This quick-reference resource is written specifically to support the professional clinician, describing the assessment and management of the common cardiac complications of cancer therapy.

Busy clinicians are confronted by increasing numbers of anticancer drug therapies with potential cardiotoxic adverse effects (e.g., targeted therapies) at the same time that the general population is experiencing significant improvements in life expectancy. These combine to create larger numbers of oncologic patients requiring long-term monitoring of potential health complications, including cardiotoxicity. This book fills the need for an easy-to-use reference that includes the concise pathophysiology, signs and symptoms, diagnostic tests, and medical and nursing management of individuals with cardiac complications of cancer therapy.

Barbara L. Summers, PhD, RN, NEA-BC, FAAN
Professor and Chair, Department of Nursing
Vice President and Chief Nursing Officer
Division Head, Nursing
University of Texas MD Anderson Cancer Center
Houston, Texas

CHAPTER 1

Cardiovascular Anatomy and Cardiac Malignancy

Monika J. Leja, MD

Overview

This chapter will cover basic cardiac anatomy and tumors that are commonly found in the heart. The heart is divided into four chambers: left atrium, right atrium, left ventricle, and right ventricle. Different cardiac chambers have a propensity to have different cardiac masses or tumors. Cardiac tumors are rare entities: metastasis to the heart from another primary cancer is 30 times more likely (Bisel, Wróblewski, & La-Due, 1953). Malignancies that are commonly associated with metastasis to the heart include breast, lung, leukemia, sarcoma, and melanoma, although almost any cancer can metastasize to the heart (Hanfling, 1960). The incidence of primary cardiac tumors ranges from 0.3%–0.7% in most autopsy series, with 75% of these being benign (Yu, Liu, Wang, Hu, & Long, 2007). Clinical presentation and treatment of cardiac tumors frequently depend on the chamber location and malignant potential. If the tumor is malignant and not resected, 90% of patients are deceased within 9–12 months; even with resection, prognosis can be poor (Reardon, 2010).

Left Atrial Structures and Masses

The left atrium is a posterior chamber of the heart. The structures of the left atrium include the pulmonary veins, left atrial ridge, left atrial appendage, and fossa ovalis. Oxygenated blood enters the chamber through one of the four pulmonary veins and proceeds through the mitral valve with each cardiac cycle. Left atrial tumors can be benign or malignant. The benign tumors include myxoma, lipoma, papillary fibroelastoma, rhabdomyoma, fibroma, and teratoma. It is more common to have a benign tumor in the left atrium. If malignant, the most common histology of the left atrium is malignant fibrous histiocytoma, also known as pleomorphic sarcoma, and leiomyosarcoma (Glancy, Morales, & Roberts, 1968) (see Figure 1-1).

Figure 1-1. Anatomy of the Heart

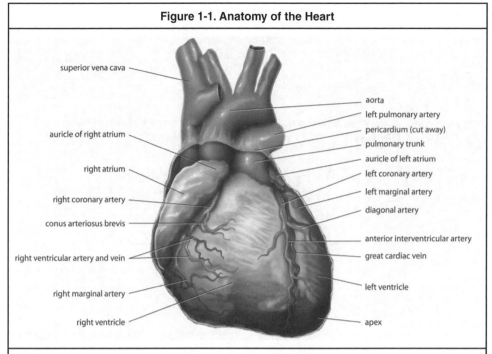

superior vena cava

auricle of right atrium

right atrium

right coronary artery

conus arteriosus brevis

right ventricular artery and vein

right marginal artery

right ventricle

aorta
left pulmonary artery
pericardium (cut away)
pulmonary trunk
auricle of left atrium
left coronary artery
left marginal artery
diagonal artery

anterior interventricular artery
great cardiac vein

left ventricle

apex

Note. Figure created by Ties van Brussel, 2010. Retrieved from Wikimedia Commons, http://en.wikipedia.org/wiki/File:Anatomy_Heart_English_Tiesworks.jpg#file. This image has been released into the public domain and may be used for any purpose, without any conditions, unless such conditions are required by law.

Myxomas: Common tumors of the left atrium include myxomas, which are mostly benign and account for up to half of the benign cardiac tumors. These usually are sporadic, left atrial, arising from the fossa ovalis, and solitary. They can, however, exist in any of the four cardiac chambers. Many are pedunculated with a 1–2 cm based attachment to the endocardial septum. Surgical resection is curative in 95% of the cases and has a low morbidity and mortality (Piazza et al., 2004). Rarely, benign myxomas are misdiagnosed and are actually malignant sarcomas or can have malignant transformation potential. Thus, the goal of excision is to remove the entire tumor and not leave remnants. About 5% of myxomas can be hereditary and present as part of the Carney syndrome consisting of myxomas, spotty pigmentation, and endocrine changes (Bireta et al., 2011) (see Figure 1-2).

Lipomas: These usually are benign tumors of adipose tissue that can be found in the subendocardium or subepicardium but also can be intramuscular. These tumors usually are well encapsulated.

Papillary fibroelastomas: These are small (less than 1 cm) benign tumors that protrude from a central stalk and usually are single and mobile. Most are located on the ventricular surface of the aortic valve, with the atrial side of the mitral valve being the second most common location. These usually can be distinguished from Lambl excrescences, as they are located on non-contact areas of the valve. Lambl excrescences are thin and elongated echoreflective structures with undulating hypermobility seen on the atrial side of the mitral and tricuspid valves and the ventricular side of the aortic valve.

Figure 1-2. Left Atrial Tumor

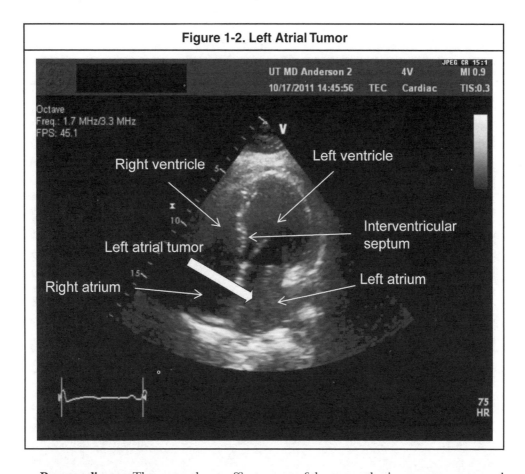

Paragangliomas: These are chromaffin tumors of the sympathetic nervous system and are fleshy tumors that can be found on the surface of the heart or the pericardium. The paragangliomas that grow into the anterior mediastinum arise from the parasympathetic chain and are relatively asymptomatic. Posterior paragangliomas arise from the sympathetic chain and can present with symptoms consistent with catecholamine response of the tumor. Some of these tumors present with severe malignant hypertension secondary to the release of catecholamines. They can be diagnosed by measuring the level of catecholamines in the urine and can be localized by computed tomography scan or metaiodobenzylguanidine scintigraphy (Lee et al., 2006). Patients should be treated with alpha- and beta-blockade combination medication followed by surgery. These are highly vascular tumors and have a characteristic appearance on cardiac angiogram (see Figure 1-3).

Lymphoma: Lymphoma can present in any of the four chambers and is best treated with chemotherapy with occasional debulking of the tumor if hemodynamic compromise occurs.

Clinical Manifestations of Patients With Cardiac Tumors

Cardiac tumors can present as constitutional symptoms, intracardiac obstruction, embolic phenomena, arrhythmias, or cardiac tamponade (Butany, Leong, Carmichael, & Komeda, 2005; Butany, Nair, et al., 2005; Weinberg, Conces, & Waller, 1989). Constitutional symptoms may be vague but include fever, malaise, weight loss,

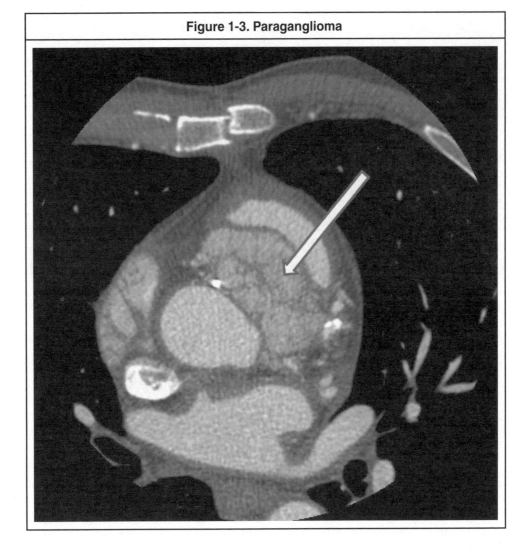

Figure 1-3. Paraganglioma

night sweats, polymyositis, and cachexia (Debourdeau, Gligorov, Teixeira, Aletti, & Zammit, 2004). These symptoms are likely promoted by the release of inflammatory cytokines from the tumor, such as interleukin-6 and antimyocardial antibodies, and often normalize once the tumors are resected from the heart (Pinede, Duhaut, & Loire, 2001).

Diagnostic Evaluation

Common laboratory abnormalities include anemia, elevated erythrocyte sedimentation rate, C-reactive protein, thrombocytosis, and hyperglobulinemia. Left atrial tumors also have presented as arrhythmias such as atrial flutter or embolic phenomena that include transient ischemic attacks or stroke (Hayes, Liles, & Sorrell, 2003). If on the left side, the emboli also can result in myocardial infarction as the tumor emboli occlude the coronary arteries (Pinede et al., 2001). Unfortunately, left-sided tumors also present with intracardiac obstruction of the mitral valve causing cardiogenic shock.

Assessment Findings

Normal heart sounds of the cardiac cycle include a first heart sound (S_1) caused by the closing of the mitral and tricuspid valves. Mitral valve closure usually occurs slightly before tricuspid valve closure. S_2, the second heart sound, is caused by closure of the aortic and pulmonic valves, with the aortic valve closure occurring slightly earlier than the pulmonic valve closure. A patient with a left atrial tumor that is large enough to obstruct the mitral valve may have a loud, widely split S_1 because of late closure of the mitral valve. This also is seen with mitral stenosis and preexcitation. A presystolic crescendo murmur may be present if the tumor obstructs the mitral valve orifice. A tumor plop may be heard early in diastole after the opening snap as the tumor protrudes through the mitral valve.

Treatment and Prognosis

Current treatment of malignant left atrial tumors includes neoadjuvant chemotherapy and resection of the tumor followed by postoperative chemotherapy. Left atrial tumors remain a surgical challenge because of the posterior location of the tumor in the chest. Cardiac autotransplantation is a relatively new technique for the removal of left atrial cardiac masses and is advocated especially for malignant left atrial tumors, as survival is very dependent on obtaining a negative margin (Hoffmeier, Schmid, & Scheld, 2004; Mery, Reardon, Haas, Lazar, & Hindenburg, 2003; Reardon, DeFelice, Sheinbaum, & Baldwin, 1999; Reardon, Malaisrie, et al., 2006; Reardon, Walkes, & Benjamin, 2006). This technique involves complete excision of the heart, ex vivo tumor removal with cardiac reconstruction, and cardiac reimplantation (Reardon, 2010; Reardon, Walkes, DeFelice, & Wojciechowski, 2006). Besides routine postoperative complications, bradycardia may result because the vagal innervations to the heart have been interrupted. The most common histology of malignant tumors of the heart is sarcoma. The majority of patients with malignant left atrial tumors die from metastatic disease rather than local recurrence. Complete resection with new techniques such as autotransplantation has improved the chance of obtaining negative surgical margins with a median survival of 36 months. Median survival of patients undergoing standard resection is 11 months versus 22 months with cardiac autotransplantation (Bakaeen et al., 2003; Blackmon et al., 2008; Murphy et al., 1990; Putnam et al., 1991; Reardon, Malaisrie, et al., 2006).

Postoperative Management

The role of neoadjuvant and postoperative chemotherapy for cardiac sarcoma is unclear. Several drug combinations are routinely used in the treatment of sarcoma, including doxorubicin and ifosfamide, gemcitabine and docetaxel, and dacarbazine. The Sarcoma Meta-Analysis Collaboration (1997) concluded that doxorubicin-based chemotherapy improved time to local recurrence and overall recurrence-free survival with a trend toward improved survival in patients with sarcoma. Pervaiz et al. (2008) also found that the addition of ifosfamide improved the efficacy of the regimen. However, this has not been evaluated in patients with sarcoma of the heart.

Left Ventricular Structures and Masses

The left ventricle receives blood through the inlet of the mitral valve. Blood then moves toward the apex, which contains fine trabeculations. Blood is then pumped with ventricular contraction toward the left ventricular outlet tract and out to the aorta through the aortic valve. Left ventricular tumors can present as left ventricular congestive heart failure (including symptoms of dyspnea, edema, and chest pain) and as deadly arrhythmias such as ventricular tachycardia, which cause sudden cardiac death (Ottaviani, Matturri, Rossi, & Jones, 2003; Schrepfer et al., 2003). Left ventricular tumors have presented with arrhythmias such as heart block if they invade the atrioventricular (AV) node. Common tumors of the left ventricle are similar to tumors of the left atrium, with sarcoma being a prominent malignant tumor. However, some unique tumors of the left ventricle include rhabdomyoma and fibroma. Treatment also is similar to that for left atrial tumors, with resection and chemotherapy as the mainstay of treatment. Chemotherapy regimens are similar to those for left atrial sarcoma. Ventricular tumors may be excised via three main techniques: through the atrioventricular valve, through the transaortic valve, and via ventricular incisions.

Rhabdomyomas: These are the most common tumors found in children and infants and are frequently found in the ventricles. They usually are multiple and are associated with tuberous sclerosis. They can produce arrhythmias such as ventricular tachycardia. Most are just observed, as they tend to regress with age. Resection is only considered for incessant, uncontrollable, life-threatening arrhythmias.

Fibromas: These are benign connective tissue tumors described as firm and circumscribed but unencapsulated and usually are found in children. They typically are intramural and almost exclusively originate in the left ventricle. Tumor calcification can frequently be seen on chest x-ray. Gorlin syndrome is a genetic condition that has been identified with cardiac fibromas, multiple basal cell carcinomas, keratocystic odontogenic (jaw) tumors, and skeletal abnormalities.

Right Atrial Structures and Masses

The right atrium consists of the inferior vena cava and superior vena cava, which receives deoxygenated blood from the systemic venous system. It also receives blood from the coronary sinus. The Eustachian valve is at the border of the inferior vena cava and helps form a fenestrated network termed the *Chiari network*. The anterolateral portion of the right atrium is made of pectinate muscle and appendage. The smooth and rough portion of the right atrium is separated by a muscle ridge called the *crista terminalis*. Blood flows through the right atrium and through the tricuspid valve. Right atrial tumors tend to be more malignant than left-sided tumors, with the most common histology being angiosarcoma. Right atrial tumors also may be the result of extension of infradiaphragmatic tumors such as renal cell carcinoma, hepatocellular tumors, or uterine tumors (see Figure 1-4).

Clinical Manifestations

Right atrial and right ventricular tumors can present with embolic phenomena. If the tumor is on the right side, the emboli usually result in a pulmonary embolism, which if left untreated can result in cor pulmonale (right-sided heart failure). If the tumor

Figure 1-4. Right Atrial Tumor

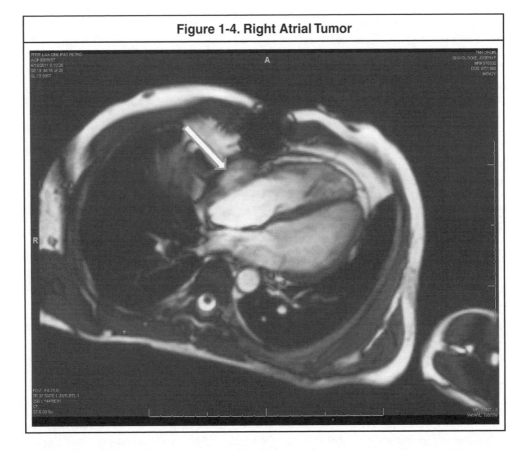

is large enough, pulmonary hypertension can occur, causing hypoxia, clubbing, and polycythemia. Right heart failure may occur, which manifests as dyspnea, increased abdominal girth, and peripheral edema. Heart failure symptoms usually present later in the disease as compared to left-sided tumors (Esaki et al., 1998). On physical examination, a diastolic (period of ventricular filling) rumble that varies with inspiration may be the result of tricuspid valve obstruction. P2, the closure of the pulmonic valve, may also be delayed.

Treatment

Complete and early resection of right atrial tumors is needed because of the aggressive nature of these tumors and the resulting symptoms and complications. Surgery may involve extensive resection including removal of a majority of the right atrium, transection of the right coronary artery with bypass graft placement, and resection of up to one-third of the right ventricle. Treatment of right atrial sarcoma involves a combination of neoadjuvant chemotherapy and surgical excision, with most of these patients dying of metastatic disease. Surgical resection resulted in survival when disease-free margins were obtained at excision (median survival 27 months versus 4 months), achieving a significantly higher overall five-year survival rate than those with positive surgical margins (Reardon, 2010; Vaporciyan & Reardon, 2010). Systemic therapy is important and is similar to regimens discussed for left-sided tumors. (See the Postoperative

Management section of left atrial tumors for common systemic chemotherapy agents.) Some unique tumors of the right atrium include lipomatous hypertrophy of the interatrial septum and angiosarcoma.

Lipomatous hypertrophy of the interatrial septum: This is a benign mass composed of adipose tissue that collects at the atrial septum and protrudes into the right atrium. It appears on imaging as a barbell shape of the septum sparing the fossa ovalis. It usually does not create symptoms and is incidentally found on routine transthoracic echocardiography. No treatment besides observation is necessary.

Angiosarcoma: Angiosarcoma is the most common malignant tumor of the right heart. Treatment and management includes resection with aggressive chemotherapy, as previously discussed (see Figure 1-5).

Right Ventricular Structures and Masses

The right ventricle receives blood through the tricuspid valve, and, similar to the left ventricle, consists of three sections. The inlet region contains the tricuspid valve apparatus. The apical region is highly trabeculated. Blood then flows with contraction into the right ventricular outflow tract and through the pulmonic valve into the pulmonary artery and on toward the lungs. Tumors of the right ventricle are similar to tumors of the right atrium and should be treated as such. A unique tumor of the right ventricle is leukemia, which has been predominantly noted in right ventricular wall lesions. This

Figure 1-5. Right Atrial Synovial Sarcoma

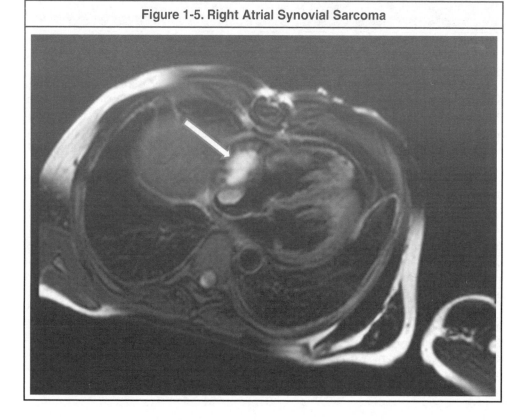

tumor regresses with chemotherapy. Many varied regimens exist for leukemia depending on the type and classification. Treatment agents include but are not limited to doxorubicin, vincristine, prednisone, and tyrosine kinase inhibitors.

Pericardium

The pericardium is the sac that surrounds the heart and has both a visceral and parietal layer. The most common tumor of the pericardium is mesothelioma (Fine, 1968). Presenting symptoms may include pericarditis or pericardial hemorrhagic effusion. This tumor can extend into the conduction pathways, primarily the AV node, which can cause complete heart block and sudden cardiac death (Strauss, Asinger, & Hodges, 1988). The prognosis for patients with mesothelioma is poor.

Metastatic Tumors to the Heart

Almost any tumor can metastasize to the heart to almost any chamber, but lung cancer is the most common metastatic tumor to the heart. Other common cancers include breast cancer, lymphoma, leukemia, and melanoma. Infradiaphragmatic tumors can extend through the inferior vena cava into the heart, usually from malignant renal or hepatic tumors (Hanfling, 1960).

Diagnosis of Cardiac Tumors

The primary modalities of choice for diagnosing cardiac tumors include transthoracic echocardiography, transesophageal echocardiography, myocardial magnetic resonance imaging (MRI), and computed tomography angiography (CTA) (Leja, Shah, & Reardon, 2011).

Transthoracic echocardiography: This is an initial noninvasive screening tool for assessing gross cardiac structure and function. However, it is not very sensitive for cardiac tumors because it can often miss structures in the posterior of the atrium and ventricles. The tumor has similar visual characteristics to myocardium and can be missed. This is a good tool for assessing pericardial effusion (fluid around the heart), which is associated with cardiac tumors.

Transesophageal echocardiography: This often is used for initial screening for a cardiac tumor but generally is not helpful for obtaining a tissue diagnosis and is an invasive test. Similar to transthoracic echocardiography, transesophageal echocardiography often misses structures in the posterior sections of the left and right atrium and apical ventricular masses. It can initially help to determine implantation site and mobility of the tumor and can discriminate between vegetation, thrombi, and tumor.

Computed tomography angiography: Ultrafast CTA is especially useful for assessing blood supply to the tumor and for assessing extrathoracic cardiac metastasis.

Magnetic resonance imaging: MRI is excellent to assess size, shape, and three-dimensional relationships to other cardiac structures (Araoz, Eklund, Welch, & Breen, 1999; Gilkeson & Chiles, 2003; Sparrow, Kurian, Jones, & Sivananthan, 2005; Thakrar et al., 2009). It is particularly useful in distinguishing among tumor, thrombus, and pseudotumor and is likely the best choice for assessing cardiac tumors because of its high contrast and spatial resolution (Hoey, Mankad, Puppala, Gopalan, & Sivananthan, 2009;

Shah, 2010). Although it can give a clue to tissue pathology, it cannot determine histology, and a cardiac biopsy may be necessary.

Angiography: Angiograms are useful for defining coronary and anomalous blood supply to the tumor, which is extremely important for surgical excision. However, the healthcare professional performing the procedure must be careful not to dislodge tumor fragments during manipulation of catheters and dye injection. Transseptal puncture and left ventriculograms are relatively contraindicated for fear of tumor dissemination but can be beneficial if safely done. The ideal imaging modality is likely a combination of all these methods, as each provides different information to the clinician.

Conclusion

Cardiac tumors are rare. Although tumors of the heart usually are benign, malignant cardiac tumors are very serious and must be diagnosed and treated early in the disease process. Advanced surgical techniques and novel systemic therapies are necessary for treatment.

References

Araoz, P.A., Eklund, H.E., Welch, T.J., & Breen, J.F. (1999). CT and MR imaging of primary cardiac malignancies. *Radiographics, 19,* 1421–1434.

Bakaeen, F.G., Reardon, M.J., Coselli, J.S., Miller, C.C., Howell, J.F., Lawrie, G.M., ... DeBakey, M.E. (2003). Surgical outcome in 85 patients with primary cardiac tumors. *American Journal of Surgery, 186,* 641–647. doi:10.1016/j.amjsurg.2003.08.004

Bireta, C., Popov, A.F., Schotola, H., Trethowan, B., Friedrich, M., El-Mehsen, M., ... Tirilomis, T. (2011). Carney-complex: Multiple resections of recurrent cardiac myxoma. *Journal of Cardiothoracic Surgery, 6,* 12. doi:10.1186/1749-8090-6-12

Bisel, H.F., Wróblewski, F., & LaDue, J.S. (1953). Incidence and clinical manifestations of cardiac metastases. *JAMA, 153,* 712–715. doi:10.1001/jama.1953.02940250018005

Blackmon, S.H., Patel, A.R., Bruckner, B.A., Beyer, E.A., Rice, D.C., Vaporciyan, A.A., ... Reardon, M.J. (2008). Cardiac autotransplantation for malignant or complex primary left-heart tumors. *Texas Heart Institute Journal, 35,* 296–300.

Butany, J., Leong, S.W., Carmichael, K., & Komeda, M. (2005). A 30-year analysis of cardiac neoplasms at autopsy. *Canadian Journal of Cardiology, 21,* 675–680.

Butany, J., Nair, V., Naseemuddin, A., Nair, G.M., Catton, C., & Yau, T. (2005). Cardiac tumours: Diagnosis and management. *Lancet Oncology, 6,* 219–228. doi:10.1016/S1470-2045(05)70093-0

Debourdeau, P., Gligorov, J., Teixeira, L., Aletti, M., & Zammit, C. (2004). [Malignant cardiac tumors]. *Bulletin du Cancer, 91*(Suppl. 3), 136–146.

Esaki, M., Kagawa, K., Noda, T., Nishigaki, K., Gotoh, K., Fujiwara, H., ... Hara, M. (1998). Primary cardiac leiomyosarcoma growing rapidly and causing right ventricular outflow obstruction. *Internal Medicine, 37,* 370–375. doi:10.2169/internalmedicine.37.370

Fine, G. (1968). Neoplasms of the pericardium and heart. In S.E. Gould (Ed.), *Pathology of the heart and blood vessels* (3rd ed., pp. 851–883). Springfield, IL: Thomas.

Gilkeson, R.C., & Chiles, C. (2003). MR evaluation of cardiac and pericardial malignancy. *Magnetic Resonance Imaging Clinics of North America, 11,* 173–186. doi:10.1016/S1064-9689(02)00047-8

Glancy, D.L., Morales, J.B., Jr., & Roberts, W.C. (1968). Angiosarcoma of the heart. *American Journal of Cardiology, 21,* 413–419. doi:10.1016/0002-9149(68)90144-6

Hanfling, S.M. (1960). Metastatic cancer to the heart. Review of the literature and report of 127 cases. *Circulation, 22,* 474–483.

Hayes, D., Jr., Liles, D.K., & Sorrell, V.L. (2003). An unusual cause of new-onset atrial flutter: Primary cardiac lymphoma. *Southern Medical Journal, 96,* 799–802. doi:10.1097/01.SMJ.0000054225.89526.BD

Hoey, E.T., Mankad, K., Puppala, S., Gopalan, D., & Sivananthan, M.U. (2009). MRI and CT appearances of cardiac tumours in adults. *Clinical Radiology, 64,* 1214–1230. doi:10.1016/j.crad.2009.09.002

Hoffmeier, A., Schmid, C., & Scheld, H.H. (2004). Reply: "Ex situ resection of primary cardiac tumors" Thorac Cardiovasc Surg 2003; 51: 293–294. *Thoracic and Cardiovascular Surgery, 52,* 125.

Lee, K.Y., Oh, Y.-W., Noh, H.J., Lee, Y.J., Yong, H.-S., Kang, E.-Y., ... Lee, N.J. (2006). Extraadrenal paragangliomas of the body: Imaging features. *American Journal of Roentgenology, 187,* 492–504. doi:10.2214/AJR.05.0370

Leja, M.J., Shah, D.J., & Reardon, M.J. (2011). Primary cardiac tumors. *Texas Heart Institute Journal, 38,* 261–262.

Mery, G.M., Reardon, M.J., Haas, J., Lazar, J., & Hindenburg, A. (2003). A combined modality approach to recurrent cardiac sarcoma resulting in a prolonged remission: A case report. *Chest, 123,* 1766–1768. doi:10.1378/chest.123.5.1766

Murphy, M.C., Sweeney, M.S., Putnam, J.B., Jr., Walker, W.E., Frazier, O.H., Ott, D.A., & Cooley, D.A. (1990). Surgical treatment of cardiac tumors: A 25-year experience. *Annals of Thoracic Surgery, 49,* 612–618. doi:10.1016/0003-4975(90)90310-3

Ottaviani, G., Matturri, L., Rossi, L., & Jones, D. (2003). Sudden death due to lymphomatous infiltration of the cardiac conduction system. *Cardiovascular Pathology, 12,* 77–81. doi:10.1016/S1054-8807(02)00168-0

Pervaiz, N., Colterjohn, N., Farrokhyar, F., Tozer, R., Figueredo, A., & Ghert, M. (2008). A systematic meta-analysis of randomized controlled trials of adjuvant chemotherapy for localized resectable soft-tissue sarcoma. *Cancer, 113,* 573–581. doi:10.1002/cncr.23592

Piazza, N., Chughtai, T., Toledano, K., Sampalis, J., Liao, C., & Morin, J.F. (2004). Primary cardiac tumours: Eighteen years of surgical experience on 21 patients. *Canadian Journal of Cardiology, 20,* 1443–1448.

Pinede, L., Duhaut, P., & Loire, R. (2001). Clinical presentation of left atrial cardiac myxoma: A series of 112 consecutive cases. *Medicine, 80,* 159–172. doi:10.1097/00005792-200105000-00002

Putnam, J.B., Jr., Sweeney, M.S., Colon, R., Lanza, L.A., Frazier, O.H., & Cooley, D.A. (1991). Primary cardiac sarcomas. *Annals of Thoracic Surgery, 51,* 906–910. doi:10.1016/0003-4975(91)91003-E

Reardon, M.J. (2010). Malignant tumor overview. *Methodist DeBakey Cardiovascular Journal, 6*(3), 35–37.

Reardon, M.J., DeFelice, C.A., Sheinbaum, R., & Baldwin, J.C. (1999). Cardiac autotransplant for surgical treatment of a malignant neoplasm. *Annals of Thoracic Surgery, 67,* 1793–1795. doi:10.1016/S0003-4975(99)00343-4

Reardon, M.J., Malaisrie, S.C., Walkes, J.-C., Vaporciyan, A.A., Rice, D.C., Smythe, W.R., ... Wojciechowski, Z.J. (2006). Cardiac autotransplantation for primary cardiac tumors. *Annals of Thoracic Surgery, 82,* 645–650. doi:10.1016/j.athoracsur.2006.02.086

Reardon, M.J., Walkes, J.-C., & Benjamin, R. (2006). Therapy insight: Malignant primary cardiac tumors. *Nature Clinical Practice: Cardiovascular Medicine, 3,* 548–553. doi:10.1038/ncpcardio0653

Reardon, M.J., Walkes, J.-C., DeFelice, C.A., & Wojciechowski, Z. (2006). Cardiac autotransplantation for surgical resection of a primary malignant left ventricular tumor. *Texas Heart Institute Journal, 33,* 495–497.

Sarcoma Meta-Analysis Collaboration. (1997). Adjuvant chemotherapy for localised resectable soft-tissue sarcoma of adults: Meta-analysis of individual data. *Lancet, 350,* 1647–1654. doi:10.1016/S0140-6736(97)08165-8

Schrepfer, S., Deuse, T., Detter, C., Treede, H., Koops, A., Boehm, D.H., ... Reichenspurner, H. (2003). Successful resection of a symptomatic right ventricular lipoma. *Annals of Thoracic Surgery, 76,* 1305–1307. doi:10.1016/S0003-4975(03)00523-X

Shah, D.J. (2010). Evaluation of cardiac masses: The role of cardiovascular magnetic resonance. *Methodist DeBakey Cardiovascular Journal, 6*(3), 4–11.

Sparrow, P.J., Kurian, J.B., Jones, T.R., & Sivananthan, M.U. (2005). MR imaging of cardiac tumors. *Radiographics, 25,* 1255–1276. doi:10.1148/rg.255045721

Strauss, W.E., Asinger, R.W., & Hodges, M. (1988). Mesothelioma of the AV node: Potential utility of pacing. *Pacing and Clinical Electrophysiology, 11,* 1296–1298. doi:10.1111/j.1540-8159.1988.tb03991.x

Thakrar, A., Farag, A., Lytwyn, M., Fang, T., Arora, R.C., & Jassal, D.S. (2009). Multimodality cardiac imaging for the noninvasive characterization of intracardiac neoplasms [Letter to the editor]. *International Journal of Cardiology, 132,* e74–e76. doi:10.1016/j.ijcard.2007.08.025

Vaporciyan, A., & Reardon, M.J. (2010). Right heart sarcomas. *Methodist DeBakey Cardiovascular Journal, 6*(3), 44–48.

Weinberg, B.A., Conces, D.J., Jr., & Waller, B.F. (1989). Cardiac manifestations of noncardiac tumors. Part I: Direct effects. *Clinical Cardiology, 12,* 289–296. doi:10.1002/clc.4960120512

Yu, K., Liu, Y., Wang, H., Hu, S., & Long, C. (2007). Epidemiological and pathological characteristics of cardiac tumors: A clinical study of 242 cases. *Interactive Cardiovascular and Thoracic Surgery, 6,* 636–639. doi:10.1510/icvts.2007.156554

CHAPTER 2

Anthracyclines, Trastuzumab, and Cardiomyopathy

Sarah Anderson, MSN, APRN, ANP-BC,
and Brenda Wimberly White, RN, BSN

Introduction

Anthracyclines have been a mainstay of typical chemotherapy regimens used to treat a wide range of malignancies, including cancers of the thyroid, breast, lung, and stomach, as well as lymphomas and leukemias ("Doxorubicin," 2011). The cardiotoxic effects of anthracyclines were first discovered in the early 1970s, and since that time, scientists and physicians alike have been feverishly trying to develop a safer yet equally effective drug (Rahman, Yusuf, & Ewer, 2007). Other formulations in the anthracycline antibiotic class have been developed, but a significant risk of cardiotoxicity still exists. Because a consistent definition of cardiotoxicity is lacking, it is difficult to establish a firm risk of cardiotoxicities. Estimates suggest anywhere from 4%–28% of patients receiving these drugs may be affected (Peng, Chen, Lim, & Sawyer, 2005; Suter, Cook-Bruns, & Barton, 2004).

The discovery of the HER2 receptor as a marker of breast cancer activity and the advent of the HER2 receptor blocker trastuzumab in 1998 ushered in a new era for patients with breast cancer and brought hope for a safer, more effective drug (Ewer & Benjamin, 2006; Peng et al., 2005). Trastuzumab has proved to be most effective against HER2+ breast cancer and is currently the only recommended chemotherapeutic treatment regimen for the disease, but it still carries the risk of cardiotoxicity (Suter et al., 2007).

As the population of the United States ages and the incidence of cancer consequently rises, it is apparent that cancer treatment may have a significant effect on the presence of heart disease. In addition, more patients are surviving after cancer treatment, largely due to the success of therapy. All of these dynamics demand that the medical community be aware of these facts.

When anthracycline-induced cardiomyopathy is detected well after substantial damage has occurred, the risk of mortality increases significantly, with only a 40% survival rate at two years (Felker et al., 2000). Although many newer cancer therapies are being developed, it is crucial to understand how accurate identification and proper use of cardioprotective treatments may have an impact on standard cancer therapies. Early identification and prompt treatment of anthracycline-induced cardiotoxicity are now thought to allow substantial recovery from toxicity, but a delay in treatment of even six months may be too late (Cardinale et al., 2010). The focus of care is shifting to prevention and early detection of cardiotoxicity when possible and prompt treatment when necessary.

Pathophysiology

Anthracycline-Induced Cardiotoxicity

Anthracycline antibiotics have an established direct toxic effect on cardiac myocytes. Anthracyclines interfere with the normal processes of DNA, RNA, and protein synthesis and result in the release of free radicals that damage the phospholipid layer of the cell membrane (Sawyer, Peng, Chen, Pentassuglia, & Lim, 2010). Apoptosis and necrosis of myocytes occur after oxidative damage results in structural changes to the myocardium (Sawyer et al., 2010). This leads to the long-term sequela of cardiomyopathy.

Trastuzumab-Induced Cardiotoxicity

Unlike the anthracyclines, trastuzumab is a monoclonal antibody. It targets the ErbB2 receptor, also called HER2, in the cancer cells that lead to cancer control (Carver, 2010; Sawyer et al., 2010). Interestingly, HER2 receptors have been detected in myocardial cells, which is the partial explanation for the unexpected high incidence of cardiotoxicity noted with initial treatment with trastuzumab (D.J. Lenihan, personal communication, August 26, 2011). These receptors are important in the regulation of the heart's response to stressors, such as exercise (Carver, 2010). When these pathways are disrupted, the heart is not able to properly respond to stressors, and cardiac dysfunction can result for the period of time that the pathways are disrupted. For this reason, trastuzumab-induced cardiotoxicity often is reversible with drug interuption (Carver, 2010).

Risk Factors for the Development of Cardiotoxicity

Some major risk factors for cardiotoxicity are hypertension (Von Hoff et al., 1979), family history, extremes of age (Bristow, 1980; Pratt, Ransom, & Evans, 1978; Von Hoff et al., 1979), diabetes (Pinder, Duan, Goodwin, Hortobagyi, & Giordano, 2007), history of coronary artery disease (Von Hoff et al., 1979), elevated brain natriuretic peptide (BNP) levels prior to initiation of treatment (Lenihan, 2011), history of mediastinal or mantle radiation (Minow, Benjamin, Lee, & Gottlieb, 1977), female gender (Gottdiener, Appelbaum, Ferrans, Deisseroth, & Ziegler, 1981; Silber, Jakacki, Larsen, Goldwein, & Barber, 1993), being female and African American (Pinder et al., 2007), and combination chemotherapy with large or repeated doses of known cardiotoxic chemotherapy (Gottdiener et al., 1981; Meinardi et al., 1999).

Patients who have a family history of coronary heart disease, hypertension, or heart failure (HF) are likely to have a greater predisposition to cardiovascular toxicity. The most common and treatable risk factor is hypertension. Vigilance in the management of hypertension or borderline hypertension should be a priority, as it can be an early indicator of cardiotoxicity in patients who are receiving antiangiogenic therapy (Lenihan, 2011). The overlap between cardiac and oncology risk factors that may predispose patients to develop cardiotoxicity is shown in Figure 2-1.

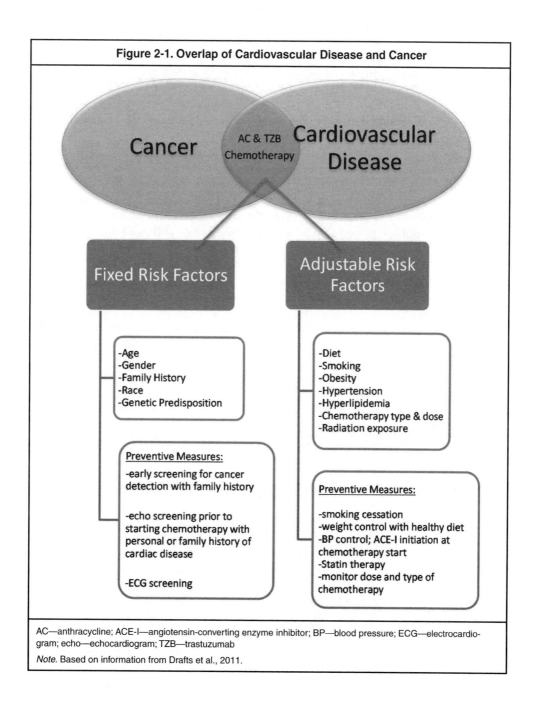

Figure 2-1. Overlap of Cardiovascular Disease and Cancer

AC—anthracycline; ACE-I—angiotensin-converting enzyme inhibitor; BP—blood pressure; ECG—electrocardiogram; echo—echocardiogram; TZB—trastuzumab

Note. Based on information from Drafts et al., 2011.

African American women, not considering other comorbidities, have a 49% greater risk of developing HF when compared with Caucasian females who receive anthracycline adjuvant chemotherapy (trastuzumab) during breast cancer therapy (C.A. Geisberg, personal communication, August 2, 2011; Pinder et al., 2007). Women between the ages of 66 and 70, regardless of race, who undergo adjuvant chemotherapy for breast cancer have a significantly higher incidence of congestive heart failure than younger women with the same condition (Pinder et al., 2007).

In a large observational study comparing long-term outcomes between patients with cancer who were treated during childhood and their nonaffected siblings, the treated siblings were found to have a threefold increased risk for developing a chronic cardiovascular disease (Mulrooney et al., 2009). They were also eight times more likely to have a severe or life-threatening event than their siblings (Mulrooney et al., 2009). Later in life, the treated group of children was found to have an increased incidence of congestive heart failure and coronary artery disease (Mulrooney et al., 2009). This group of patients has had documented occurrences of cardiotoxicities up to 30 years after completion of cancer chemotherapy (Drafts et al., 2011).

The role of anthracyclines as a causative agent for cardiotoxicity has been documented since the late 1960s; however, the exact dosage at which the toxicity occurs is still being researched. The cardiotoxic effects are thought to be due to the cumulative effect of the drug over time. The higher the dose, the greater the risk for developing cardiotoxicity. Currently, opinions differ regarding at what dose this occurs, at what point during the chemotherapy regimen a patient is most at risk, and in whom HF will most likely occur. The consensus among practitioners is that anthracycline dosages at or below 500 mg/m^2 seem to carry less risk of cardiotoxicity than previously used higher doses (Legha et al., 1982; Meinardi et al., 1999; Shan, Lincoff, & Young, 1996; Torti et al., 1983; Von Hoff et al., 1979). Figure 2-2 shows the correlation between increasing doses of anthracyclines and increasing incidence of cardiotoxicities.

Unlike anthracycline-induced toxicity, trastuzumab-associated cardiotoxicity is not thought to be due to a cumulative drug effect; however, the cumulative dose effect of trastuzumab has not yet been studied (D.J. Lenihan, personal communication, November 30, 2011). Although the drug does carry a risk of cardiotoxicity when given as monotherapy, this risk is generally low. The risk of cardiotoxicity increases when trastuzumab is used in combination with other chemotherapeutic agents. The combination of trastuzumab with anthracyclines, cyclophosphamide, or paclitaxel carries a significantly increased risk of cardiotoxicity (Cardinale et al., 2006; Gottdiener et al., 1981; Suter & Ewer, 2006).

Clinical Presentation of Cardiomyopathy in Patients With Cancer

The classic presenting signs and symptoms of HF are discussed in Chapter 10. The earliest sign of cardiac dysfunction resulting from cardiotoxicity in a patient with cancer is persistent tachycardia after mild or moderate activity (Ewer & Benjamin, 2006). Early symptoms of cardiotoxicity may be more difficult to discern as to their origin because patients may be experiencing similar symptoms secondary to chemotherapy side effects (Lenihan, 2006; Yusuf, Razeghi, & Yeh, 2008). Figure 2-3 shows other major mechanisms in which cardiotoxicities can present in the oncology population. Differential diagnoses for these presenting symptoms are listed in Figure 2-4.

Although several symptoms such as orthopnea and paroxysmal nocturnal dyspnea are late hallmark signs specific to HF, the clinician must explore these symp-

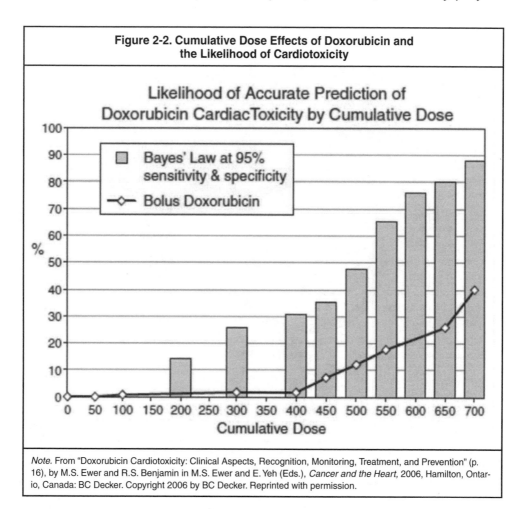

Figure 2-2. Cumulative Dose Effects of Doxorubicin and the Likelihood of Cardiotoxicity

Note. From "Doxorubicin Cardiotoxicity: Clinical Aspects, Recognition, Monitoring, Treatment, and Prevention" (p. 16), by M.S. Ewer and R.S. Benjamin in M.S. Ewer and E. Yeh (Eds.), *Cancer and the Heart,* 2006, Hamilton, Ontario, Canada: BC Decker. Copyright 2006 by BC Decker. Reprinted with permission.

toms because they are often missed during physical examination if they are not specifically addressed. Dyspnea and fatigue are the most common presenting symptoms for HF (West, Hernandez, O'Connor, Starling, & Califf, 2010) and often are attributed to the disease process in patients with cancer. Often, clinicians fail to accurately report patients' symptoms. A study of 37 men with metastatic prostate cancer compared clinician reporting to patient reporting of symptoms using a quality-of-life questionnaire. Results showed that the symptoms of dyspnea and fatigue were missed by physicians 77% and 38% of the time, respectively, when compared with patients' reporting of the same symptoms (Fromme, Eilers, Mori, Hsieh, & Beer, 2004). The use of a symptom assessment instrument such as a visual analog scale (VAS) may be helpful for patients to better describe their symptoms. A validation study of a VAS for dyspnea assessment that included 190 patients seeking care for dyspnea in the emergency department showed that using the VAS was helpful in distinguishing HF-related dyspnea from non-HF-related dyspnea (Ekman, Granger, Swedberg, Stenlund, & Boman, 2011). Based on the findings of these studies, perhaps routinely using a symptom assessment instrument such as the MD Anderson Symptom Inventory–Heart Failure questionnaire (Fadol et al., 2008; see Figure 10-13 in Chapter 10) would be useful for early detection and management of cardiotoxicity in patients with cancer.

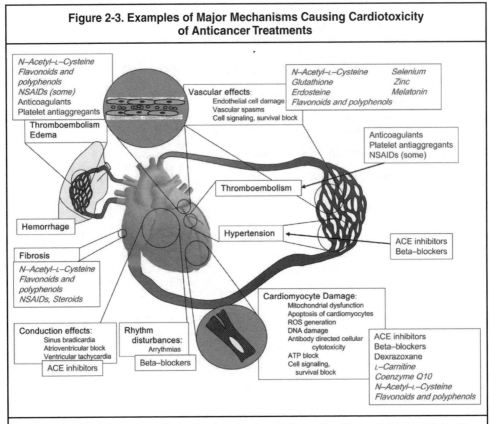

Figure 2-3. Examples of Major Mechanisms Causing Cardiotoxicity of Anticancer Treatments

Examples of major mechanisms causing cardiotoxicity of anticancer treatments, clinically used therapeutic agents, and potential protective agents (italicized text).

ACE—angiotensin-converting enzyme; NSAIDs—nonsteroidal anti-inflammatory drugs; ROS—reactive oxygen species

Note. From "Cardiotoxicity of Anticancer Drugs: The Need for Cardio-Oncology and Cardio-Oncological Prevention," by A. Albini, G. Pennesi, F. Donatelli, R. Cammarota, S. De Flora, and D.M. Noonan, 2010, *Journal of the National Cancer Institute, 102,* p. 21. Copyright 2010 by Oxford University Press. Reprinted with permission.

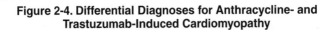

Figure 2-4. Differential Diagnoses for Anthracycline- and Trastuzumab-Induced Cardiomyopathy

- Heart failure
- Hypertension
- Anemia
- Myocardial infarction
- Pulmonary edema
- Pulmonary embolism
- Asthma

Early cardiotoxicity symptoms are frequently missed, perhaps due, in part, to the way patients' symptoms are reported in the oncology setting. The symptoms of early cardiomyopathy are categorized as separate adverse events in the *Common Terminology Criteria for Adverse Events* (CTCAE) (i.e., respiratory, cardiovascular, and constitutional) rather than the constellation of symptoms comprising a single disease process (National Cancer Institute Cancer Therapy Evaluation Program [NCI CTEP], 2010). Furthermore, according to the CTCAE, in order to diagnose HF at grade 1, diagnostic testing must occur (NCI CTEP, 2010). Biomarker testing would indeed be the earliest sign of cardiotoxicity development (Cardinale et al., 2010); however, biomarker testing is currently not routine practice for patients receiving chemotherapy. CTCAE grade 2 criteria require mild symptoms that are often overlooked. It is not until grade 3 toxicity that severe symptoms specific to HF become evident. At this point in the disease progression, there may be little or no reversibility. For these reasons, the early diagnosis of cardiomyopathy in patients with cancer is challenging, and the need for definitive diagnostic measures is ever greater (Ederhy et al., 2011).

Laboratory and Diagnostic Tests

Common Cardiac Diagnostic Tests

Echocardiogram: An echocardiogram is an ultrasound of the heart that is used to assess heart function, ventricular wall motion, and valve function. Normal left ventricular ejection fraction (LVEF) is 55% or greater. A decline in LVEF from baseline can be indicative of cardiomyopathy.

Multigated acquisition (MUGA) scan: MUGA is a scan of the heart using technetium-99 to assess cardiac function and wall motion. Similar to echocardiogram, a MUGA scan can determine LVEF.

Cardiac magnetic resonance imaging (MRI): A scan that produces detailed images of the heart and surrounding structures. LVEF, as well as ischemia, can be measured using cardiac MRI.

Electrocardiogram (ECG): An ECG is a representation of the electrical conduction system of the heart. Abnormalities present on ECG may be a late sign of cardiac dysfunction.

Cardiac biomarkers: Cardiac biomarkers are laboratory tests that are cardiac specific. The utilization of troponin I and BNP in patients with cancer is currently being studied. Abnormalities may represent acute or chronic injury to the heart. Troponin I is used clinically to help diagnose acute coronary syndrome. BNP trending is used clinically to help assess volume status in patients with HF.

Laboratory and Diagnostic Testing in Patients With Cancer

Current guidelines from the American Heart Association (AHA), the American College of Cardiology (ACC), the Heart Failure Society of America, and the American Society of Clinical Oncology recommend baseline LVEF measurement and a repeated measurement at some time point after chemotherapy initiation (Lenihan, 2010). A decline in LVEF by 15% from baseline or LVEF lower than 55% is an important clue of impending cardiotoxicity (Meinardi et al., 1999).

The most accurate LVEF measurement method has been debated for many years. The two most common methods for measuring LVEF are echocardiography and MUGA scan. Both methods have advantages and disadvantages. Measurements obtained via echocardiogram may better represent volume and structural deficits that may not be acquired by MUGA scan (Lenihan, 2011). The use of strain measurements proves useful in obtaining a more accurate LVEF (Plana, 2011). An additional benefit of echocardiography over MUGA scan is that it does not expose the patient to radiation. Limitations of echocardiography are related to reader variability and anatomic configurations such as truncal obesity, barrel chest, or severe lung disease that may cloud images (Ewer, Ewer, & Suter, 2011; Meinardi et al., 1999). The use of contrast agents during echocardiography can provide better definition of the borders of the heart and therefore a more accurate LVEF measurement with improved inter- and intra-observer reliability (Chuang et al., 2000; Plana, 2011). Other available methods for measuring LVEF are the use of three-dimensional (3-D) echocardiography. The 3-D image may provide more precise measurements because of the high-resolution quality of the images produced. This technology may have limited accessibility for smaller facilities and usually is found in large clinics or hospital settings.

Volume measurements that are limited during echocardiography are better visualized during MUGA scanning, but it may not actually reveal true myocyte damage (Lenihan, 2011). MUGA scans have less variability between readers and give a consistent measurement between patients. Given these benefits, it is important to emphasize that MUGA does require additional exposure to radiation.

Cardiac MRI is an alternative method to measure cardiac function. It provides high-quality resolution of the heart but has limitations of expense and institutional availability (Ewer et al., 2011). Additionally, patients with metal implants are not eligible for C-MRI (Plana, 2011), and patients with severe claustrophobia may not be able to tolerate the confinement (Meinardi et al., 1999).

The inadequacy of depending on echocardiography, MUGA scan, or cardiac MRI as the sole method to diagnose cardiomyopathy is that a reduced LVEF is most often considered a latent sign of cardiotoxicity (Ewer & Lenihan, 2008; Meinardi et al., 1999). Cardio-oncology pioneers are studying the role of cardiac biomarkers in terms of early and preclinical detection of cardiotoxicity. Laboratory testing offers the benefits of relatively low cost combined with noninvasive testing and immediate results (Cardinale, 2010; Lenihan et al., 2006; Monsuez, Charniot, Vignat, & Artigou, 2010).

Since the mid- to late-1990s, troponin I levels have been the gold standard in detecting myocardial damage created by myocardial infarction (Apple et al., 1995). In recent years, researchers have looked at the validity of using the same biomarkers in the detection of myocardial damage from causes other than infarct. Evidence shows that troponin I has predictive value for cardiotoxicity (Cardinale et al., 2004). In recent history, BNP has proved useful in guiding HF therapy. Increased laboratory values have shown a direct correlation of HF symptom severity. BNP results of patients who are undergoing chemotherapy have provided insight into possible cardiotoxicity detection (Lenihan et al., 2007).

In a small study monitoring BNP level during therapy in patients with cancer, researchers found that those with elevated BNP levels were 44 times more likely to develop cardiotoxicity than those whose BNP levels were not elevated (Lenihan et al., 2007). Still, no general consensus exists regarding the value of serial testing of biomarkers in the oncology population; however, clinical studies are in progress with the intent to establish standards that will be beneficial to the management and early detection of potential cardiac events in this population (Lenihan, 2010).

As a standard, many oncologists may order an ECG as part of the initial workup. ECGs have limited predictive value in the detection of cardiotoxicity because changes are common after chemotherapy administration. The presence of HF may be noted in diminished QRS on ECG, but, again, this is often a sign of late HF. The specificity and sensitivity of ECG are low for the diagnosis of cardiotoxicity (Meinardi et al., 1999) (see Table 2-1).

Table 2-1. Diagnostic Testing to Detect Cardiotoxicity

Test/Procedure	Definition	Advantages	Disadvantages	Clinical Considerations
Two-dimensional transthoracic echocardiogram (2-D TTE)	Ultrasound of the heart used to measure wall motion and heart/valve function	Cost-effective Noninvasive No radiation No iodine contrast needed	Reader variability Body habitus may limit image quality	Non-iodine contrast available for improved image quality
Three-dimensional transthoracic echocardiogram (3-D TTE)	Ultrasound of the heart used to measure wall motion and heart/valve function with enhanced 3-D images	Improved image quality over 2-D TTE Noninvasive Accurate volume measurement of heart chambers	Limited accessibility	Non-iodine contrast available for improved image quality
Multigated acquisition (MUGA) scan	Scan of the heart using technetium-99 with gamma camera to assess heart wall motion and function	Consistent measurements Reduced reader variability	Radiation required Requires IV contrast agent More expensive than echocardiogram	Cautious use in patient with renal dysfunction
Cardiac magnetic resonance imaging (MRI)	Powerful magnetic field, radiofrequency pulses, and a computer to produce detailed images of the heart and surrounding structures	Noninvasive Superior image quality and detail Consistent measurements	High cost Limited accessibility Requires IV contrast agent	Cautious use in patients with renal dysfunction Patients with metal objects, devices, or implants not candidates for MRI Claustrophobic patients may not tolerate scanner.
Electrocardiogram (ECG)	Snapshot of the electrical conduction system of the heart	Cost-effective Immediate results Readily available	Limited predictive value for cardiotoxicity ECG changes often latent sign of cardiotoxicity Low clinical specificity and sensitivity for cardiotoxicity	–

(Continued on next page)

Table 2-1. Diagnostic Testing to Detect Cardiotoxicity *(Continued)*

Test/Procedure	Definition	Advantages	Disadvantages	Clinical Considerations
Cardiac biomarkers	Laboratory test indicating injury to myocardium	Noninvasive Cost-effective Immediate results Cardiac specific Readily available	Validation of use in detecting cardiotoxicity is ongoing in clinical trials.	Laboratory values may be elevated with other disease processes, such as kidney failure or diabetes.
• Troponin I	Used clinically to differentiate myocardial damage during acute coronary syndrome			
• Brain natriuretic peptide (BNP)	Used clinically to indicate heart failure severity and volume status			

Management of Cardiomyopathy in Patients With Cancer

Pharmacologic Therapies

Historically, anthracycline-induced cardiomyopathy has been considered to cause irreversible damage, whereas trastuzumab-induced cardiomyopathy has been considered to be reversible. Recent studies are challenging both of these notions. Although it is known that anthracycline-associated cardiotoxicity may manifest up to 20 years after completion of therapy (Geisberg & Sawyer, 2010), recent studies have shown reversal of symptomatology with prompt treatment (Cardinale et al., 2010) and that it may even be somewhat preventable (Cardinale et al., 2006). When detected, trastuzumab-induced cardiotoxicity usually receives prompt treatment, and therefore symptom reversal is often seen (Carver, 2010). This is not always the case; in a recent study in which pharmacologic treatment was withheld in patients with trastuzumab-induced cardiomyopathy, not all patients had reversal of symptoms (Telli, Hunt, Carlson, & Guardino, 2007). This calls into question the current understanding of reversibility of the disease process as a whole. What both studies do show is that prevention and early treatment are paramount to symptom reduction and disease reversal independent of the chemotherapeutic agent.

Treatment Guidelines

Currently, no standard guidelines exist for the treatment of anthracycline- or trastuzumab-induced cardiomyopathy. ACC/AHA guidelines recommend treating chemotherapy-induced HF similarly to HF from other causes (Hunt et al., 2009). Keystone HF therapies include the use of beta-blockers and angiotensin-converting enzyme (ACE) inhibitors (Hunt et al., 2009). These same therapies have been studied in patients with cancer and have been shown to be beneficial for the treatment and prevention of cardiotoxicity (Albini et al., 2010; Lenihan, 2006). As early as 2000, a small retrospective study showed the positive effects of beta-blockers in patients with anthracycline-induced cardiomyopathy (Noori et al., 2000). ACE inhibitors were shown to aid in the reversal of anthracycline-induced cardiotoxicity in a 2010 landmark study by Cardinale et al. The most commonly used medications today in the cancer population are enalapril and carvedilol (Bosch et al., 2011; Lenihan, 2006). ACE inhibitors are thought to have a class effect and can be used interchangeably (Lenihan, 2006). Carvedilol is the preferred beta-blocker, but metoprolol and bisoprolol also may be used (Hunt et al., 2009; Kveiborg, Major-Petersen, Christiansen, & Torp-Pedersen, 2007; Lenihan, 2006).

Pharmacologic Protection During Chemotherapy

ACE inhibitors and beta-blockers not only are the mainstay therapies in treating cardiotoxicity but also may play a role in preventing cardiotoxicity due to chemotherapy. In a small study, carvedilol was found to have antioxidant properties in addition to its beta-adrenergic blocking effects (Oliveira et al., 2004). Carvedilol has also been shown to be cardioprotective in patients receiving anthracycline chemotherapy (Kalay et al., 2006). In a study where patients received either carvedilol 12.5 mg daily or placebo, the treatment group demonstrated preserved LVEF, whereas the control group showed diminished LVEF (Kalay et al., 2006). Enalapril has also been shown to be cardioprotective for patients receiving high-dose chemotherapy (Cardinale et al., 2006). Additionally, lipid-lowering medications such as statins may have cardioprotective properties as well. They decrease the anti-inflammatory responses caused by anthracyclines (Geisberg & Sawyer, 2010) and have antineoplastic value (Albini et al., 2010).

Current Notions

Because of these newly discovered pharmacologic properties of drugs, studies are now beginning to challenge the concept that damage from anthracycline-induced cardiomyopathy is nonreversible. A recent study demonstrated that if treatment with enalapril and carvedilol was initiated within six months of diagnosis, there was a 28% response to medical therapy, and if treatment was started within one to two months, the response rate increased to 68% (Cardinale & Sandri, 2010). This is the largest study to date that has demonstrated reversibility of anthracycline-associated cardiomyopathy. More studies are needed to confirm this finding. This shows how vital it is to detect cardiomyopathy early and initiate treatment immediately to maximize the chance of reversibility of the disease process.

Trastuzumab-related cardiomyopathy generally is thought to be reversible (Ewer & Lippman, 2005; Suter et al., 2007). It is believed that withholding trastuzumab therapy for a period of two to four months will allow the myocyte cells to repair from the dysfunction and allow for continuation of the chemotherapy at a later date (Ewer & Lippman, 2005). Treatment with typical HF medications will enhance recovery during the holding period, but not all patients have reversal of cardiac dysfunction (Telli et al., 2007). Thus, it is important that patients be followed closely during this period to ensure resolution of the cardiac event prior to reinitiating therapy (Jones et al., 2009).

Use of Dexrazoxane

Dexrazoxane is an iron-chelating agent that is thought to be cardioprotective against anthracycline-induced cardiomyopathy and is given concomitantly with anthracyclines.

Recent studies have shown that the risks of using the drug may outweigh its potential benefits (van Dalen, Caron, Dickinson, & Kremer, 2011). For this reason, the American Society of Clinical Oncology has changed its recommended guidelines on the use of this drug. It is no longer recommended for routine use along with anthracycline therapy but can be considered when patients are receiving doses of doxorubicin higher than 300 mg/m^2 (Hensley et al., 2009).

Medical Management

The Team Approach

A collaborative approach among all members of the healthcare team, including the patient, is the best way to recognize symptoms early. Several interdisciplinary approaches recently have been presented in the literature as examples of how to facilitate a partnership between the oncologist and the cardiologist (Albini et al., 2010; Ederhy et al., 2011; Hong, Iimura, Sumida, & Eager, 2010; Raschi et al., 2010). Generally, these management strategies focus on identifying those who are at high risk for developing chemotherapy-induced cardiomyopathy followed by recommendations for a cardiac evaluation prior to beginning chemotherapy and interim monitoring throughout the treatment period. Figure 2-5 is an example of the cardio-oncology approach to care for a patient receiving chemotherapy.

It is suggested that for all patients a complete history and physical examination be performed by both an oncologist and cardiologist, particularly for high-risk patients (Albini et al., 2010). Recommended cardiac screening testing includes baseline ejection fraction measurement (echocardiogram or MUGA scan), biomarker testing, blood pressure assessment, and chest x-ray (Albini et al., 2010; Lenihan, 2006; Raschi et al., 2010). Patients should receive treatment for underlying comorbid conditions such as hypertension, hyperlipidemia, and diabetes, if present, prior to beginning anthracycline or trastuzumab to reduce risk factors for the development of toxicity during chemotherapy (Geisberg & Sawyer, 2010; Harbeck, Ewer, De Laurentiis, Suter, & Ewer, 2011). All of these diagnostics are an effort of prevention and early recognition of cardiotoxicity (see Figure 2-6).

Follow-Up Testing

The follow-up for an oncology patient with cardiac side effects has not been clearly defined in the literature. Harbeck et al. (2011) recommended repeat LVEF measurements for patients receiving anthracycline or trastuzumab to occur "every 3–6 months during therapy and every 6–12 months for at least 2 years following cessation" of therapy (pp. 1255–1256). With several trials currently ongoing using testing of biomarkers (troponin I, BNP) before, during, and after anthracycline and trastuzumab therapy, outcomes will provide guidelines as to when biomarker testing is most clinically useful during a chemotherapy regimen for the early detection of cardiotoxicity.

Management After Diagnosis

Basic management of patients with HF includes a combination of lifestyle changes and medical therapies. If the patient is still smoking, tobacco cessation should be strong-

Figure 2-5. Example of Cardio-Oncology Team Approach

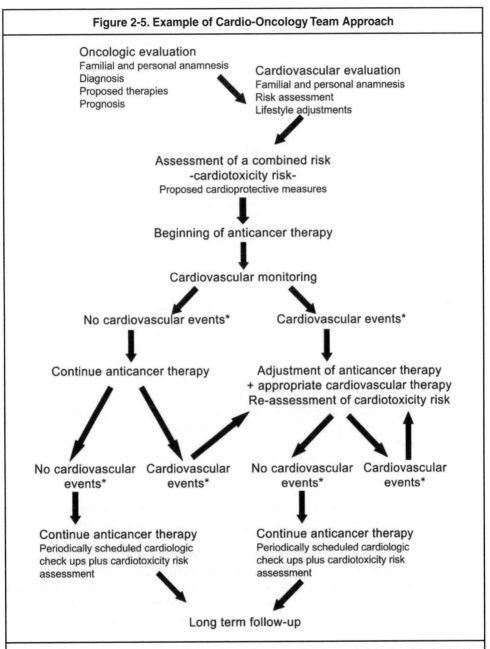

A possible cardio-oncology team flowchart. In a cardio-oncology team effort, the oncologist and cardiologist should work together, evaluating the patient's cardiovascular risk level as an integral part of the choice of cancer therapy. In addition, the patient is monitored throughout therapy and follow-up so that eventual cardiovascular alterations can be detected in a timely manner and treated either by intervention on the cardiovascular side or by modulation of the cancer therapy.

*Substantial changes in cardiovascular risk assessment; for example, a reduction in left ventricular ejection fraction (LVEF) from baseline greater than 5% to less than 55% with accompanying signs or symptoms of HF or a reduction in LVEF greater than 10% to less than 55%, without accompanying signs or symptoms.

Note. From "Cardiotoxicity of Anticancer Drugs: The Need for Cardio-Oncology and Cardio-Oncological Prevention," by A. Albini, G. Pennesi, F. Donatelli, R. Cammarota, S. De Flora, and D.M. Noonan, 2010, *Journal of the National Cancer Institute, 102,* p. 19. Copyright 2009 by A. Albini. Reprinted with permission of Oxford University Press.

Figure 2-6. Assessing for Cardiotoxicity With Cancer Treatment

Pretreatment Phase
- Identify risk factors.
  - Hypertension, obesity, older age
  - Prior exposure to cardiotoxic agents
  - Previous coronary artery disease
- Initiate baseline studies.
  - Multigated acquisition (MUGA) scan/echocardiogram
  - Lipid, diabetes mellitus screening
- Serum markers
  - Brain natriuretic peptide
  - Troponin I
- Lifestyle modifications
  - Smoking cessation
  - Exercise as tolerated

Treatment Phase
- Assess for symptoms of heart failure.
  - Fatigue
  - Dyspnea
  - Orthopnea
  - Paroxysmal nocturnal dyspnea
- Examine for physical signs.
  - Weight gain, edema, S_3, jugular venous distension, ascites, lung sounds
- Repeat baseline studies.
  - After completion of first cycle of doxorubicin (Adriamycin®) or greater than 300 mg/m²
  - Signs and symptoms develop
- Lifestyle modifications

Post-Treatment Phase
- Ongoing awareness/symptom monitoring
  - Patient and family education regarding symptom monitoring
- Cardiovascular assessment
  - Identify early signs and symptoms of heart failure.
- Cardiac studies
  - Repeat MUGA scan/echocardiogram if clinically indicated.
  - Stress test/cardiac catheterization
- Lifestyle modifications

Note. Based on information from Carver et al., 2007; Lenihan & Esteva, 2008.

---

ly advocated. Dietary changes such as moderate sodium restriction combined with fluid restriction of 2 L/day and monitoring weight daily will help to control excess fluid retention that can occur in patients with HF (Hobbs & Boyle, 2010; Hunt et al., 2009). If the patient is taking a diuretic, compliance with these tactics also may allow for a lower dose of diuretic (Hunt et al., 2009). Daily home blood pressure monitoring is encouraged. A nurse can monitor the patient's daily weight and blood pressure with reports of highs or lows brought to the clinician's attention (Hunt et al., 2009). Although routine moderate exercise is encouraged in patients with HF (Albert, 2006; Hobbs & Boyle, 2010; Hunt et al., 2009), the role of exercise in patients receiving anthracyclines and trastuzumab anticancer therapies has not yet been elucidated and continues to be explored (Dickey et al., 2011).

Additionally, close monitoring of electrolytes, such as potassium, is essential. The pharmacologic therapies can work synergistically to increase or decrease serum potassium to the point of necessitating treatment (Albert, 2006). This is especially a concern with patients taking diuretics, ACE inhibitors, and aldosterone antagonists, as these drugs have a direct effect on the body's absorption or excretion of potassium.

Conclusion

With improved therapy for cancer, patients are left in the wake of surviving the cancer only to face cardiotoxicity and possible heart failure. Hope is on the horizon with early detection of cardiotoxicity and the development of new cancer therapies that may possess fewer cardiotoxic risks. To further this endeavor, continued research is necessary to eradicate the cardiotoxic effects on this patient population.

The authors thank Dr. Daniel J. Lenihan, director of clinical research and professor of medicine at the Vanderbilt Heart and Vascular Institute, for his invaluable assistance and review of the manuscript.

References

Albert, N.M. (2006). Evidence-based nursing care for patients with heart failure. *AACN Advanced Critical Care, 17,* 170–185. Retrieved from http://www.aacn.org

Albini, A., Pennesi, G., Donatelli, F., Cammarota, R., De Flora, S., & Noonan, D.M. (2010). Cardiotoxicity of anticancer drugs: The need for cardio-oncology and cardio-oncological prevention. *Journal of the National Cancer Institute, 102,* 14–25. doi:10.1093/jnci/djp440

Apple, F.S., Voss, E., Lund, L., Preese, L., Berger, C.R., & Henry, T.D. (1995). Cardiac troponin, CK-MB and myoglobin for the early detection of acute myocardial infarction and monitoring of reperfusion following thrombolytic therapy. *Clinica Chimica Acta, 237,* 59–66. doi:10.1016/0009-8981(95)06064-K

Bosch, X., Esteve, J., Sitges, M., de Caralt, T.M., Domènech, A., Ortiz, J.T., … Rovira, M. (2011). Prevention of chemotherapy-induced left ventricular dysfunction with enalapril and carvedilol: Rationale and design of the OVERCOME trial. *Journal of Cardiac Failure, 17,* 643–648. doi:10.1016/j.cardfail.2011.03.008

Bristow, M.R. (1980). Anthracycline cardiotoxicity. In M.R. Bristow (Ed.), *Drug-induced heart disease* (pp. 191–215). New York, NY: Elsevier.

Cardinale, D. (2010, October). Cardiac biomarkers and preclinical detection of cardiotoxicity. In D.J. Lenihan (Chair), *Cardiology and Oncology Partnership: IV Annual International Symposium.* Symposium conducted at the meeting of Cardiology and Oncology Partnership, Nashville, TN.

Cardinale, D., Colombo, A., Lamantia, G., Colombo, N., Civelli, M., De Giacomi, G., … Cipolla, C.M. (2010). Anthracycline-induced cardiomyopathy: Clinical relevance and response to pharmacologic therapy. *Journal of the American College of Cardiology, 55,* 213–220. doi:10.1016/j.jacc.2009.03.095

Cardinale, D., Colombo, A., Sandri, M.T., Lamantia, G., Colombo, N., Civelli, M., … Cipolla, C.M. (2006). Prevention of high-dose chemotherapy–induced cardiotoxicity in high-risk patients by angiotensin-converting enzyme inhibition. *Circulation, 114,* 2474–2481. doi:10.1161/CIRCULATIONAHA.106.635144

Cardinale, D., & Sandri, M.T. (2010). Role of biomarkers in chemotherapy-induced cardiotoxicity. *Progress in Cardiovascular Diseases, 53,* 121–129. doi:10.1016/j.pcad.2010.04.002

Cardinale, D., Sandri, M.T., Colombo, A., Colombo, N., Boeri, M., Lamantia, G., … Cipolla, C.M. (2004). Prognostic value of troponin I in cardiac risk stratification of cancer patients undergoing high-dose chemotherapy. *Circulation, 109,* 2749–2754. doi:10.1161/01.CIR.0000130926.51766.CC

Carver, J.R. (2010). Management of trastuzumab-related cardiac dysfunction. *Progress in Cardiovascular Diseases, 53,* 130–139. doi:10.1016/j.pcad.2010.07.001

Carver, J.R., Shapiro, C.L., Ng, A., Jacobs, L., Schwartz, C., Virgo, K.S., … Vaughn, D.J. (2007). American Society of Clinical Oncology clinical evidence review on the ongoing care of adult cancer survivors: Cardiac and pulmonary late effects. *Journal of Clinical Oncology, 25,* 3991–4008. doi:10.1200/JCO.2007.10.9777

Chuang, M.L., Hibberd, M.G., Salton, C.J., Beaudin, R.A., Riley, M.F., Parker, R.A., … Manning, W.J. (2000). Importance of imaging method over imaging modality in noninvasive determination of left ventricular volumes and ejection fraction: Assessment by two- and three-dimensional echocardiography and magnetic resonance imaging. *Journal of the American College of Cardiology, 35,* 477–484. doi:10.1016/S0735-1097(99)00551-3

Dickey, A.K., Geisberg, C., Su, Y.R., Mayer, I.A., Means-Powell, J.A., Silverstein, X., … Sawyer, D. (2011). Strategies for protecting patients from anthracycline-induced cardiac dysfunction. *Journal of Clinical Oncology, 29*(Suppl.), Abstract 591. Retrieved from http://www.asco.org/ascov2/Meetings/Abstracts?&vmview=abst_detail_view&confID=102&abstractID=77608

Doxorubicin: Drug information. (2011). Retrieved from http://www.uptodate.com

Drafts, B.C., Carr, D., Chaosuwannakit, N., Twomley, K.M., Castellino, S., Ntim, W.O., … Hundley, W.G. (2011). *Cardiovascular events in cancer survivors: A review of risk, surveillance, prevention and therapeutics.* Manuscript submitted for publication.

Ederhy, S., Izzedine, H., Massard, C., Dufaitre, G., Spano, J.P., Milano, G., … Soria, J.C. (2011). Cardiac side effects of molecular targeted therapies: Towards a better dialogue between oncologists and cardiologists. *Critical Reviews in Oncology/Hematology, 80,* 369–379. doi:10.1016/ j.critrevonc.2011.01.009

Ekman, I., Granger, B., Swedberg, K., Stenlund, H., & Boman, K. (2011). Measuring shortness of breath in heart failure (SOB-HF): Development and validation of a new dyspnea assessment tool. *European Journal of Heart Failure, 13,* 838–845. doi:10.1093/eurjhf/hfr062

Ewer, M.S., & Benjamin, R.S. (2006). Doxorubicin cardiotoxicity: Clinical aspects, recognition, monitoring, treatment, and prevention. In M.S. Ewer & E. Yeh (Eds.), *Cancer and the heart* (pp. 9–32). Hamilton, Ontario, Canada: BC Decker.

Ewer, M.S., Ewer, S.M., & Suter, T. (2011). *Cardiac complications.* Manuscript submitted for publication.

Ewer, M.S., & Lenihan, D.J. (2008). Left ventricular ejection fraction and cardiotoxicity: Is our ear really to the ground? *Journal of Clinical Oncology, 26,* 1201–1203. doi:10.1200/JCO.2007.14.8742

Ewer, M.S., & Lippman, S.M. (2005). Type II chemotherapy-related cardiac dysfunction: Time to recognize a new entity. *Journal of Clinical Oncology, 23,* 2900–2902. doi:10.1200/JCO.2005.05.827

Fadol, A., Mendoza, T., Gning, I., Kernicki, J., Symes, L., Cleeland, C.S., & Lenihan, D. (2008). Psychometric testing of the MDASI-HF: A symptom assessment instrument for patients with cancer and concurrent heart failure. *Journal of Cardiac Failure, 14,* 497–507. doi:10.1016/j.cardfail.2008.01.012

Felker, G.M., Thompson, R.E., Hare, J.M., Hruban, R.H., Clemetson, D.E., Howard, D.L., ... Kasper, E.K. (2000). Underlying causes and long-term survival in patients with initially unexplained cardiomyopathy. *New England Journal of Medicine, 342,* 1077–1084. Retrieved from http://www.nejm.org/ doi/pdf/10.1056/NEJM200004133421502

Fromme, E.K., Eilers, K.M., Mori, M., Hsieh, Y., & Beer, T.M. (2004). How accurate is clinician reporting of chemotherapy adverse effects? A comparison with patient-reported symptoms from the quality-of-life questionnaire C30. *Journal of Clinical Oncology, 22,* 3485–3490. doi:10.1200/JCO.2004.03.025

Geisberg, C.A., & Sawyer, D.B. (2010). Mechanisms of anthracycline cardiotoxicity and strategies to decrease cardiac damage. *Current Hypertension Reports, 12,* 404–410. doi:10.1007/s11906-010-0146-y

Gottdiener, J.S., Appelbaum, F.R., Ferrans, V.J., Deisseroth, A., & Ziegler, J. (1981). Cardiotoxicity associated with high-dose cyclophosphamide therapy. *Archives of Internal Medicine, 141,* 758–763.

Harbeck, N., Ewer, M.S., De Laurentiis, M., Suter, T.M., & Ewer, S.M. (2011). Cardiovascular complications of conventional and targeted adjuvant breast cancer therapy. *Annals of Oncology, 22,* 1250–1258. doi:10.1093/annonc/mdq543

Hensley, M.L., Hagerty, K.L., Kewalramani, T., Green, D.M., Meropol, N.J., Wasserman, T.H., ... Schuchter, L.M. (2009). American Society of Clinical Oncology 2008 clinical practice guideline update: Use of chemotherapy and radiation therapy protectants. *Journal of Clinical Oncology, 27,* 127–145. doi:10.1200/JCO.2008.17.2627

Hobbs, R., & Boyle, A. (2010, August 1). Heart failure. Retrieved from http://www.clevelandclinicmeded .com/medicalpubs/diseasemanagement/cardiology/heart-failure

Hong, R.A., Iimura, T., Sumida, K.N., & Eager R.M. (2010). Cardio-oncology/onco-cardiology. *Clinical Cardiology, 33,* 733–737. doi:10.1002/clc.20823

Hunt, S.A., Abraham, W.T., Chin, M.H., Feldman, A.M., Francis, G.S., Ganiats, T.G., ... Yancy, C.W. (2009). 2009 focused update incorporated into the ACC/AHA 2005 guidelines for the diagnosis and management of heart failure in adults. *Circulation, 119,* e391–e479. doi:10.1161/CIRCULATIONAHA .109.192065

Jones, A.L., Barlow, M., Barrett-Lee, P.J., Canney, P.A., Gilmour, I.M., Robb, S.D., ... Verrill, M.W. (2009). Management of cardiac health in trastuzumab-treated patients with breast cancer: Updated United Kingdom National Cancer Research Institute recommendations for monitoring. *British Journal of Cancer, 100,* 684–692. doi:10.1038/sj.bjc.6604909

Kalay, N., Basar, E., Ozdogru, I., Er, O., Cetinkaya, Y., Dogan, A., ... Ergin, A. (2006). Protective effects of carvedilol against anthracycline-induced cardiomyopathy. *Journal of the American College of Cardiology, 48,* 2258–2262. doi:10.1016/j.jacc.2006.07.052

Kveiborg, B., Major-Petersen, A., Christiansen, B., & Torp-Pedersen, C. (2007). Carvedilol in the treatment of chronic heart failure: Lessons from the Carvedilol Or Metoprolol European Trial. *Vascular Health and Risk Management, 3,* 31–37. Retrieved from http://www.dovepress.com

Legha, S.S., Benjamin, R.S., Mackay, B., Yap, H.Y., Wallace, S., Ewer, M., ... Freireich, E.J. (1982). Adriamycin therapy by continuous intravenous infusion in patients with metastatic breast cancer. *Cancer, 49,* 1762–1766. doi:10.1002/1097-0142(19820501)49:9<1762::AID-CNCR2820490905>3.0.CO;2-Q

Lenihan, D.L. (2006). Diagnosis and management of heart failure in the cancer patient. In M.S. Ewer & E. Yeh (Eds.), *Cancer and the heart* (pp. 129–138). Hamilton, Ontario, Canada: BC Decker.

Lenihan, D.J. (2010, October). PREDICT trial: Prospective point of care cardiac biomarkers to detect cardiotoxicity. In D.J. Lenihan (Chair), *Cardiology and Oncology Partnership: IV Annual International*

Symposium. Symposium conducted at the meeting of Cardiology and Oncology Partnership, Nashville, TN.

Lenihan, D.J. (2011, Spring). Cardiovascular side effects of antiangiogenic therapy. *Targeting Tumor Angiogenesis.* Retrieved from http://www.angio.org/cme/cvside.php

Lenihan, D.J., & Esteva, F.J. (2008). Multidisciplinary strategy for managing cardiovascular risks when treating patients with early breast cancer. *Oncologist, 13,* 1224–1234. doi:10.1634/theoncologist .2008-0112

Lenihan, D.J., Massey, M.R., Baysinger, K.B., Adorno, C.L., Warneke, C.L., Steinert, D., ... Yeh, E. (2007). Superior detection of cardiotoxicity during chemotherapy using biomarkers [Abstract 265]. *Journal of Cardiac Failure, 13*(6, Suppl. 2), S151.

Lenihan, D.J., Massey, M.R., Isabel, J., Baysinger, K., Steinert, D., Fayad, L., ... Yeh, E.T.H. (2006). Early detection of cardiotoxicity during chemotherapy using biomarkers [Abstract 297]. *Journal of Cardiac Failure, 12*(6, Suppl. 1), S92. doi:10.1016/j.cardfail.2006.06.313

Meinardi, M.T., van der Graaf, W.T.A., van Veldhuisen, D.J., Gietema, J.A., de Vries, E.G.E., & Sleijfer, D.T. (1999). Detection of anthracycline-induced cardiotoxicity. *Cancer Treatment Reviews, 25,* 237–247. doi:10.1053/ctrv.1999.0128

Minow, R.A., Benjamin, R.S., Lee, E.T., & Gottlieb, J.A. (1977). Adriamycin cardiomyopathy—Risk factors. *Cancer, 39,* 1397–1402.

Monsuez, J., Charniot, J., Vignat, N., & Artigou, J. (2010). Cardiac side-effects of cancer chemotherapy. *International Journal of Cardiology, 144,* 3–15. doi:10.1016/j.ijcard.2010.03.003

Mulrooney, D.A., Yeazel, M.W., Kawashima, T., Mertens, A.C., Mitby, P., Stovall, M., ... Leisenring, W.M. (2009). Cardiac outcomes in a cohort of adult survivors of childhood and adolescent cancer: Retrospective analysis of the Childhood Cancer Survivor Study cohort. *BMJ, 339,* b4606. doi:10.1136/bmj.b4606

National Cancer Institute Cancer Therapy Evaluation Program. (2010, June 14). *Common terminology criteria for adverse events* [v.4.03]. Retrieved from http://evs.nci.nih.gov/ftp1/CTCAE/ CTCAE_4.03_2010-06-14_QuickReference_8.5x11.pdf

Noori, A., Lindenfeld, J., Wolfel, E., Ferguson, D., Bristow, M.R., & Lowes, B.D. (2000). Beta-blockade in Adriamycin-induced cardiomyopathy. *Journal of Cardiac Failure, 6,* 115–119. doi:10.1054/jcaf.2000.7505

Oliveira, P.J., Bjork, J.A., Santos, M.S., Leino, R.L., Froberg, M.K., Moreno, A.J., & Wallace, K.B. (2004). Carvedilol-mediated antioxidant protection against doxorubicin-induced cardiac mitochondrial toxicity. *Toxicology and Applied Pharmacology, 200,* 159–168. doi:10.1016/j.taap.2004.04.005

Peng, X., Chen, B., Lim, C.C., & Sawyer, D.B. (2005). The cardiotoxicology of anthracycline chemotherapeutics: Translating molecular mechanism into preventative medicine. *Molecular Interventions, 5,* 163–171. doi:10.1124/mi.5.3.6

Pinder, M.C., Duan, Z., Goodwin, J.S., Hortobagyi, G.N., & Giordano, S.H. (2007). Congestive heart failure in older women treated with adjuvant anthracycline chemotherapy for breast cancer. *Journal of Clinical Oncology, 25,* 3808–3815. doi:10.1200/JCO.2006.10.4976

Plana, J.C. (2011). Chemotherapy and the heart. *Revista Española de Cardiología, 64,* 409–415. doi:10.1016/j.rec.2010.12.019

Pratt, C.B., Ransom, J.L., & Evans, W.E. (1978). Age-related adriamycin cardiotoxicity in children. *Cancer Treatment Reports, 62,* 1381–1385.

Rahman, A.M., Yusuf, S.W., & Ewer, M.S. (2007). Anthracycline-induced cardiotoxicity and the cardiac-sparing effect of liposomal formulation. *International Journal of Nanomedicine, 2,* 567–583. doi:10.2147/IJN.S

Raschi, E., Vasina, V., Ursino, M.G., Boriani, G., Martoni, A., & De Ponti, F. (2010). Anticancer drugs and cardiotoxicity: Insights and perspectives in the era of targeted therapy. *Pharmacology and Therapeutics, 125,* 196–218. doi:10.1016/j.pharmthera.2009.10.002

Sawyer, D.B., Peng, X., Chen, B., Pentassuglia, L., & Lim, C.C. (2010). Mechanisms of anthracycline cardiac injury: Can we identify strategies for cardioprotection? *Progress in Cardiovascular Diseases, 53,* 105–113. doi:10.1016/j.pcad.2010.06.007

Shan, K., Lincoff, A.M., & Young, J.B. (1996). Anthracycline-induced cardiotoxicity. *Annals of Internal Medicine, 125,* 47–58. Retrieved from http://www.annals.org/content/125/1/47.abstract

Silber, J.H., Jakacki, R.I., Larsen, R.L., Goldwein, J.W., & Barber, G. (1993). Increased risk of cardiac dysfunction after anthracyclines in girls. *Medical and Pediatric Oncology, 21,* 477–479.

Suter, T.M., Cook-Bruns, N., & Barton, C. (2004). Cardiotoxicity associated with trastuzumab (Herceptin) therapy in the treatment of metastatic breast cancer. *Breast, 13,* 173–183. doi:10.1016/j .breast.2003.09.002

Suter, T.M., & Ewer, M.S. (2006). Trastuzumab-associated cardiotoxicity. In M.S. Ewer & E. Yeh (Eds.), *Cancer and the heart* (pp. 67–74). Hamilton, Ontario, Canada: BC Decker.

Suter, T.M., Proctor, M., van Veldhuisen, D.J., Muscholl, M., Bergh, J., Caromagno, C., ... Piccart-Gebhart, M.J. (2007). Trastuzumab-associated cardiac adverse effects in the Herceptin adjuvant trial. *Journal of Clinical Oncology, 25*, 3859–3865. doi:10.1200/JCO.2006.09.1611

Telli, M.L., Hunt, S.A., Carlson, R.W., & Guardino, A.E. (2007). Trastuzumab-related cardiotoxicity: Calling into question the concept of reversibility. *Journal of Clinical Oncology, 25*, 3525–3533. doi:10.1200/JCO.2007.11.0106

Torti, F.M., Bristow, M.R., Howes, A.E., Aston, D., Stockdale, F.E., Carter, S.K., ... Billingham, M.E. (1983). Reduced cardiotoxicity of doxorubicin delivered on a weekly schedule: Assessment by endomyocardial biopsy. *Annals of Internal Medicine, 99*, 745–749. Retrieved from http://annals.org/article.aspx?articleid=697360

van Dalen, E.C., Caron, H.N., Dickinson, H.O., & Kremer, L.C.M. (2011). Cardioprotective interventions for cancer patients receiving anthracyclines. *Cochrane Database of Systematic Reviews, 2011*(6). doi:10.1002/14651858.CD003917.pub4

Von Hoff, D.D., Layard, M.W., Basa, P., Davis, H.L., Jr., Von Hoff, A.L., Rozencweig, M., & Muggia, F.M. (1979). Risk factors for doxorubicin-induced congestive heart failure. *Annals of Internal Medicine, 91*, 710–717. Retrieved from http://www.annals.org/content/91/5/710.short

West, R.L., Hernandez, A.F., O'Connor, C.M., Starling, R.C., & Califf, R.M. (2010). A review of dyspnea in acute heart failure syndromes. *American Heart Journal, 160*, 209–214. doi:10.1016/j.ahj.2010.05.020

Yusuf, S.W., Razeghi, P., & Yeh, E.T.H. (2008). The diagnosis and management of cardiovascular disease in cancer patients. *Current Problems in Cardiology, 33*, 163–196. doi:10.1016/j.cpcardiol.2008.01.002

CHAPTER 3

Targeted Therapies and Cardiomyopathy

Courtney L. Bickford, PharmD, BCPS

Introduction

Targeted cancer therapies inhibit the growth of cancer cells by interfering with specific molecules required for tumor growth and progression (Gerber, 2008). The use of targeted therapies has increased tremendously over the past decade because of their ability to prolong survival and decrease cancer recurrence. In the initial design of these newer agents, the hope was that they would target molecules such as tyrosine kinases overexpressed in only cancer cells (Chen, 2009). However, the fact remains that these molecules are biologically active in noncancerous tissues as well, and several play an important role in the normal physiology of diverse organ systems, including the cardiovascular system. Hence, inhibiting these molecules may lead to cardiac toxicity (Chen, 2009). The term *cardiotoxicity* encompasses a number of side effects, including arrhythmias, myocardial ischemia, hypertension, and thromboembolism, as well as left ventricular dysfunction (LVD) and heart failure (HF), which will be the focus of this chapter.

Classically, chemotherapy-induced LVD has been described with anthracyclines; however, recent data suggest that cardiotoxicity caused by some of the targeted agents is generated through mechanisms distinct from that of anthracyclines, which has led some to propose the terms *type I* and *type II* cardiotoxicity (Jones & Ewer, 2006). Type I cardiotoxicity, which is exemplified by anthracycline therapy, is associated with dose-dependent and irreversible damage to cardiomyocytes, leading to cell death. Because of its progressive nature, initiation of HF therapy may stabilize the natural course of the disease but does not necessarily reverse the underlying damage (Jones & Ewer, 2006). As a result, rechallenge with anthracycline therapy is not always possible. In contrast, type II cardiotoxicity, which is modeled by trastuzumab therapy, often is due to cardiomyocyte dysfunction and therefore may be reversible with discontinuation of the targeted agent and initiation of HF therapy. It does not appear to be cumulative-dose dependent, and rechallenge often is tolerated after recovery (Jones & Ewer, 2006).

Incidence of Left Ventricular Dysfunction Associated With Targeted Anticancer Therapy

Currently, six targeted therapies have been implicated in the development of LVD (see Table 3-1). It is important to keep in mind that LVD was unanticipated in clinical trials and is a relatively recent finding (Chen, 2009). Therefore, routine monitoring of left ventricular function was not part of the U.S. Food and Drug Administration (FDA) preapproval process for most agents currently on the market. As a result, very little cardiac data exist for most targeted therapies in use today. Consequently, the incidences presented in Table 3-1 come from both prospective and retrospective reviews, as well as the package inserts (Yeh & Bickford, 2009).

Mechanism of Action of Targeted Therapies

Trastuzumab

HER2 is a type I receptor tyrosine kinase belonging to a family of receptor proteins that includes epidermal growth factor receptor (EGFR/HER1), HER2, HER3, and HER4.

Table 3-1. Targeted Therapies and Incidence of Left Ventricular Dysfunction		
Agent	**Incidence (%)**	**FDA-Approved Indications**
Bevacizumab	1–3.8	Glioblastoma multiforme of brain Metastatic breast cancer, colorectal cancer, and renal cell carcinoma Nonsquamous non-small cell lung cancer
Dasatinib	2	Chronic myeloid leukemia Acute lymphoid leukemia
Imatinib	0.5–1.7	Acute lymphoid leukemia Chronic eosinophilic leukemia Chronic myeloid leukemia Dermatofibrosarcoma protuberans Gastrointestinal stromal tumor Hypereosinophilic syndrome Myelodysplastic syndrome Myeloproliferative disorder Systemic mast cell disease
Lapatinib	1.5–2.2	Breast cancer
Sunitinib	2.7–11	Gastrointestinal stromal tumor Pancreatic neuroendocrine tumor Renal cell carcinoma
Trastuzumab	2–28	Glioblastoma multiforme of brain Metastatic breast, colorectal, and renal cell cancer Nonsquamous non-small cell lung cancer

FDA—U.S. Food and Drug Administration
Note. Based on information from Yeh & Bickford, 2009.

HER2 is overexpressed in an estimated 25%–30% of patients with breast cancer and is associated with a high rate of cancer recurrence and poor prognosis (Dhillon & Wagstaff, 2007). Trastuzumab is a human anti-HER2 monoclonal antibody approved for use in patients with HER2+ breast cancer as a single agent or in combination with chemotherapy (Genentech, Inc., 2010). Despite its success in the treatment of breast cancer, concerns exist regarding its potential to cause cardiotoxicity. The reported incidence of LVD associated with trastuzumab ranges from 2%–28% (Yeh & Bickford, 2009). Trastuzumab-induced cardiomyopathy is discussed further in Chapter 2.

Lapatinib

Lapatinib is a newer, oral, reversible inhibitor of both EGFR and HER2 approved for use in patients with advanced or metastatic HER2+ breast cancer in combination with capecitabine after prior therapies have been utilized, and also in postmenopausal women with HER2+ breast cancer in combination with letrozole (GlaxoSmithKline, 2010). In contrast to trastuzumab, cardiotoxicity associated with lapatinib has been observed less frequently.

A retrospective analysis evaluated the cardiac safety of this agent using prospective data from 44 clinical trials involving 3,689 patients with breast cancer and solid tumors treated with lapatinib (Perez et al., 2008). Cardiac events were defined as symptomatic (grade 3 or 4 LVD) or asymptomatic (left ventricular ejection fraction [LVEF] decreases of 20% or greater relative to baseline and below the institution's lower limit of normal; no symptoms). The authors reported that overall LVEF declined in 1.6% of patients treated with lapatinib. Patients with prior anthracycline exposure had the highest incidence of LVD and also a higher incidence of symptomatic reduction in ejection fraction. LVEF decline in those who received prior anthracycline therapy was 0.5% as compared to 0.1% observed in those who were anthracycline naïve. In patients treated with prior anthracyclines, trastuzumab, or neither, the overall incidence of cardiac events was 2.2%, 1.7%, and 1.5%, respectively. The mean time to onset of cardiac events was 13 weeks. No predictive factors for change in LVEF were identified. Cardiac outcomes were similar whether lapatinib was discontinued per trial protocol or continued per the investigators' decision. Almost all patients had partially or fully recovered their ejection fraction after a mean duration of 7.3 weeks. This finding suggests that lapatinib-induced LVD, similar to trastuzumab-induced LVD, may be reversible (Perez et al., 2008).

The mechanism of trastuzumab- and lapatinib-induced cardiotoxicity is not fully understood. However, significant evidence suggests that HER2 has an important role in promoting cardiomyocyte proliferation, contractile function, and survival (Crone et al., 2002; Ewer & O'Shaughnessy, 2007; Ozcelik et al., 2002). This concept originated from animal studies in which ErbB2 knockout mice developed dilated cardiomyopathy and poor contractility, had impaired ability to withstand stress, and showed enhanced susceptibility to anthracycline-induced cardiotoxicity (Sawyer, Zuppinger, Miller, Eppenberger, & Suter, 2002). In addition, reduction of ErbB2 signaling induces cardiomyocyte apoptosis. Thus, inhibition of ErbB2 by trastuzumab and lapatinib may reduce the heart's ability to respond to stress, which leads to the development of cardiotoxicity (Force, Krause, & Van Etten, 2007).

Because both trastuzumab and lapatinib inhibit ErbB2, there have been questions as to why a higher incidence of LVD has been observed with trastuzumab as compared to lapatinib. One consideration is that lapatinib studies had stricter exclusion criteria, as well as prospective cardiac monitoring employed because of the cardiac effects observed with trastuzumab; consequently, this may have reduced the number of cardiac events seen with lapatinib. In addition, a mechanism of cardiotoxicity independent of ErbB2 signaling may be involved. One mechanism that has been proposed for trastuzumab-induced cardiac toxicity includes its immune-mediated effects on the heart cells (Force et al., 2007). Trastuzumab is an immunoglobulin G1 (IgG1) monoclonal antibody, which, compared to other isotypes of IgG, is most effective for mediating complement-dependent cell lysis and antibody-dependent, cell-mediated cytotoxicity. As a result, when trastuzumab binds to ErbB2 located on the surface of both cancer and heart cells, it can induce cancer cell death and destruction of cardiomyocytes through these immune-mediated mechanisms via the actions of T lymphocytes and natural killer cells (Force et al., 2007).

Bevacizumab

Bevacizumab is a recombinant humanized monoclonal IgG1 antibody that binds to vascular endothelial growth factor (VEGF), blocking kinase activation and thereby preventing the proliferation of endothelial cells and formation of new blood vessels. Bevacizumab is FDA approved for the treatment of several malignancies, including glioblastoma multiforme, metastatic breast cancer, metastatic colorectal cancer, metastatic renal cell carcinoma, and nonsquamous non-small cell neoplasm of the lung (Genentech, Inc., 2011). HF associated with bevacizumab has been sporadically reported in several trials in patients with advanced solid tumors; however, few trials have included prospective monitoring, and therefore the true extent of LVD cannot be fully assessed.

In a recent meta-analysis of five randomized, multicenter, phase 3 trials including 3,784 patients, bevacizumab therapy significantly increased the relative risk of HF in patients with metastatic breast cancer (Choueiri et al., 2011). The overall incidence of HF associated with regimens containing bevacizumab compared to regimens without bevacizumab was 1.6% versus 0.4%. Furthermore, the overall relative risk of developing high-grade HF with bevacizumab therapy was 4.74 (95% CI [1.84, 12.19]; p = 0.001). No significant differences in HF incidence or relative risk were found between the low-dose (2.5 mg/week) and high-dose (5 mg/week) bevacizumab regimens. When looking at the influence of concomitant chemotherapy (taxanes, capecitabine, and anthracyclines), the incidence of HF was highest with concomitant anthracycline therapy. However, this was not found to be statistically significant (Choueiri et al., 2011).

According to the package insert, the incidence of grade 3 or higher LVD was 1% in patients receiving bevacizumab compared to 0.6% in the control arm across all indications (Genetech, Inc., 2011). In patients with metastatic breast cancer, the incidence of grade 3–4 HF was 2.2% in patients who received bevacizumab plus paclitaxel compared to 0.3% in the control arm. Among patients who had received prior anthracyclines for metastatic breast cancer, the rate of HF was 3.8% in patients receiving bevacizumab compared to 0.6% in patients receiving paclitaxel alone. The safety of continuation or resumption of bevacizumab in patients with cardiac dysfunction has not been studied (Genentech, Inc., 2011). Therefore, the cardiologist and oncologist should discuss the risks and benefits of continuing bevacizumab therapy, and the decision should be made on a case-by-case basis.

Bevacizumab may cause HF through inhibition of VEGF, which is the main mechanism implicated in the development of hypertension as well (Chen, Kerkelä, & Force, 2008). The VEGF pathway is thought to have an important role in cardiac physiology. Mice lacking the VEGF gene have thinned myocardial walls and depressed contractile function. Animal studies have shown that VEGF is important for normal tissue growth and angiogenesis, which play a key role in the normal adaptive response to pressure load. Therefore, blocking this pathway disrupts the normal adaptive response to pressure load. Pressure overload may then result in a reduction of myocardial capillary density, global contractile dysfunction, cardiac fibrosis, and eventually decompensated HF (Chen et al., 2008).

Imatinib

Imatinib inhibits the activity of the fusion protein Bcr-Abl, which arises from the chromosomal translocation that creates the Philadelphia chromosome and is the fundamental defect observed in nearly 90% of cases of chronic myeloid leukemia (CML) and some cases of B-cell acute lymphoblastic leukemia (ALL). The true incidence of imatinib-induced LVD is unknown because cardiac function was not prospectively measured in clinical trials. Kerkelä and colleagues (2006) were the first to propose the association between cardiotoxicity and imatinib when they reported 10 patients who developed severe HF while on imatinib therapy. In addition, they showed that imatinib-treated mice developed left ventricular contractile dysfunction and cellular abnormalities suggestive of toxic myopathy (Kerkelä et al., 2006). After this report was published, three retrospective analyses and two randomized controlled trials were published, suggesting that the overall incidence of imatinib-induced LVD is low, ranging from 0.2%–1.7% (Atallah, Durand, Kantarjian, & Cortes, 2007; Hatfield, Owen, & Pilot, 2007; O'Brien et al., 2003; Trent et al., 2010; Verweij et al., 2007). Risk factors for imatinib-induced cardiotoxicity have not been defined.

The mechanism by which imatinib induces HF is unknown. Research by Kerkelä et al. (2006) suggested that inhibition of the Abl protein, the main target of imatinib in CML, seems to be the key mechanism involved in causing cardiotoxicity. Abl protein maintains endoplasmic reticulum (ER) homeostasis by regulating the ER stress response. Therefore, when imatinib is administered and inhibits Abl, excessive stress is placed upon the ER, leading to cell apoptosis and necrosis. In addition, inhibition of platelet-derived growth factor receptor (PDGFR) by imatinib also may contribute to the development of LVD, as PDGFR may possess a cardioprotective role in response to stress as well (Force et al., 2007; Kerkelä et al., 2006).

Sunitinib

Sunitinib is an oral, small-molecule, multitargeted receptor tyrosine kinase inhibitor that was approved by the FDA for the treatment of renal cell carcinoma and imatinib-resistant gastrointestinal stromal tumor. Sunitinib targets VEGFR1–3, PDGFR alpha and beta, c-Kit, FMS-like tyrosine kinase-3, colony-stimulating factor-1 receptor, and the product of the human *RET* gene (RET, mutated in medullary thyroid carcinomas) (Krause & Van Etten, 2005). Although sunitinib generally is well tolerated, HF has been reported with its use.

The exact incidence of HF with sunitinib is unknown. According to the package insert (Pfizer Inc., 2012), in metastatic renal cell carcinoma, more patients treated with sunitinib compared with interferon alfa (27% versus 15%) experienced a decline in LVEF to below the lower limit of normal. In patients with gastrointestinal stromal tumor, 11% of those treated with sunitinib compared to 3% treated with placebo developed LVEF values below the lower limit of normal. Additionally, based on data from five clinical trials of sunitinib, the incidence of HF ranges from 0% seen in both prospective studies to 2.7%–15% seen in retrospective reviews. The inconsistent findings are most likely explained by the differences in patient populations, study duration, and methods for obtaining the data. In one study, the only significant risk factor associated with the development of HF was coronary artery disease (Chu et al., 2007). The mean time to development of HF was variable, ranging from 22 days to 27 weeks (Chu et al., 2007; Khakoo et al., 2008). Sunitinib-induced HF appears to respond well to medical therapy; however, cardiomyopathy may not be completely reversible (Khakoo et al., 2008).

Several mechanisms have been proposed for sunitinib-induced LVD. Animal studies have shown that sunitinib induces mitochondrial injury and cardiomyocyte apoptosis (Chu et al., 2007). Sunitinib also may cause HF through inhibition of VEGF, which may lead to hypertension, thereby causing HF. Force et al. (2007) suggested that sunitinib may cause cardiotoxicity through inhibition of ribosomal S6 kinase (known as RSK), leading to the activation of the intrinsic apoptotic pathway and adenosine triphosphate depletion. Khakoo and colleagues (2008) hypothesized that hypertension also may play an important role because sunitinib inhibits PDGFR, which helps to regulate the response of cardiomyocytes in the setting of hypertensive stress. Lastly, sunitinib is associated with hypothyroidism in 4%–16% of patients, which is a rare cause of cardiomyopathy and is also associated with an increased risk of HF, which should be ruled out in all patients treated with sunitinib as a potential cause as well (Yeh & Bickford, 2009).

According to the package insert, all patients on sunitinib therapy should be monitored for clinical signs and symptoms of HF, and baseline and periodic evaluations for LVEF should be performed. Sunitinib should be discontinued in the presence of clinical HF. The dose should be interrupted or reduced if the patient's LVEF drops to below 50% and more than 20% below baseline (Pfizer Inc., 2012).

Dasatinib

Dasatinib is an inhibitor of multiple tyrosine kinases and is indicated for the treatment of CML or Philadelphia chromosome–positive ALL with resistance or intolerance to prior therapy. It suppresses the growth and proliferation of leukemic cell lines overexpressing Bcr-Abl and inhibits alternate signaling pathways involving the Src family kinases. The incidence of HF reported with dasatinib therapy is 2%. In patients with leukemia across all dasatinib studies (n = 2,182), HF or cardiac dysfunction (all grades) occurred in 2%, with grade 3 or 4 dysfunction occurring in 1% of these patients (Bristol-Myers Squibb Co., 2011).

The mechanism of dasatinib-induced cardiotoxicity may be similar to that with imatinib because they are both inhibitors of Abl. Besides Abl, dasatinib also inhibits Src and a number of other kinases, which may be involved in the development of cardiotoxicity as well (Chen et al., 2008).

Monitoring of Left Ventricular Dysfunction With Targeted Therapy

The current national cardiology guidelines recommend regular cardiac function assessment by evaluation of LVEF by either echocardiogram or multigated acquisition scan in patients receiving cardiotoxic chemotherapy. However, more than one-third of patients with HF have a normal LVEF; therefore, monitoring LVEF is not sensitive or specific enough to predict late declines in cardiac function. In addition, there are currently no firm recommendations for biomarker testing or preventive therapy, but hopefully future studies will help to clarify their role. Therefore, symptoms are the mainstay of the diagnosis of HF.

For targeted anticancer treatments specifically, no universally accepted guidelines exist for monitoring LVEF. However, the manufacturers of trastuzumab and lapatinib have published recommendations in the package inserts regarding the frequency of cardiac evaluation. For trastuzumab, LVEF should be evaluated at baseline, every three months, upon completion of therapy, and every six months for at least two years after (Genentech, Inc., 2010) (see Chapter 2). For lapatinib, LVEF should be measured at baseline and periodically while on active treatment. According to the package insert, if the LVEF drops below normal or if the LVEF drops and is greater than grade 2, which includes a patient with mild to moderate symptoms with activity or exertion, then lapatinib should be discontinued. The LVEF should then be rechecked in at least two weeks. Once the LVEF returns to normal and the patient is asymptomatic, the lapatinib should be restarted at a decreased dose (GlaxoSmithKline, 2010).

The package inserts for imatinib and dasatinib do not include specific recommendations. According to the package insert for sunitinib, all patients should be monitored for clinical signs and symptoms of HF, and baseline and periodic evaluations for LVEF should be performed. The drug should be discontinued in the presence of clinical HF. The dose should be interrupted or reduced if the patient's LVEF drops to below 50% and more than 20% below baseline (Pfizer Inc., 2012).

Treatment

Please see Chapter 10: Heart Failure in Patients With Cancer.

Conclusion

Targeted therapies have made tremendous advances in oncology, but much is still unknown about predicting, preventing, and reducing the occurrence of cardiotoxicity. From a pharmacologic perspective, eventual understanding of the primary mechanisms involved in the development of cardiotoxicity is essential, and from a clinical perspective, it is necessary to define the clinical end points of cardiotoxicity and standardize cardiac monitoring. Until then, each patient should be managed on a case-by-case basis, weighing the therapeutic gains versus the cardiovascular risks.

References

Atallah, E., Durand, J.B., Kantarjian, H., & Cortes, J. (2007). Congestive heart failure is a rare event in patients receiving imatinib therapy. *Blood, 110*, 1233–1237. doi:10.1182/blood-2007-01-070144

Bristol-Myers Squibb Co. (2011). *Sprycel®* [Package insert]. Princeton, NJ: Author.

Chen, M.H. (2009). Cardiac dysfunction induced by novel targeted anticancer therapy: An emerging issue. *Current Cardiology Reports, 11*, 167–174. doi:10.1007/s11886-009-0025-9

Chen, M.H., Kerkelä, R., & Force, T. (2008). Mechanisms of cardiac dysfunction associated with tyrosine kinase inhibitor cancer therapeutics. *Circulation, 118*, 84–95. doi:10.1161/CIRCULATIONAHA.108.776831

Choueiri, T.K., Mayer, E.L., Je, Y., Rosenberg, J.E., Nguyen, P.L., Azzi, G.R., ... Schutz, F.A.B. (2011). Congestive heart failure risk in patients with breast cancer treated with bevacizumab. *Journal of Clinical Oncology, 29,* 632–638. doi:10.1200/JCO.2010.31.9129

Chu, T.F., Rupnick, M.A., Kerkelä, R., Dallabrida, S.M., Zurakowski, D., Nguyen, L., ... Chen, M.H. (2007). Cardiotoxicity associated with tyrosine kinase inhibitor sunitinib. *Lancet, 370,* 2011–2019. doi:10.1016/S0140-6736(07)61865-0

Crone, S.A., Zhao, Y.Y., Fan, L., Gu, Y., Minamisawa, S., Liu, Y., ... Lee, K.F. (2002). ErbB2 is essential in the prevention of dilated cardiomyopathy. *Nature Medicine, 8,* 459–465. doi:10.1038/nm0502-459

Dhillon, S., & Wagstaff, A.J. (2007). Lapatinib. *Drugs, 67,* 2101–2108. doi:10.2165/00003495-200767140 -00008

Ewer, M.S., & O'Shaughnessy, J.A. (2007). Cardiac toxicity of trastuzumab-related regimens in HER2-overexpressing breast cancer. *Clinical Breast Cancer, 7,* 600–607. doi:10.3816/CBC.2007.n.017

Force, T., Krause, D.S., & Van Etten, R.A. (2007). Molecular mechanisms of cardiotoxicity of tyrosine kinase inhibition. *Nature Reviews Cancer, 7,* 332–344. doi:10.1038/nrc2106

Genentech, Inc. (2010). *Herceptin®* [Package insert]. South San Francisco, CA: Author.

Genentech, Inc. (2011). *Avastin®* [Package insert]. South San Francisco, CA: Author.

Gerber, D.E. (2008). Targeted therapies: A new generation of cancer treatments. *American Family Physician, 77,* 311–319.

GlaxoSmithKline. (2010). *Tykerb®* [Package insert]. Research Triangle Park, NC: Author.

Hatfield, A., Owen, S., & Pilot, P.R. (2007). In reply to 'Cardiotoxicity of the cancer therapeutic agent imatinib mesylate.' *Nature Medicine, 13,* 13. doi:10.1038/nm0107-13a

Jones, R.L., & Ewer, M.S. (2006). Cardiac and cardiovascular toxicity of nonanthracycline anticancer drugs. *Expert Review of Anticancer Therapy, 6,* 1249–1269. doi:10.1586/14737140.6.9.1249

Kerkelä, R., Grazette, L., Yacobi, R., Iliescu, C., Patten, R., Beahm, C., ... Force, T. (2006). Cardiotoxicity of the cancer therapeutic agent imatinib mesylate. *Nature Medicine, 12,* 908–916. doi:10.1038/nm1446

Khakoo, A.Y., Kassiotis, C.M., Tannir, N., Plana, J.C., Halushka, M., Bickford, C., ... Lenihan, D.J. (2008). Heart failure associated with sunitinib malate: A multitargeted receptor tyrosine kinase inhibitor. *Cancer, 112,* 2500–2508. doi:10.1002/cncr.23460

Krause, D.S., & Van Etten, R.A. (2005). Tyrosine kinases as targets for cancer therapy. *New England Journal of Medicine, 353,* 172–187. doi:10.1056/NEJMra044389

O'Brien, S.G., Guilhot, F., Larson, R.A., Gathmann, I., Baccarani, M., Cervantes, F., ... Druker, B.J. (2003). Imatinib compared with interferon and low-dose cytarabine for newly diagnosed chronic-phase chronic myeloid leukemia. *New England Journal of Medicine, 348,* 994–1004. doi:10.1056/ NEJMoa022457

Ozcelik, C., Erdmann, B., Pilz, B., Wettschureck, N., Britsch, S., Hübner, N., ... Garratt, A.N. (2002). Conditional mutation of the ErbB2 (HER2) receptor in cardiomyocytes leads to dilated cardiomyopathy. *Proceedings of the National Academy of Sciences of the USA, 99,* 8880–8885. doi:10.1073/pnas.122249299

Perez, E.A., Koehler, M., Byrne, J., Preston, A.J., Rappold, E., & Ewer, M.S. (2008). Cardiac safety of lapatinib: Pooled analysis of 3689 patients enrolled in clinical trials. *Mayo Clinic Proceedings, 83,* 679–686.

Pfizer Inc. (2012). *Sutent®* [Package insert]. New York, NY: Author.

Sawyer, D.B., Zuppinger, C., Miller, T.A., Eppenberger, H.M., & Suter, T.M. (2002). Modulation of anthracycline-induced myofibrillar disarray in rat ventricular myocytes by neuregulin-1beta and anti-erbB2: Potential mechanism for trastuzumab-induced cardiotoxicity. *Circulation, 105,* 1551–1554. doi:10.1161/01.CIR.0000013839.41224.1C

Trent, J.C., Patel, S.S., Zhang, J., Araujo, D.M., Plana, J.C., Lenihan, D.J., ... Khakoo, A.Y. (2010). Rare incidence of congestive heart failure in gastrointestinal stromal tumor and other sarcoma patients receiving imatinib mesylate. *Cancer, 116,* 184–192. doi:10.1002/cncr.24683

Verweij, J., Casali, P.G., Kotasek, D., Le Cesne, A., Reichard, P., Judson, I.R., ... Blay, J.-Y. (2007). Imatinib does not induce cardiac left ventricular failure in gastrointestinal stromal tumours patients: Analysis of EORTC-ISG-AGITG study 62005. *European Journal of Cancer, 43,* 974–978. doi:10.1016/ j.ejca.2007.01.018

Yeh, E.T., & Bickford, C.L. (2009). Cardiovascular complications of cancer therapy: Incidence, pathogenesis, diagnosis, and management. *Journal of the American College of Cardiology, 53,* 2231–2247. doi:10.1016/j.jacc.2009.02.050

CHAPTER 4

Radiation Therapy and the Heart

*Virginia Beggs, MSc, FNP-C, APRN,
and Claire Pace, MSN, FNP-C, ACHPN*

Introduction

The goal of radiation therapy is a balance of prescribing a dose of ionizing radiation that is adequate to kill tumor cells with a dose that can be tolerated by normal tissue so that harm is avoided. As more patients survive long after their cancer treatments, the late effects of treatment have become evident and require understanding and care.

Radiation therapy has been an effective modality for the treatment of cancer for decades. As with other cancer treatments, ionizing radiation has early and late effects. Boerma and Hauer-Jensen (2011) coined the term *radiation-induced heart disease* (RIHD) to describe the potentially severe side effect of radiation to thoracic and chest wall tumors. Patients who have been treated for cancer involving the chest incur an increased risk. This high-risk group includes those who received radiation for left-sided breast cancer, lung cancer, lymphomas involving the chest, and esophageal cancer. The effects of ionizing radiation on the heart include accelerated atherosclerosis, pericardial and myocardial fibrosis, conduction abnormalities, and injury to cardiac valves (Boerma & Hauer-Jensen, 2011). Except for pericarditis, pericardial effusions, and arrhythmias, which can occur during treatment, most toxicities are late effects that can develop 10 or more years after the completion of treatment (Constine et al., 2008). As the science of radiation oncology has evolved over the recent decade, new radiation oncology techniques have reduced the incidence of cardiac toxicities. However, the risk continues to exist if any part of the heart is in the radiation field. RIHD is not reversible and can only be minimized through careful planning by radiation oncologists to limit cardiac exposure. Nurses who care for patients who have received ionizing radiation to the chest need to be knowledgeable about not only the care of patients as they undergo radiation therapy but also the late effects of these treatments.

Epidemiology

The incidence of cancers that involve the chest is significant. The American Cancer Society estimated that in 2012, more than 550,000 patients will be diagnosed with a cancer that involves the chest (American Cancer Society, 2012). Of these, the largest numbers are patients with lung and breast cancer (see Table 4-1). Considering that nearly two-thirds of all patients with cancer receive radiation therapy and that two of the three most frequently treated cancers that utilize radiation therapy are breast and lung, the patient population at risk for the development of RIHD is significant (American Society for Radiation Oncology, 2011).

Radiation Oncology Basics

Radiation therapy has been used as a cancer treatment for more than 100 years and has greatly evolved as a result of increasing knowledge related to cell biology and the ongoing development of new technologies. In the 1970s when Godfrey Hounsfield developed computed tomography (CT), radiation therapy took a leap forward, enabling radiation oncologists to perform three-dimensional (3-D) planning versus two-dimensional (2-D) planning and thus achieve better dose distribution. The advent of new imaging technologies, including magnetic resonance imaging in the 1970s and positron-emission tomography in the 1980s, has moved radiation therapy from 3-D conformal to intensity-modulated radiation therapy (IMRT) and image-guided radiation therapy. These advances allowed radiation oncologists to better see and target tumors, which resulted in better treatment outcomes, more organ preservation, and fewer side effects. IMRT, which enables the delivery of different doses of radiation to specific areas in a single fraction, also reduces cardiac exposure. Additional techniques such as respiratory-gated and respiration synchronized radiation therapy are used to limit the effect of the motion created by respiration, thus minimizing unintentional exposure of the heart within the treatment volume (Halperin, Perez, & Brady, 2008).

Ionizing radiation is defined as radiation with sufficient energy to disrupt atomic structures by ejecting orbital electrons (Iwamoto, Haas, & Gosselin, 2006; Kahn, 2003), leading to DNA damage in the targeted cells. Ionizing radiation is composed of electromagnetic and particulate radiation. Electromagnetic radiation includes photons, and particulate radiation includes electrons, protons, and neutrons. All tissues have a cer-

Table 4-1. Types of Cancer Most Commonly Treated With Radiation Therapy	
Type of Cancer	**Estimated New Cases in 2012**
Breast	229,060
Lung	226,160
Non-Hodgkin lymphoma	70,130
Esophagus	17,460
Hodgkin lymphoma	9,060
Note. Based on information from American Cancer Society, 2012.	

tain tolerance level, that is, a maximum dose that can be administered without causing harm. The unit of measurement for radiation therapy is the absorbed dose from a beam of radiation per unit of mass. Radiation therapy is given in units designated as gray (Gy), and 1 radiation absorbed dose (rad; often seen in medical records) is equal to 1 centigray (cGy), and 100 cGy equals 1 Gy (Coia & Moylan, 1998).

Radiobiology

Radiosensitivity varies by tissue and is affected by the cell-cycle phase. Some tissues are more radiosensitive and thus are more likely to respond to treatment. Variables exist that either alone or in combination account for the different radiosensitivities of tumors. Generally, rapidly dividing cells are more sensitive to radiation therapy, and the presence of oxygen enhances radiation damage. Cells that have high hypoxic fractions are less radiosensitive (Halperin et al., 2008). Tumor cells also are known to have inherent radiosensitivity (Iwamoto et al., 2012).

Radiation oncologists thus consider numerous factors in planning radiation therapy. Figure 4-1 shows the variables that are considered in planning radiation (Halperin et al., 2008). Other variables include determining if radiosensitizing chemotherapy will be used with drugs such as anthracyclines and trastuzumab (Fadol & Lech, 2011). To reduce radiation risk to the heart, planning for radiation therapy includes minimizing the volume of the heart that is included in the radiation field.

Delivery of Radiation Therapy

Radiation therapy is delivered using several different methods depending on the source of the radiation. Radiation to the chest generally uses external beam radiation, which is delivered using linear accelerators to create x-ray (photons) and electron beams (most common type of machine used). A few centers in the United States have a new technology for the delivery of proton therapy. External beam radiation is delivered in *fractions*, generally five times a week for several weeks. The purpose of fractionation is to allow for repair of normal tissues. The dose usually is limited to 180–200 cGy for each fraction. Fraction size is the dominant factor in determining late effects on tissues because large doses and fractions increase the risk of late effects (Iwamoto et al., 2012). Another method of radiation therapy is known as *brachytherapy*, which uses sealed isotopes placed within or near the targeted tumor. This technique has not been used extensively for tumors involving the chest but has been used with patients who have breast cancer and for palliative radiation therapy involving the airways. Little documentation exists in the literature regarding brachytherapy and RIHD.

Figure 4-1. Variables Considered in Planning Radiation Therapy

- Indication for treatment
- Site of tumor
- Size of tumor (treatment volume)
- Goal of treatment: palliative versus curative
- Normal tissue that needs to be protected
- Cumulative tolerable dose to involved tissue(s)
- Patient comorbidities
- The effect of radiation if provided before or after surgery
- Depth of tumor
- Organ motion
- Radiation fraction dose

Note. Based on information from Halperin et al., 2008.

Pathophysiology

The pathophysiologic pathway responsible for the manifestations of RIHD after ionizing radiation involves damage to blood vessels. This injury results in disruption of DNA strands, causing inflammatory changes that lead to fibrosis. Microscopically, the hallmarks of radiation-associated cardiotoxicity are diffuse fibrosis in the interstitium of the myocardium, normal-appearing myocytes, and narrowing of capillary and arterial lumens (Cuzick et al., 1994). Irregularities of the endothelial cell membranes, cytoplasmic swelling, thrombosis, and rupture of the walls are evident microscopically. The ratio of capillaries to myocytes is reduced by approximately 50%; this leads to myocardial ischemia, cell death, and ultimately fibrosis. Dense collagen and fibrin replace the normal adipose tissue of the outer layer of the heart, leading to pericardial fibrosis, effusion, and (rarely) tamponade. As a result, ionizing radiation damage to the heart leads to coronary artery disease, damage to the cusp and/or leaflets of the valves of the heart, dysrhythmias, and diastolic dysfunction (Adams, Hardenbergh, Constine, & Lipshultz, 2003). The hallmark of RIHD is fibrosis leading to cardiac injury. The pathophysiologic mechanisms of the different RIHDs will be discussed in the next sections.

Pericardial Damage

Fibrosis of the pericardium is both microscopic and macroscopic. At a microscopic level, collagen and fibrin replace normal pericardial fat tissue and cause a thickening of the fibrous layer of the pericardial sac. Injured microvasculature results in increased permeability, which leads to tissue ischemia and eventual fibrosis. This results in stiff, noncompliant tissue that can lead to constrictive pericarditis. At a macroscopic level, adhesions may occur, as well as effusions from exudative fluid that cannot negotiate its normal passage through the pericardial sac and drainage system. Fibrosis of the venous and lymphatic channels of the heart and mediastinum decreases the ability to drain extracellular fluid, including the fluid in the pericardium (Darby, McGale, Taylor, & Peto, 2005).

Self-limited, asymptomatic, small pericardial effusions have been reported in as many as 30% of patients treated with mediastinal radiation. Symptomatic effusions are less common. Total doses greater than 41 Gy and daily fractionation in excess of 1.8–2 Gy have been associated with an increased incidence of effusion (Byhardt et al., 1975).

Myocardial Damage

Microvascular damage seems to lead to progressive obstruction of blood vessels and replacement of healthy tissue with fibrin, leading to ischemia and ultimately cell death. Myocardial muscle cells that have received radiation exhibit bands of collagen that have replaced myocytes; deposits of collagen can form between cells with deposits ranging from a few millimeters to centimeters. This leads to diffuse nonspecific myocardial fibrosis. Fibrosis can lead to diastolic dysfunction, which is an abnormality during the relaxation, or diastolic, phase of the cardiac cycle. Extensive fibrosis can lead to heart failure (Darby et al., 2005; Heidenreich, Hancock, Lee, Mariscal, & Schnittger, 2003).

Conduction System Defects

The conduction system comprises cells that are sensitive to radiation injury. The injury is related to fibrosis, which can lead to arrhythmias or conduction defects years after therapy. Although bradycardia and different degrees of heart block and sick sinus syndrome are the common abnormalities seen, ventricular tachycardia and a prolonged QT interval have been observed more often in patients who received radiation, or radiation and anthracyclines, than in healthy controls (Adams, Lipshultz, et al., 2003; Larsen et al., 1992; Orzan et al., 1993).

Coronary Artery Disease

Radiation appears to cause an accelerated rate of development of atherosclerosis. Microvascular damage appears to play a role in altering smooth muscle in the media of the coronary artery as seen in autopsy studies (Brosius, Waller, & Roberts, 1981). Changes show extensive fibrosis as compared with typical coronary artery disease. The pathology believed to be responsible for coronary artery disease is microvascular injury with intimal hyperplasia leading to thrombus formation (Adams, Hardenbergh, et al., 2003). A cascade of events occurs, with damaged cardiac muscle cells being replaced by myofibroblasts and concomitant deposition of platelets. The left anterior descending artery and the right coronary artery are most commonly involved; disease is often in the proximal portion of the blood vessels and ostia. The plaques seen in the arteries have been found to be fibrotic and are difficult to distinguish from lesions not induced by radiation (Early Breast Cancer Trialists' Collaborative Group, 2000).

Valvular Changes

Few studies about radiation-associated valvular disease are available, and little information exists regarding the echocardiographic appearance of RIHD compared with valvular disease of other origins (Hering, Faber, & Horstkotte, 2003). In a study of survivors of Hodgkin disease, valvular disease was noted up in to 43% with a median survival of 15 years (Heidenreich et al., 2003). The most commonly affected valves were the tricuspid, mitral, and aortic valves with incidences of 26%, 21%, and 19%, respectively. The lesions were most often regurgitant. Another study reported a sevenfold increase in the risk of clinically significant valve disease in a cohort of 294 asymptomatic Hodgkin disease survivors (Heidenreich et al., 2003). Observation over time in serial follow-up studies showed the disease to be progressive in nature (Hull, Morris, Pepine, & Mendenhall, 2003; Wethal et al., 2009). The manifestations of RIHD are summarized in Table 4-2.

Late Cardiovascular Effects in Patients With Cancer

Patients who have been treated with radiation therapy present with a spectrum of risk factors for developing late cardiotoxic adverse effects, related to treatment and/or individual risk. Risks related to specific cancers will be reviewed.

Hodgkin Disease

Numerous studies have shown that patients who survived Hodgkin disease and had received mediastinal irradiation are at increased risk for RIHD compared with the general population matched for age and gender, and the risk becomes significant 5–10 years after completion of radiation therapy (Galper et al., 2011; Hull et al., 2003; Marks et al., 2005).

Table 4-2. Radiation-Induced Cardiac Damage

Manifestation	Notes	Risk Factors
Pericarditis	During therapy, it can be associated with mediastinal or cardiac tumors; associated with certain chemotherapies such as cyclophosphamide. Post-therapy, acute or chronic effusion, pericarditis, or constrictive pericarditis may be seen.	Higher total dose > 30–35 Gy Fractionated dose (2 Gy/day) Increased volume of heart exposed Relative weighting of radiation portals—not using subcarinal blocking Presence of tumor next to heart Type of radiation source
Fibrosis of myocardium	Fibrosis is secondary to microvascular changes. Left ventricle is often normal on echocardiogram. May be progressive, restrictive cardiomyopathy with fibrosis. Can also cause pulmonary vascular changes and pulmonary hypertension. Diastolic dysfunction can occur, alone or with systolic dysfunction.	Higher total dose > 30–35 Gy Fractionated dose (2 Gy/day) Increased volume of heart exposed Relative weighting of radiation portals—not using subcarinal blocking Younger age at exposure Increased time since exposure Use of adjuvant cardiotoxic chemotherapy
Coronary artery disease	Premature fibrosis and acceleration of atherosclerosis can occur. Anterior distribution of effects with anterior weighted therapy. Rates of silent ischemia and silent myocardial infarction (MI) increase, as well as symptomatic MI. Lesions tend to be proximal or ostial.	Higher total dose > 30–35 Gy Fractionated dose (2 Gy/day) Increased volume of heart exposed Relative weighting of radiation portals—not using subcarinal blocking Younger age at exposure Increased time since exposure Type of radiation source Presence of other known risk factors such as current age, weight, lipid profile, smoking, inactivity
Valvular changes	Predominantly mitral and aortic valves are affected. Regurgitation and stenosis increase with increase in time since therapy. Despite normal valves at completion of therapy, progression to significant disease can occur 10–20 years later.	Higher total dose > 30–35 Gy Increased time since exposure Use of adjuvant cardiotoxic chemotherapy *Likely associated with:* Fractionated dose (2 Gy/day) Increased volume of heart exposed Relative weighting of radiation portals—not using subcarinal blocking Younger age at exposure Type of radiation source
Arrhythmias/conduction problems	Right bundle branch block may be due to fibrosis of right bundle branch. May progress to complete heart block, requiring a pacemaker. Complete heart block can occur without other radiation-induced cardiac abnormalities, although rarely. Changes in left ventricle are associated with high-grade ventricular ectopy. Increased right atrial pressure can lead to increased risk of atrial arrhythmias.	Higher total dose > 30–35 Gy Increased time since exposure Use of adjuvant cardiotoxic chemotherapy *Likely associated with:* Fractionated dose (2 Gy/day) Increased volume of heart exposed Relative weighting of radiation portals—not using subcarinal blocking Younger age at exposure Type of radiation source

(Continued on next page)

Table 4-2. Radiation-Induced Cardiac Damage *(Continued)*		
Manifestation	**Notes**	**Risk Factors**
Autonomic dysfunction	Tachycardia, loss of circadian rhythm, and respirophasic heart rate variability Decreased perception of angina	–
Cardiomyopathy	Can cause both systolic and diastolic dysfunction May be subclinical, which is common	Higher total dose Use of adjuvant cardiotoxic chemotherapy Concomitant coronary artery disease
Vascular changes	Significant pulmonary artery stenosis, especially in those treated in early childhood Increase in incidence of carotid, aortic, and renal artery fibrosis and atherosclerosis	–

Note. From "Cardiac Responses to Environmental Stress: Radiation" (p. 8.15.3), by M.J. Adams, L.S. Constine, and S.E. Lipshultz in M.H. Crawford and J.P. DiMarco (Eds.), *Cardiology*, 2001, London, England: Mosby International. Copyright 2001 by Mosby International. Adapted with permission.

High prevalence rates have been reported for abnormal myocardial perfusion and stress-induced radionuclide perfusion defects or wall motion abnormalities noted on stress echocardiography (Galper et al., 2011). These findings led to identification of severe three-vessel or left main coronary disease that prompted revascularization in asymptomatic patients after mediastinal irradiation for Hodgkin disease. Conventional risk factors for coronary disease were uncommon and did not predict coronary disease. These findings suggest that screening for coronary artery disease should be considered during follow-up care for asymptomatic patients who have received mediastinal irradiation with doses of 35 Gy or more (Galper et al., 2011; Heidenreich et al., 2003, 2007).

A study of 294 participants with Hodgkin disease who received radiation therapy from 1960 to 1995 were screened for coronary artery disease using stress echocardiography and radionuclide perfusion imaging (Heidenreich et al., 2007). Among the participants, 21.4% had abnormal ventricular images at rest, suggesting prior myocardial injury, and 14% developed perfusion defects, impaired wall motion, or both abnormalities during the stress test. Coronary angiography showed coronary artery stenosis greater than 50% in more than half of the patients and no stenosis in 22.5%. Screening led to coronary artery bypass graft surgery in seven patients. Twenty-three patients developed coronary events, with 10 acute myocardial infarctions during a median of 6.5 years of follow-up. Galper et al. (2011) reviewed the cardiac events for 1,279 patients who had mediastinal irradiation from 1969 to 1998 (median of 14.7 years of follow-up) and compared them with a healthy matched population for excess risk. Before 1995, the participants were treated mostly with 2-D radiation planning, whereas participants treated from 1995 onward had 3-D planning with CT. The radiation dose that may affect the heart was estimated at a median of 40 Gy. The excess risks compared to the general population in the 5-, 10-, 15-, and 20-year cumulative incidence rates of cardiac events were 2.2%, 4.5%, 9.6%, and 16%, respectively.

Schellong et al. (2010) analyzed the impact of mediastinal irradiation on the incidence of late cardiac effects in 1,132 long-term survivors of pediatric Hodgkin disease who had received treatment before 18 years of age and had maintained remission for 3.1–29.4 years. The mediastinal radiation dose received was 36, 30, 25, or 20 Gy or no radiation in addition to chemotherapy with doxorubicin at a uniform cumulative dose of 160 mg/m². After a median interval of 19.5 years since therapy, valvular defects were diagnosed most frequently, followed by coronary artery diseases, cardiomyopathies, conduction disorders, and pericardial abnormalities. After 25 years, the incidence of cardiac disease was highest in the group that had received the most radiation therapy at 36 Gy (21%) and decreasing (10%, 6%, 5%, and 3%, respectively) in the groups that had received lower radiation doses or no radiation ($p < 0.001$).

Breast Cancer

Cardiac complications in patients with breast cancer who received radiation therapy vary depending on the era in which they received their radiation treatment. A meta-analysis was performed on 10-year and 20-year results from 40 randomized trials of radiation therapy for early breast cancer involving 20,000 women, half with node-positive disease (Early Breast Cancer Trialists' Collaborative Group, 2000). The radiation fields included not only the chest wall (or breast) but also the axillary, supraclavicular, and internal mammary nodes. Results showed that approximately two-thirds of patients experienced a reduction in local recurrence of breast cancer independent of the type of patient or radiation received. Breast cancer mortality was reduced ($p = 0.0001$); however, vascular mortality was increased ($p = 0.0003$). Those who received radiation to the breast/chest wall and regional lymph nodes were at higher risk of death not attributed to breast cancer.

In the analysis of 40 randomized trials encompassing 178,000 person years of follow-up, annual mortality from breast cancer was reduced by 13.2%; however, mortality from other causes was increased by 21% (Early Breast Cancer Trialists' Collaborative Group, 2000). A number of early reviews showed an excess of cardiac deaths in the irradiated groups of patients with breast cancer. Gutt et al. (2008) showed that although overall survival was similar in both groups, radiation was associated with a higher incidence of cardiac death in patients with left-sided breast cancer. Efforts should be made to minimize cardiac exposure and also to promote more vigilant risk factor modification in this group of women. The excess mortality appears to be confined to heart disease, and for this cause, the risk appears to be related to the dose and the fields used. In a study of 20,000 women with breast cancer diagnosed between 1971 and 1988, those receiving radiation to the left breast had a 25% higher cardiovascular mortality rate at 15 years after diagnosis than women who received radiation to the right breast (Roychoudhuri et al., 2007). Correa et al. (2007) conducted an analysis of 961 medical records from patients with early breast cancer to evaluate long-term (median 12 years since radiation therapy) radiation-associated coronary damage. Results showed that among the 46 patients with left-sided and 36 patients with right-sided disease who had undergone cardiac stress testing, patients treated with left-sided chest radiation therapy had significant stress test abnormalities (59% versus 8%, respectively; $p = 0.001$) (Lenihan & Esteva, 2008).

In contrast, analysis of data from the Surveillance, Epidemiology, and End Results (SEER) Medicare database of 16,000 patients with breast cancer diagnosed between 1986 and 1993 revealed no difference in cardiac morbidity—including ischemic heart disease—between women with left- and right-sided breast cancer (Darby et al., 2005). A later study (Hooning et al., 2006) of 4,414 patients with breast cancer at a median follow-up of 17.7 years suggested that radiation to either side of the mammary chain was correlated with a higher risk for cardiovascular disease, with an overall hazard ratio (HR) of 1.41. Although the risk for myocardial infarction was lower in women treated after 1979 (because of the introduction of breast-conserving therapy), the risk of developing heart failure persisted (HR = 2.66). The risk for myocardial infarction was higher in women receiving radiation to the left chest regardless of treatment period or regimen (HR = 3.54; 95% CI) versus no radiation or negligible dose to the heart (Hooning et al., 2007; Patt et al., 2005).

With current radiation techniques, less radiation is delivered to the heart, both in volume (of heart irradiated) and dose. The more current literature examining contemporary radiation techniques does not describe the cardiotoxicity seen in earlier studies but lacks the extended time span to look at late effects. Newer echocardiographic and radiologic techniques have evolved and may be useful to describe changes in wall motion, myocardial perfusion defects, and changes in myocardial strain before patients report any cardiac symptoms.

Lung Cancer

The literature looking at the cardiotoxicity of radiation in patients with lung cancer is sparse, with the overall mortality from lung cancer and competing cardiovascular comorbidities making it difficult to clearly determine the cause of specific changes to the heart. However, current therapeutic modalities are improving the mortality for patients with treated lung cancer. Several studies suggest up to a threefold increase in cardiac mortality in irradiated versus nonirradiated patients. The doses of radiation used to treat lung cancer are often high (45 Gy and above), and treating tumors of the chest often requires radiation fields that involve some degree of heart volume (Prosnitz, Chen, & Marks, 2005). Over time, it is plausible that very aggressively and successfully treated patients with lung cancer will develop RIHD.

Esophageal Cancer

The esophagus lies close to the heart; thus, exposure of cardiac structures is unavoidable when irradiating portions of the esophagus. Pericardial effusions have been reported in 25%–30% of patients receiving radiation, with a median onset of approximately five months. One small study using multigated acquisition scan to evaluate change in overall ejection fraction following treatment with radiation showed a very small drop that was not considered clinically significant (Tripp et al., 2005). As patients treated for esophageal cancer with newer techniques and therapies survive longer, more information about this cohort will be available (Osawa et al., 2009; Sasamoto et al., 2007; Tripp et al., 2005). Table 4-3 summarizes radiation dosing by type of cancer.

Nursing Implications

Awareness of the potential for RIHD in patients who have received radiation to the heart is key to identifying patients who are at risk and providing education regarding symptoms they might experience. Although most survivors do not experience cardi-

Table 4-3. Radiation Dosing by Site			
Type of Cancer	Prescription	Dose Limitations	Comment
Breast	45–50 Gy increasing to 60–66 Gy with boost to tumor bed	For left breast cancer, need to minimize heart volume in the field.	Coronary artery disease (CAD), arrhythmia
Esophagus	50.4 Gy	Limit 50% of ventricles, < 25 Gy.	Pericarditis, CAD
Hodgkin disease	30–40 Gy	Entire cardiac silhouette < 15 Gy, block at apex; after 30–35 Gy, add subcarinal block (5 cm below the carina).	CAD
Lung	50–70 Gy with fractionation every day	Limit 50% of volume of the heart so that the dose is < 25–40 Gy.	Subacute—pericarditis Late effect—CAD
Non-Hodgkin lymphoma	25–36 Gy	Entire cardiac silhouette < 15 Gy, block at apex; after 30–35 Gy, add subcarinal block (5 cm below the carina).	CAD

Note. Based on information from Chen et al., 2007; Chung & Bevan, 2007a, 2007b; Dai, 2007; Hansen & Haas-Kogan, 2007; Missett & Haas-Kogan, 2007.

ac problems, knowing the signs and symptoms of the possible late effects will help patients to take steps to care for their heart. The late effects of radiation therapy, corresponding signs and symptoms, screening and diagnostic tests, and management are outlined in Table 4-4.

Obtaining a comprehensive patient history will help to identify patients at increased cardiovascular risk, especially when there is a prior history of chest irradiation. Identifying the doses of radiation and chemotherapies that patients have received and documenting this information in the medical record will enable providers to understand the risks and monitor for the long-term cardiovascular effects of radiation therapy in patients. These risk factors are summarized in Figure 4-2. Survivorship care plans are becoming more important for patients to keep and use as a tool for ensuring appropriate surveillance of long-term or late effects and to help inform their providers.

Patients and survivors who have undergone cancer therapy should be educated on the management of modifiable risk factors and early identification of symptoms of the cardiovascular complications that can potentially result from radiation therapy. This would include primary and secondary prevention strategies such as lipid and blood pressure control, a healthy diet, and regular exercise as recommended by the approved national guidelines (Greenland et al., 2010; Lindenfeld al., 2010; Mosca et al., 2011). Collaboration between primary care providers, oncologists, and cardiologists is of utmost importance in the long-term follow-up of these patients.

Table 4-4. Cardiovascular Late Effects of Radiation Therapy

Late Effects	Treatment	Signs and Symptoms	Screening and Diagnostic Tests	Management
Pericarditis	> 35 Gy	Fatigue, dyspnea on exertion, chest pain, cyanosis, ascites, peripheral edema, hypotension, friction rub, muffled heart sounds, venous distension, pulsus paradoxus, Kussmaul sign	Electrocardiogram (ECG) Chest x-ray Echocardiogram	Pericardiocentesis Pericardiectomy
Cardiomyopathy/heart failure due to systolic or diastolic dysfunction	> 35 Gy or > 25 Gy and anthracycline	Heart failure symptoms Fatigue, cough, dyspnea on exertion, orthopnea, peripheral edema, hyper/hypotension, tachypnea, rales, murmur, elevated jugular venous pressure, tachycardia, S_3, hepatomegaly, syncope	Echocardiogram ECG proBNP (brain natriuretic peptide) test Possibly angiography	Heart failure education Beta-blockers, angiotensin-converting enzyme inhibitors or angiotensin receptor blockers, aldosterone antagonists, digoxin for symptom relief, diuretics as needed for volume control Possibly cardiac resynchronization therapy Low-sodium diet Advanced therapies as appropriate, including ventricular assist devices or cardiac transplant
Coronary artery disease	> 30 Gy	Anginal symptoms such as chest, neck, or jaw pain, dyspnea, diaphoresis, nausea, arrhythmia	Exercise stress test with or without radionuclide angiography or dobutamine stress echocardiogram Echocardiogram Possibly coronary angiogram	Risk factor modification: smoking cessation, exercise, dietary modification Cardiac medications and lipid-lowering agents as appropriate Coronary interventions as appropriate, including angioplasty, stenting, coronary artery bypass grafting

(Continued on next page)

Table 4-4. Cardiovascular Late Effects of Radiation Therapy *(Continued)*

Late Effects	Treatment	Signs and Symptoms	Screening and Diagnostic Tests	Management
Valvular disease	> 40 Gy	Cough, shortness of breath, anginal symptoms, syncope, murmurs, heart failure signs and/or symptoms such as fatigue, dyspnea on exertion	Echocardiogram Cardiac catheterization	Valvular replacement
Arrhythmia	–	Palpitations, lightheadedness, syncope, heart failure	ECG 24-hour Holter monitor	Pacemaker for bradycardia

Note. From "Cardiac Responses to Environmental Stress: Radiation" (p. 8.15.2), by M.J. Adams, L.S. Constine, and S.E. Lipshultz in M.H. Crawford and J.P. DiMarco (Eds.), *Cardiology,* 2001, London, England: Mosby International. Copyright 2001 by Mosby International. Adapted with permission.

Figure 4-2. Risk Factors for Radiation-Induced Heart Disease

Radiation-Related Factors
• Total radiation dose
• Dose per fraction
• Volume of heart irradiated
• Concomitant administration of cardiotoxic systemic agents (e.g., anthracyclines, trastuzumab)

Patient-Related Factors
• Younger age at the time of treatment
• Hypertension
• Diabetes
• Metabolic syndrome
• Obesity
• Hyperlipidemia
• Primary cardiac tumors are rare but put a patient at high risk.

Note. From "Cardiac Responses to Environmental Stress: Radiation" (p. 8.15.3), by M.J. Adams, L.S. Constine, and S.E. Lipshultz in M.H. Crawford and J.P. DiMarco (Eds.), *Cardiology,* 2001, London, England: Mosby International. Copyright 2001 by Mosby International. Adapted with permission.

Conclusion

Radiation therapy has been an important tool in the management of a number of cancers and remains a mainstay of treatment for many types of cancer that involve the chest. Radiation continues to evolve with respect to treatment benefit and safety profile. Certain patient populations, such as patients with breast cancer, exhibit fewer cardiotoxic effects with more contemporary radiation treatment. Other populations, such as patients with lung cancer and esophageal cancer, are living longer, and the cardiotoxicity profiles need to be quantified.

Nurses have the opportunity and the obligation to influence survivorship care by assessing pretreatment cardiovascular risk, as well as assessing the specific treatments their patients have received for risk of cardiac disease. Cancer survivors need to be educated about the symptoms that indicate cardiac toxicities and warrant further evaluation. Ongoing coaching regarding lifestyle choices and cardiovascular risk assessment is within the nurse's role and can improve quality of life and reduce cardiac morbidity.

References

Adams, M.J., Hardenbergh, P.H., Constine, L.S., & Lipshultz, S.E. (2003). Radiation-associated cardiovascular disease. *Critical Reviews in Oncology/Hematology, 45,* 55–75. doi:10.1016/S1040-8428(01)00227-X

Adams, M.J., Lipshultz, S.E., Schwartz, C., Fajardo, L.F., Coen, V., & Constine, L.S. (2003). Radiation-associated cardiovascular disease: Manifestations and management. *Seminars in Radiation Oncology, 13,* 346–356.

American Cancer Society. (2012). Cancer facts and figures 2012. Retrieved from http://www.cancer.org/Research/CancerFactsFigures/index

American Society for Radiation Oncology. (2011). ASTRO FAQs: Fast facts about radiation therapy. Retrieved from https://astro.org/News-and-Media/Media-Resources/FAQs/Fast-Facts-About-Radiation-Therapy/Index.aspx

Boerma, M., & Hauer-Jensen, M. (2011). Preclinical research into basic mechanisms of radiation-induced heart disease. *Cardiology Research and Practice, 2011,* Article ID 858262. doi:10.4061/2011/858262

Brosius, F.C., 3rd, Waller, B.F., & Roberts, W.C. (1981). Radiation heart disease: Analysis of 16 young (aged 15 to 33 years) necropsy patients who received over 3,500 rads to the heart. *American Journal of Medicine, 70,* 519–530. doi:10.1016/0002-9343(81)90574-X

Byhardt, R., Brace, K., Ruckdeschel, J., Chang, P., Martin, R., & Wiernik, P. (1975). Dose and treatment factors in radiation-related pericardial effusion associated with the mantle technique for Hodgkin's disease. *Cancer, 35,* 795–802.

Chen, A., Park, C., Bevans, A., & Margolis, L.W. (2007). Breast cancer. In E.K. Hansen & M. Roach III (Eds.), *Handbook of evidence-based radiation oncology* (pp. 182–207). New York, NY: Springer.

Chung, H.T., & Bevan, A. (2007a). Hodgkin's lymphoma. In E.K. Hansen & M. Roach III (Eds.), *Handbook of evidence-based radiation oncology* (pp. 381–393). New York, NY: Springer.

Chung, H.T., & Bevan, A. (2007b). Non-Hodgkin's lymphoma. In E.K. Hansen & M. Roach III (Eds.), *Handbook of evidence-based radiation oncology* (pp. 394–401). New York, NY: Springer.

Coia, L.R., & Moylan, D.J. (1998). *Introduction to clinical radiation oncology* (3rd ed.). Madison, WI: Medical Physics Publishing.

Constine, L.S., Milano, M.T., Friedman, D., Morris, M., Williams, J.P., Rubin, P., & Okunieff, P. (2008). Late effects of cancer treatment on normal tissues. In E.C. Halperin, C.A. Perez, & L.W. Brady (Eds.), *Perez and Brady's principles and practice of radiation oncology* (5th ed., pp. 320–355). Philadelphia, PA: Wolters Kluwer/Lippincott Williams & Wilkins.

Correa, C.R., Litt, H.I., Hwang, W.T., Ferrari, V.A., Solin, L.J., & Harris, E.E. (2007). Coronary artery findings after left-sided compared with right-sided radiation treatment for early-stage breast cancer. *Journal of Clinical Oncology, 25,* 3031–3037. doi:10.1200/JCO.2006.08.6595

Cuzick, J., Stewart, H., Rutqvist, L., Houghton, J., Edwards, R., Redmond, C., ... Host, H. (1994). Cause-specific mortality in long-term survivors of breast cancer who participated in trials of radiotherapy. *Journal of Clinical Oncology, 12,* 447–453.

Dai, C.Y. (2007). Esophageal cancer. In E.K. Hansen & M. Roach III (Eds.), *Handbook of evidence-based radiation oncology* (pp. 208–218). New York, NY: Springer.

Darby, S.C., McGale, P., Taylor, C.W., & Peto, R. (2005). Long-term mortality from heart disease and lung cancer after radiotherapy for early breast cancer: Prospective cohort study of about 300,000 women in US SEER cancer registries. *Lancet Oncology, 6,* 557–565. doi:10.1016/S1470-2045(05)70251-5

Early Breast Cancer Trialists' Collaborative Group. (2000). Favourable and unfavourable effects on long-term survival of radiotherapy for early breast cancer: An overview of the randomised trials. *Lancet, 355,* 1757–1770. doi:10.1016/S0140-6736(00)02263-7

Fadol, A., & Lech, T. (2011). Cardiovascular adverse events associated with cancer therapy. *Journal of the Advanced Practitioner in Oncology, 2,* 229–242.

Galper, S.L., Yu, J.B., Mauch, P.M., Strasser, J.F., Silver, B., Lacasce, A., ... Ng, A.K. (2011). Clinically significant cardiac disease in patients with Hodgkin lymphoma treated with mediastinal irradiation. *Blood, 117,* 412–418. doi:10.1182/blood-2010-06-291328

Greenland, P., Alpert, J.S., Beller, G.A., Benjamin, E.J., Budoff, M.J., Fayad, Z.A., ... Wenger, N.K. (2010). 2010 ACCF/AHA guideline for assessment of cardiovascular risk in asymptomatic adults: A report of the American College of Cardiology Foundation/American Heart Association Task Force on Practice Guidelines. *Journal of the American College of Cardiology, 56,* e50–e103. doi:10.1016/j.jacc.2010.09.001

Gutt, R., Correa, C.R., Hwang, W.T., Solin, L.J., Litt, H.I., Ferrari, V.A., & Harris, E.E. (2008). Cardiac morbidity and mortality after breast conservation treatment in patients with early-stage breast cancer and preexisting cardiac disease. *Clinical Breast Cancer, 8,* 443–448. doi:10.3816/CBC.2008.n.054

Halperin, E.C., Perez, C.A., & Brady, L.W. (2008). The discipline of radiation oncology. In E.C. Halperin, C.A. Perez, & L.W. Brady (Eds.), *Perez and Brady's principles and practice of radiation oncology* (5th ed., pp. 2–75). Philadelphia, PA: Wolters Kluwer/Lippincott Williams & Wilkins.

Hansen, E.K., & Haas-Kogan, D.A. (2007). Non-small cell lung cancer. In E.K. Hansen & M. Roach III (Eds.), *Handbook of evidence-based radiation oncology* (pp. 157–173). New York, NY: Springer.

Heidenreich, P.A., Hancock, S.L., Lee, B.K., Mariscal, C.S., & Schnittger, I. (2003). Asymptomatic cardiac disease following mediastinal irradiation. *Journal of the American College of Cardiology, 42,* 743–749. doi:10.1016/S0735-1097(03)00759-9

Heidenreich, P.A., Schnittger, I., Strauss, H.W., Vagelos, R.H., Lee, B.K., Mariscal, C.S., ... Hancock, S.L. (2007). Screening for coronary artery disease after mediastinal irradiation for Hodgkin's disease. *Journal of Clinical Oncology, 25,* 43–49. doi:10.1200/JCO.2006.07.0805

Hering, D., Faber, L., & Horstkotte, D. (2003). Echocardiographic features of radiation-associated valvular disease. *American Journal of Cardiology, 92,* 226–230. doi:10.1016/S0002-9149(03)00546-0

Hooning, M.J., Aleman, B.M., van Rosmalen, A.J., Kuenen, M.A., Klijn, J.G., & van Leeuwen, F.E. (2006). Cause-specific mortality in long-term survivors of breast cancer: A 25-year follow-up study. *International Journal of Radiation Oncology, Biology, Physics, 64,* 1081–1091. doi:10.1016/j.ijrobp.2005.10.022

Hooning, M.J., Botma, A., Aleman, B.M., Baaijens, M.H., Bartelink, H., Klijn, J.G., ... van Leeuwen, F.E. (2007). Long-term risk of cardiovascular disease in 10-year survivors of breast cancer. *Journal of the National Cancer Institute, 99,* 365–375. doi:10.1093/jnci/djk064

Hull, M.C., Morris, C.G., Pepine, C.J., & Mendenhall, N.P. (2003). Valvular dysfunction and carotid, subclavian, and coronary artery disease in survivors of Hodgkin lymphoma treated with radiation therapy. *JAMA, 290,* 2831–2837. doi:10.1001/jama.290.21.2831

Iwamoto, R.R., Haas, M.L., & Gosselin, T.K. (Eds.). (2012). *Manual for radiation oncology nursing practice and education* (4th ed.). Pittsburgh, PA: Oncology Nursing Society.

Kahn, F.M. (2003). *Physics of radiation therapy* (3rd ed.). Philadelphia, PA: Lippincott Williams & Wilkins.

Larsen, R.L., Jakacki, R.I., Vetter, V.L., Meadows, A.T., Silber, J.H., & Barber, G. (1992). Electrocardiographic changes and arrhythmias after cancer therapy in children and young adults. *American Journal of Cardiology, 70,* 73–77. doi:10.1016/0002-9149(92)91393-I

Lenihan, D.J., & Esteva, F.J. (2008). Multidisciplinary strategy for managing cardiovascular risks when treating patients with early breast cancer. *Oncologist, 13,* 1224–1234. doi:10.1634/theoncologist .2008-0112

Lindenfeld, J., Albert, N.M., Boehmer, J.P., Collins, S.P., Ezekowitz, J.A., Givertz, M.M., ... Walsh, M.N. (2010). HFSA 2010 comprehensive heart failure practice guideline. *Journal of Cardiac Failure, 16*(6), e1–e194. doi:10.1016/j.cardfail.2010.04.004

Marks, L.B., Yu, X., Prosnitz, R.G., Zhou, S.M., Hardenbergh, P.H., Blazing, M., ... Borges-Neto, S. (2005). The incidence and functional consequences of RT-associated cardiac perfusion defects. *International Journal of Radiation Oncology, Biology, Physics, 63,* 214–223. doi:10.1016/j.ijrobp.2005.01.029

Missett, B., & Haas-Kogan, D.A. (2007). Small cell lung cancer. In E.K. Hansen & M. Roach III (Eds.), *Handbook of evidence-based radiation oncology* (pp. 153–156). New York, NY: Springer.

Mosca, L., Benjamin, E.J., Berra, K., Bezanson, J.L., Dolor, R.J., Lloyd-Jones, D.M., ... Wenger, N.K. (2011). Effectiveness-based guidelines for the prevention of cardiovascular disease in women—2011 update: A guideline from the American Heart Association. *Circulation, 123,* 1243–1262. doi:10.1161/CIR.0b013e31820faaf8

Orzan, F., Brusca, A., Gaita, F., Giustetto, C., Figliomeni, M.C., & Libero, L. (1993). Associated cardiac lesions in patients with radiation-induced complete heart block. *International Journal of Cardiology, 39,* 151–156. doi:10.1016/0167-5273(93)90027-E

Osawa, S., Furuta, T., Sugimoto, K., Kosugi, T., Terai, T., Yamade, M., ... Ikuma, M. (2009). Prospective study of daily low-dose nedaplatin and continuous 5-fluorouracil infusion combined with radiation for the treatment of esophageal squamous cell carcinoma. *BMC Cancer, 9,* 408. doi:10.1186/1471-2407-9-408

Patt, D.A., Goodwin, J.S., Kuo, Y.F., Freeman, J.L., Zhang, D.D., Buchholz, T.A., ... Giordano, S.H. (2005). Cardiac morbidity of adjuvant radiotherapy for breast cancer. *Journal of Clinical Oncology, 23,* 7475–7482. doi:10.1200/JCO.2005.13.755

Prosnitz, R.G., Chen, Y.H., & Marks, L.B. (2005). Cardiac toxicity following thoracic radiation. *Seminars in Oncology, 32*(2, Suppl. 3), S71–S80. doi:10.1053/j.seminoncol.2005.03.013

Roychoudhuri, R., Robinson, D., Putcha, V., Cuzick, J., Darby, S., & Møller, H. (2007). Increased cardiovascular mortality more than fifteen years after radiotherapy for breast cancer: A population-based study. *BMC Cancer, 7,* 9. doi:10.1186/1471-2407-7-9

Sasamoto, R., Sakai, K., Inakoshi, H., Sueyama, H., Saito, M., Sugita, T., ... Sasai, K. (2007). Long-term results of chemoradiotherapy for locally advanced esophageal cancer, using daily low-dose 5-fluorouracil and cis-diammine-dichloro-platinum (CDDP). *International Journal of Clinical Oncology, 12,* 25–30. doi:10.1007/s10147-006-0617-y

Schellong, G., Riepenhausen, M., Bruch, C., Kotthoff, S., Vogt, J., Bölling, T., ... Dörffel, W. (2010). Late valvular and other cardiac diseases after different doses of mediastinal radiotherapy for Hodgkin disease in children and adolescents: Report from the longitudinal GPOH follow-up project of the German-Austrian DAL-HD studies. *Pediatric Blood and Cancer, 55,* 1145–1152. doi:10.1002/pbc.22664

Tripp, P., Malhotra, H.K., Javle, M., Shaukat, A., Russo, R., De Boer, S., ... Yang, G.Y. (2005). Cardiac function after chemoradiation for esophageal cancer: Comparison of heart dose-volume histogram parameters to multiple gated acquisition scan changes. *Diseases of the Esophagus, 18,* 400–405. doi:10.1111/j.1442-2050.2005.00523.x

Wethal, T., Lund, M.B., Edvardsen, T., Fosså, S.D., Pripp, A.H., Holte, H., ... Fosså, A. (2009). Valvular dysfunction and left ventricular changes in Hodgkin's lymphoma survivors: A longitudinal study. *British Journal of Cancer, 101,* 575–581. doi:10.1038/sj.bjc.6605191

CHAPTER 5

Acute Coronary Syndromes in Patients With Cancer

Allison E. Fee, MSN, RN, ANP, and Cezar Iliescu, MD

Introduction

Cardiovascular disease and cancer remain the two leading causes of morbidity and mortality among the adult U.S. population. According to the 2011 American Heart Association update, cardiovascular disease accounted for more than one-third of adult deaths and was the overall leading cause of death in the United States (Roger et al., 2011). Each year, approximately 785,000 individuals will experience their first coronary event, and more than 450,000 will suffer a recurrent one (Roger et al., 2011). Cancer is the second leading cause of death in the United States, resulting in more than $263 billion in overall healthcare costs yearly (Centers for Disease Control and Prevention [CDC] National Program of Cancer Registries, 2011). The National Institutes of Health estimated that more than 11.7 million individuals in 2007 were living with a personal history of invasive cancer (CDC National Program of Cancer Registries, 2011). Amid medical and surgical advances in both cardiology and oncology, individuals living with either of these diseases are surviving many years longer than they once would have. Acute coronary syndrome (ACS) in cancer survivors or those undergoing therapy for cancer presents a major challenge to healthcare providers. This chapter will discuss ACS in patients with cancer, including its pathophysiology, associated risk factors, signs and symptoms, and diagnostic criteria, as well as both the nursing and medical management of these patients.

Pathophysiology and Mechanisms of Coronary Artery Disease

Coronary artery disease results from the process of atherosclerosis, which is a progressive, systemic disease of the arteries. Although it was traditionally believed to be primarily a process of aging, much more is now understood about atherosclerosis (Swee-ny & Fuster, 2009).

Coronary artery plaques stem from lipid-rich deposits inside the artery. This process begins early in life and progresses with aging. Risk factors such as elevated levels of low-density lipoprotein (LDL), tobacco use, elevated blood glucose, and hypertension cause oxidative stress to the inner lining of arteries, the endothelium (Davignon & Ganz, 2004). This stress leads to endothelial dysfunction and injury, accelerating the process of plaque formation and weakening the structure of existing coronary plaques. Lipid-rich plaques with large amounts of inflammatory cells and thin fibrous caps typically are the most vulnerable to rupture. Any endothelial injury results in a cascade of events, including disruption of the vulnerable plaque, platelet activation, and platelet aggregation (Davignon & Ganz, 2004). Ultimately, thrombus formation in a coronary artery causes total or partial blockage of the artery, resulting in myocardial ischemia and ACS (Sweeny & Fuster, 2009).

Risk Factors and Precipitating Factors

It is common for cancer and coronary artery disease to coexist, as these diseases share many common risk factors (Ewer & Yeh, 2006). Traditional risk factors for coronary artery disease and associated ACS include both modifiable and nonmodifiable factors (see Figure 5-1). Modifiable risk factors include obesity, physical inactivity, tobacco use, hypertension, hyperlipidemia, and diabetes (World Heart Federation, n.d.). Of note, diabetes carries such an elevated all-cause mortality rate that it is among the highest of the coronary artery disease risk factors and is actually considered to be a coronary heart disease equivalent. This means that a patient who has diabetes but has never had a myocardial infarction (MI) is considered to have the same mortality risk as a patient without diabetes who has had a previous MI. Nonmodifiable risk factors include family history of heart disease, age, and gender. Specifically, women older than 55 and men older than 45 are considered to be at higher risk for coronary artery disease (Huang, Maron, Ridker, Grundy, & Pearson, 2009).

Patients with cancer have additional risk factors unique to their disease process and treatments. Cancer itself is known to be a prothrombotic state, and both venous and ar-

---

Figure 5-1. Risk Factors for Coronary Artery Disease and Acute Coronary Syndrome in Patients With Cancer

Modifiable	Nonmodifiable
• Obesity (body mass index greater than 30)	• Family history of premature heart disease (first-degree male relatives with heart disease before age 55 or females with heart disease before age 65)
• Physical inactivity	
• Tobacco use	
• Elevated lipid levels	
• Hypertension	• Age (older than 45 for men, older than 55 for women)
• Diabetes mellitus	
• Certain types of chemotherapy	• Gender (men have greater risk than premenopausal women; male risk = postmenopausal female risk)
• Radiation therapy, with fields involving the heart	
• Anemia	• Ethnicity (African or Asian ancestry)

Note. Based on information from Ewer & Yeh, 2006; World Heart Federation, n.d.

terial thromboembolisms in patients with cancer have been reported (Khorana et al., 2006). In a recent review of embolic events in these patients, the incidence of arterial thromboembolism was 1.5% (Khorana et al., 2006). Cytotoxic chemotherapy may play a role in arterial thromboembolism, and endothelial injury caused by chemotherapeutic agents may alter the normal anticoagulant properties of the vessel, leading to a prothrombotic state (Blann & Dunmore, 2011). The cancer sites with greatest proportion of arterial embolic events include prostate, bladder, lung, and leukemia and non-Hodgkin lymphoma (Khorana et al., 2006).

Patients with cancer often receive antineoplastic agents that can cause myocardial ischemia (see Table 5-1). The antimetabolite drug 5-fluorouracil (5-FU) has been associated with angina-like chest pain and, in rare cases, MI and sudden cardiac death (Yeh & Bickford, 2009). The reported incidence of ischemia is as high as 68%. Cardiotoxicity occurs more frequently in patients receiving continuous infusions of 5-FU than in those receiving bolus injections. It is suspected that coronary artery vasospasm may be involved in cases of 5-FU myocardial ischemia (Yeh & Bickford, 2009). Although most recognized for causing cardiomyopathy, doxorubicin and daunorubicin have been known to cause acute MI (Ewer & Yeh, 2006). Myocardial ischemia and infarction with the antimicrotubule agents paclitaxel and docetaxel have been reported in 1.7%–5% of patients (Yeh & Bickford, 2009). Monoclonal antibody–based tyrosine kinase inhibitors, such as bevacizumab, have been associated with a higher incidence of arterial thrombotic events, thought possibly to be mediated by inhibition of vascular endothelial growth factor (Yeh & Bickford, 2009). Finally, small-molecule tyrosine kinase inhibitors, such as erlotinib and sorafenib, have been associated with a 2.3%–3% incidence of myocardial ischemia (Yeh & Bickford, 2009).

Patients who have received external beam radiation therapy to the chest may be at higher risk for coronary artery disease. The proposed mechanism includes damage to the endothelium of the coronary arteries, thickening of the irradiated vessels, and acceleration of the process of atherosclerosis (Yusuf, Sami, & Daher, 2010). A cohort study in 2003 that followed patients with breast cancer for an average of 28 years after treatment found that those who received radiation therapy, especially to the left chest, had a

Table 5-1. Antineoplastic Agents Associated With Myocardial Ischemia	
Agent	**Incidence of Ischemia**
Antimetabolite 5-fluorouracil	1%–68%
Antimicrotubules Paclitaxel Docetaxel	1%–5% 1.7%
Monoclonal antibody–based tyrosine kinase inhibitors Bevacizumab	0.6%–1.5%
Small-molecule tyrosine kinase inhibitors Erlotinib Sorafenib	2.3% 2.7%–3%
Note. Based on information from Fadol & Lech, 2011.	

1.33-fold higher risk of dying of cardiac disease than those who did not receive radiation (Bouillon et al., 2011). Although it generally is accepted that cardiac doses greater than 30 gray (Gy) are associated with late cardiovascular effects, newer data show the potential for increased cardiac risk at even much lower doses (Cutter, Darby, & Yusuf, 2011).

Situations that increase myocardial oxygen demand or decrease myocardial oxygen supply are common in patients with cancer and can lead to myocardial ischemia. Anemia, hypoxia, fever, and infection can contribute to a supply-demand mismatch of myocardial oxygen (Matulevicius, Rohatgi, & de Lemos, 2009). These situations place a physiologic stress on the heart. Anemia can decrease the myocardial oxygen supply secondary to low hemoglobin levels. Tachycardia may contribute to ischemia because of decreased coronary filling times (decreased supply) during a shortened diastolic period. Fever and infection increase the metabolic demands of the body. All of these stressors can cause what is called *demand ischemia* and can occur in patients with or without established coronary artery disease (Matulevicius et al., 2009). The 2007 Joint European Society of Cardiology/American College of Cardiology/American Heart Association/World Heart Federation Task Force deemed this phenomenon a *type 2* MI when it causes ischemia severe enough to meet the traditional definition of an MI (Thygesen, Alpert, & White, 2007). This definition will be discussed later in this chapter.

Signs and Symptoms of Acute Coronary Syndrome

Prompt recognition and early risk stratification of ACS is vital. Staff nurses play a crucial role in the identification, triage, and care of patients with ACS, as nurses often are the first responders to a patient's complaints of discomfort or a change in the patient's status.

The classic symptom of ACS is chest pain, which usually is retrosternal or precordial in nature. It may begin upon exertion or while at rest. It often is described as pressure, crushing, aching, or even burning. After gradually intensifying over several minutes, the discomfort usually reaches maximal intensity and persists. It may radiate to the arm, shoulder, jaw, or back. Associated symptoms often include nausea, diaphoresis, shortness of breath, and anxiety. Some patients describe "indigestion-like" pain (Morrow & Boden, 2012). Female, elderly, and diabetic patients are more likely to present with atypical symptoms, including shortness of breath, fatigue, syncope, or altered mental status, and may not complain of any chest discomfort at all (Matulevicius et al., 2009). Patients with cancer often present with subtle or atypical symptoms and may have multiple ongoing symptoms, such as nausea, pain, or shortness of breath secondary to chemotherapy or recent surgery, that can blur their presentation. Bearing this in mind, nurses need to have a low threshold for suspicion of ischemic heart disease and consider the number and degree of risk factors for coronary disease when evaluating any patient (see Table 5-2).

Diagnostic Criteria and Testing

The World Health Organization's traditional definition of MI involves at least two of the following criteria: a history of ischemic-type chest pain symptoms, evolutionary electrocardiogram (ECG) changes, and a rise and fall of serial cardiac biomarkers (Antman, 2012). However, a 2007 joint expert consensus reported that the diagnosis of MI should be based upon the presence of a rise and fall of cardiac biomarkers plus one

Table 5-2. Signs and Symptoms of Acute Coronary Syndrome		
Organ System	**Symptoms**	**Signs**
General	Anxiety, generalized fatigue and weakness	Restlessness, agitation
Neurologic	Light-headedness	Near-syncope, syncope
Pulmonary	Dyspnea, wheezing	Tachypnea, pulmonary rales
Cardiovascular	Retrosternal chest discomfort, tachycardia	Tachycardia, new murmur or S_3 or S_4, congestive heart failure symptoms, hyper- or hypotension
Gastrointestinal	Nausea, abdominal pain, "indigestion"	Vomiting
Integumentary	Diaphoresis	Cool, clammy skin, pallor

Note. Based on information from Matulevicius et al., 2009.

of the following: ischemic symptoms, ischemic ECG changes, development of pathologic Q waves in the ECG, or imaging evidence of wall motion abnormalities or new loss of viable myocardium (Thygesen et al., 2007). Clinically, the spectrum of ACS encompasses unstable angina, MI without ST elevation on ECG (non-ST-elevation MI, referred to as *NSTEMI*), and MI with ST elevation on ECG (ST-elevation MI, or *STEMI*). In clinical practice, the diagnosis of ACS or MI is based on a combination of these criteria and will be discussed in more detail throughout this chapter.

Cardiac Biomarkers

Patients with symptoms suggestive of ACS should have cardiac biomarkers drawn, including creatine kinase-MB (CK-MB) and troponin I levels (see Table 5-3). Cardiac biomarkers should be checked upon presentation. If initially normal, these should be drawn again in about six to eight hours for one or two more sets. If all are normal, they can be discontinued at this point. If any cardiac enzymes are elevated, they should continue to be checked every six to eight hours until they peak and begin to trend downward (Sabatine & Cannon, 2012). Abnormal results should be promptly communicated to the ordering clinician.

Table 5-3. Cardiac Biomarkers in Acute Coronary Syndrome			
Biomarker	**Initial Appearance After Myocardial Injury**	**Peak**	**Return to Baseline Value**
Myoglobin	1–2 hours	1–4 hours	24 hours
Creatine kinase-MB	3 hours	12–24 hours	1–3 days
Troponin I	3–12 hours	12–24 hours	7–14 days

Note. Based on information from Yang & Gersh, 2009.

CK-MB is the isoenzyme of creatine kinase found in highest concentrations in the myocardium. It is released into the bloodstream from injured myocardium. After an infarct, levels of CK-MB will appear elevated in three hours, peak in 12–24 hours, and return to normal within one to three days (Matulevicius et al., 2009).

Troponin I exists in the myocardium to regulate the interaction of cardiac actin and myosin. It begins to elevate 3–12 hours after the onset of an infarct and peaks in 12–24 hours. It remains elevated for 7–14 days, so it can be helpful in the diagnosis of a patient who complains of angina symptoms that occurred several days prior (Antman, 2012). Furthermore, troponin I is more cardiac specific than CK-MB, and its degree of elevation correlates to patient prognosis (higher levels equal a poorer prognosis) (Matulevicius et al., 2009).

Electrocardiogram

All patients complaining of chest pain should have an ECG performed. ECG changes associated with ACS are detailed later in the section on classification of ACS. Of note, a normal resting ECG in a patient with symptoms of ACS does not rule out the possibility of an evolving episode of myocardial ischemia. Therefore, it is recommended that ECGs be obtained serially with cardiac enzymes, typically every six to eight hours, to evaluate for any changes from baseline (Matulevicius et al., 2009).

Noninvasive Imaging

Noninvasive imaging studies to evaluate patients with ACS include echocardiography; exercise, chemical, or echocardiograph stress imaging; coronary computed tomography angiography (CTA); cardiac magnetic resonance imaging; and cardiac positron-emission tomography (PET).

Two-Dimensional Echocardiography

Two-dimensional echocardiography is a readily available and quick diagnostic tool that is able to assess possible mechanical disruptions in the ischemic heart. Left ventricular function, wall motion abnormalities (which may be associated with ischemia), and valvular dysfunction can be evaluated (Sabatine & Cannon, 2012).

Stress echocardiography assesses the heart both at rest and immediately after exercise or pharmacologically induced stress. A negative (normal) stress echocardiography should show a hyperdynamic, or increased muscle contraction, response to stress with no stress-induced wall motion abnormalities of the myocardium (O'Rourke, 2009).

Myocardial Perfusion Imaging

The most common type of cardiac stress test is a nuclear scan called single-photon emission computed tomography (SPECT) myocardial perfusion imaging (Udelson, Dilsizian, & Bonow, 2012). This is commonly referred to as a *nuclear stress test*. The patient undergoes injection of a radioisotope tracer both while at rest and after stress (chemical or exercise induced). SPECT imaging under a gamma camera is taken after each injection, and the subsequent images compare the myocardial perfusion from at rest to after stress (Udelson et al., 2012). Gated images, guided by the patient's ECG, allow the reader to evaluate the perfusion of the heart in motion in both two- and three-dimensional images. Areas of reversible ischemia (viable myocardium) can be evaluated, as can areas of fixed ischemia (nonviable myocardium from previous infarct). Cardiac contractility and ejection fraction, as well as wall motion, are also seen (Ewer & Yeh, 2006).

Coronary Computed Tomography Angiography

Coronary CTA is a type of CT scan to noninvasively evaluate the coronary arteries. Coronary artery CT can identify both soft and calcified coronary plaques. A quantitative measurement called the *coronary artery calcium score* provides further information into the severity of a particular plaque but has been found to correlate only modestly to what is seen on coronary angiography in the cardiac catheterization laboratory (Raggi & Berman, 2005). However, coronary CTA has a high negative predictive value and can be a useful filter test for select patients prior to consideration of cardiac catheterization (Udelson et al., 2012). A normal coronary calcium score is zero, and a score higher than 400 is considered abnormal. A score of 80–400 represents intermediate risk. Scores higher than 1,000 have been associated with a 20% occurrence of MI or cardiac death within one year (Hoffmann, Brady, & Muller, 2003).

Cardiac Positron-Emission Tomography

A cardiac PET scan uses rubidium-82 and [^{13}N]ammonia as tracers to create rest and stress perfusion images. Its advantages over SPECT imaging are greater detection of mild abnormalities in myocardial blood flow, a higher sensitivity and specificity, and higher spatial resolution. Its use is limited by cost, availability, and the inability to use exercise as a stress modality (Udelson et al., 2012).

Cardiac Catheterization and Coronary Angiography

Cardiac catheterization and coronary angiography are minimally invasive imaging strategies that allow for visualization and evaluation of the coronary arteries, as well as measurements of ejection fraction and intracardiac pressures. This imaging technique is considered the gold standard to evaluate coronary artery disease (Costa & Jozic, 2009).

Performed in a cardiac catheterization laboratory, this procedure involves advancing a small catheter up an artery into the aorta. The femoral artery of the leg and the radial or brachial arteries of the arm are the most common access sites. Local anesthetic is injected around the arterial site, and a small puncture is made. The catheter, with the assistance of a guidewire, is inserted over an introducer sheath and advanced up to the ascending aorta and to the heart. From there, radiopaque contrast is injected into each coronary artery. X-ray images under fluoroscopy allow for visualization of the coronary arteries (Costa & Jozic, 2009) (see Figure 5-2). Interventions to open the blocked coronary artery and restore perfusion, such as balloon angioplasty (percutaneous transluminal coronary angioplasty) or stenting, can be performed during this procedure (Morrow & Boden, 2012). Intracardiac pressure and hemodynamic measurements can also be recorded (Costa & Jozic, 2009). Occasionally, patients are found to have severe multivessel coronary artery disease or significant left main artery stenosis on cardiac catheterization and are subsequently referred for coronary artery bypass surgery (Morrow & Boden, 2012). Traditionally, patients with thrombocytopenia have been excluded from interventional cardiac procedures because of the concern for serious bleeding complications. However, given the large population of patients with cancer who suffer from ACS

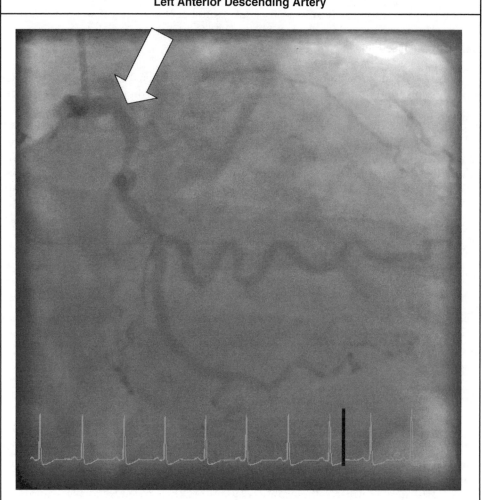

Figure 5-2. Coronary Angiography Image of Totally Occluded Left Anterior Descending Artery

while thrombocytopenic, withholding interventional procedures may mean withholding life-saving treatment. Approximately 140,000 patients are diagnosed with leukemia, lymphoma, and myeloma each year, and the majority of them will become thrombocytopenic during cancer treatment (Iliescu, Durand, & Kroll, 2011). Although platelets play an important role in the development of ACS, thrombocytopenia does not protect patients from ischemic events. The first consecutive case series of patients with thrombocytopenia who underwent endovascular procedures has shown that with meticulous access and careful hemostasis, thrombocytopenic patients can be safely treated with cardiovascular interventions with limited complications (Iliescu et al., 2011) (see Table 5-4).

Differential Diagnosis

Multiple non-ACS conditions can mimic the presentation of ACS, and many are common among patients with cancer. Gastrointestinal and musculoskeletal etiologies encompass more than 50% of patients with chest pain in the outpatient setting (Cayley, 2005). However, more than 65% of patients presenting to the emergency department with chest pain had serious cardiovascular or pulmonary disease (Cayley, 2005). Pulmonary embolism and pneumonia often cause chest discomfort, which typically is described as pleuritic. A thoracic tumor can cause inflammation and local discomfort. Aortic dissection may cause chest pain, often described as "tearing" and associated with hemodynamic instability. Chest wall pain or musculoskeletal chest pain is a di-

Table 5-4. Diagnostic Procedures for Acute Coronary Syndrome		
Diagnostic Test	**Capabilities**	**Special Considerations**
Two-dimensional echocardiogram	Quick, portable. Evaluates left ventricular function, ventricular wall motion, and valves.	Requires adequate acoustic windows (may be limited in obese or mechanically ventilated patients). Variability based on reader and operator.
Stress echocardiogram	Less expensive than myocardial perfusion imaging. Compares global and regional left ventricular function from rest to stress. Stress can be achieved via exercise or chemically with dobutamine (for patients unable to exercise).	Patient should not eat 4–8 hours prior to test. No caffeine, beta-blockers, or non-dihydropyridine calcium channel blockers 24–48 hours prior to test. Remove nitroglycerin patch 4 hours prior to test.
Myocardial perfusion imaging (nuclear stress test)	Allows for visual evaluation of myocardial perfusion at rest and after stress. Can assess size, severity, and reversibility of defects.	Same as stress echocardiogram. Patient must be able to lie flat under nuclear camera with arms above head for 30 minutes.
Cardiac computed tomography angiography	Allows noninvasive evaluation of native and bypassed coronary arteries. It has high negative predictive value and is a good filter study prior to cardiac catheterization in some patients.	Less sensitive in patient with fast (> 70 bmp) heart rates, irregular heart rhythms, or body mass index > 40. Requires the use of IV contrast (caution with renal dysfunction or iodine allergy).
Cardiac positron-emission tomography	Allows for quantitative measurements of myocardial perfusion.	Expensive; not widely available.
Cardiac catheterization	Definitive diagnosis and precise assessment of coronary artery disease. Ability to intervene with angioplasty or stenting to reperfuse an obstructed artery.	Minimally invasive, with risks such as bleeding, infection, stroke, or even death. Requires the use of contrast medium (caution in renal dysfunction or iodine allergy).
Electrocardiogram (ECG)	Evaluates for ischemic ST segment and T-wave changes.	A normal ECG does not rule out the possibility of acute coronary syndrome.

Note. Based on information from Cannon & Braunwald, 2012; Matulevicius et al., 2009.

agnosis of exclusion, which should be reserved once the previously described conditions have been ruled out (Cayley, 2005). Chest radiography and computed tomography may also be used in the initial evaluation of chest pain to rule out the aforementioned conditions (see Table 5-5).

Table 5-5. Differential Diagnoses of Chest Pain		
System	**Diagnosis**	**Features**
Cardiovascular	Angina (stable)	Retrosternal chest pressure, burning or heaviness; may radiate to left arm, neck, or jaw. Precipitated by exertion, stress, or cold weather. Lasts less than 10 minutes.
	Unstable angina, acute coronary syndrome, myocardial infarction	The same as with stable angina but typically more severe, lasting 20–30 minutes or more, and may be associated with nausea and vomiting or shortness of breath. Unlike stable angina, may have a sudden onset without obvious precipitating factors.
	Aortic dissection	Sudden-onset, excruciating "tearing" or "ripping" anterior chest pain, often radiating to the back. May be associated with hypertension or connective tissue disorders.
Pulmonary	Pneumonia or pleuritis	Pleuritic pain, often unilateral. May have cough/sputum production.
	Pulmonary embolism	Usually sudden-onset pleuritic pain, associated with dyspnea, tachycardia, and signs of right-sided heart failure.
	Spontaneous pneumothorax	Sudden onset of unilateral pleuritic pain and dyspnea.
Gastrointestinal	Gastrointestinal/esophageal reflux	Burning epigastric and substernal pain. Aggravated by large meals or recumbent position. Relieved by antacids.
	Peptic ulcer	Similar to reflux, but may be more prolonged or severe.
	Gallbladder (biliary) colic	Right upper quadrant pain with radiation to right shoulder and back. May be unprovoked or occur following a meal.
	Pancreatitis	Intense, prolonged, localized epigastric pain with radiation to back.
Musculoskeletal	Costochondritis	Sudden-onset, very brief, fleeting pain. May be reproduced with palpation over affected area.
	Trauma or strain	Constant aching or pain. Worse with movement or palpation over the affected area.
Psychological	Anxiety/panic disorder	Chest tightness or aching, often associated with dyspnea and tachypnea/hyperventilation. Unrelated to exertion or activity.

Note. Based on information from Morrow & Boden, 2012.

Classification of Acute Coronary Syndromes

ACS encompasses three major diagnoses: STEMI, NSTEMI, and unstable angina. These three disease processes can be viewed along a continuum, with STEMI requiring the most immediate intervention and generally conferring the highest risk of mortality (see Figure 5-3).

In STEMI, plaque rupture causes occlusion of a coronary artery, which ceases forward circulatory flow through it. Resulting ischemia is severe enough to cause necrosis of myocardial tissue, seen as Q waves, new left bundle branch block, and/or ST segment elevation on the surface ECG and as elevations in the cardiac biomarkers CK-MB and troponin I. The distribution of ECG changes provides information regarding the territory of the myocardium involved and the culprit vessel. The ECG of patients with STEMI will show ST segment elevation in two or more contiguous leads with reciprocal changes (see Figure 5-4). A new left bundle branch block in the setting of chest pain should be considered STEMI until proved otherwise (Yang & Gersh, 2009).

STEMI is a medical emergency. Patients with STEMI generally appear very anxious and acutely ill. They usually present with severe chest pain often described as viselike, crushing, or squeezing. Hemodynamic instability, including hypotension and tachycardia, is common. Cardiac arrhythmias may occur, including ventricular tachycardia, ventricular fibrillation, or complete heart block, depending on the site of the infarct. These patients typically are managed with urgent cardiac catheterization or thrombolytics to restore perfusion to the affected myocardial region. American College of Cardiology/ American Heart Association standards direct a 90-minute "door to balloon time" for cardiac catheterization or a 30-minute "door to drug" time for thrombolysis in patients

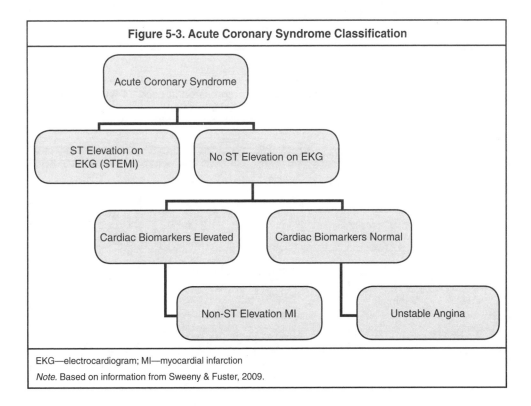

Figure 5-3. Acute Coronary Syndrome Classification

EKG—electrocardiogram; MI—myocardial infarction

Note. Based on information from Sweeny & Fuster, 2009.

with STEMI. This means that the standard of care for patients with STEMI is a 90-minute window from the time of patient presentation to intervention of the culprit vessel in the cardiac catheterization laboratory or a 30-minute window from symptom onset to administration of thrombolytics (Antman, 2012).

NSTEMI results when myocardial injury is severe enough to cause elevation in cardiac biomarkers but no ST segment elevation is present on ECG. It can be caused by occlusion of a coronary artery, demand ischemia, or coronary vasospasm. Although the ECG shows no ST segment elevation, ischemic changes such as T-wave inversions or ST segment depression may be seen (see Figure 5-5). Transient ST segment depression during

Figure 5-4. ST Segment Elevation in Lead 1, aVL, V2, V3, Suggestive of High Anterolateral Wall Myocardial Infarction

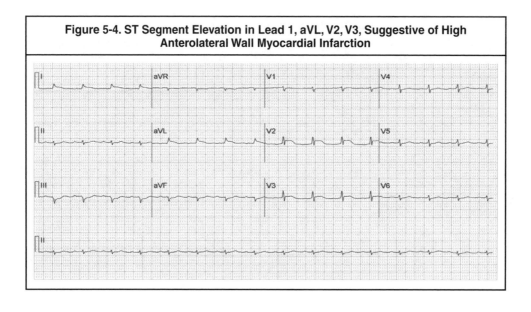

Figure 5-5. Transient Anterolateral ST Segment Depression in Lead V4–V6 and I, II, III (Non-ST-Elevation Myocardial Infarction)

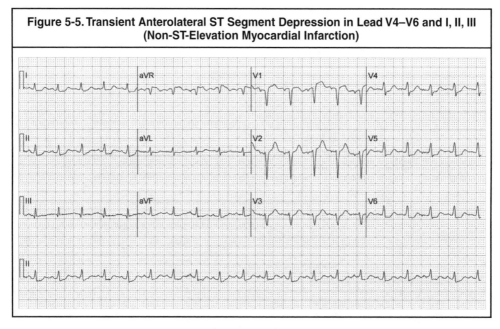

periods of chest pain that disappears with resolution of chest discomfort is highly suggestive of myocardial ischemia (Matulevicius et al., 2009). Cardiac biomarkers will be elevated in patients with NSTEMI. These patients may be treated medically or with cardiac catheterization but are not candidates for thrombolytics (Cannon & Braunwald, 2012).

Finally, unstable angina is a syndrome generally caused by nonocclusive thrombus formation. These patients typically present with chest pain similar to that of NSTEMI. In fact, the only distinguishing difference between NSTEMI and unstable angina is the absence of elevated cardiac biomarkers in unstable angina (Anderson et al., 2007). Ischemic ECG changes may or may not be seen. T-wave inversions are a common ECG finding among patients with unstable angina (Matulevicius et al., 2009). Much like patients with NSTEMI, these patients may be managed medically or brought to the cardiac catheterization laboratory for definitive diagnosis and possibly intervention with angioplasty or stenting (Cannon & Braunwald, 2012).

Further details of the nursing and medical management of each subgroup of patients with ACS will be discussed later in this chapter.

Pharmacologic Therapy

Medications used in the management of ACS can generally be divided into the following categories: antiplatelets, antithrombotics, anti-ischemics, and analgesics.

Aspirin is an antiplatelet agent that irreversibly inhibits platelet cyclooxygenase and, hence, prevents formation of thromboxane A2. Administration of 162–325 mg of chewed aspirin followed by 75–100 mg of aspirin daily by mouth is a grade 1A recommendation for all patients with no clear aspirin allergy or contraindications (Harrington et al., 2008). Nevertheless, it is important to note that patients with cancer have generally been excluded from ACS research trials, and thus far, no clear guidelines on pharmacologic management of these patients with ACS exist.

The issue of antiplatelet agents and anticoagulation presents a particularly difficult challenge in many patients with cancer who may have thrombocytopenia as a result of cancer therapy side effects, bone marrow infiltration, disseminated intravascular coagulation, sepsis, or hepatopathy. Often, antiplatelet therapy is withheld when patients have platelet counts of less than 30,000. A recent prospective study on 70 patients with cancer and ACS found that patients with thrombocytopenia had worse outcomes than those with normal platelet counts. However, patients with thrombocytopenia had much improved overall survival (90% versus only 6%) with the addition of aspirin therapy in the first seven days after an ACS event (Sarkiss et al., 2007). Furthermore, no incidences of acute major gastrointestinal bleed, intracranial bleed, or fatal hemorrhage occurred with the addition of aspirin (Sarkiss et al., 2007).

Clopidogrel (Plavix®) is a thienopyridine derivative that acts as an antiplatelet agent by inhibiting platelet aggregation induced by adenosine diphosphate. The landmark Clopidogrel in Unstable Angina to Prevent Recurrent Events (CURE) trial in 2001 demonstrated improved outcomes and an 18%–20% relative risk reduction in patients with NSTEMI when clopidogrel was combined with aspirin versus aspirin therapy alone (CURE Trial Investigators, 2001). Administration of clopidogrel with a 300 mg oral loading dose followed by 75 mg oral daily dose is a grade 1A recommendation for all patients with ACS without allergy or contraindications (Harrington et al., 2008). Patients who receive a bare metal stent must continue clopidogrel for at least six weeks to six months or more, and patients receiving drug-eluting stents must continue clopidogrel uninterrupted for at least 12 months. Early discontinuation of clopidogrel has been associated with in-stent thrombosis and recurrent MI (Brilakis, Banerjee, & Berger, 2007). In recent years, there has been much discussion about a possible pharmacodynamic interaction between proton pump inhibitors (PPIs) and clopidogrel. In particular, it appears that the PPI omeprazole can significantly reduce the inhibitory effect that clopidogrel has on platelet aggregation (Wright et al., 2011). Patients should be instructed to discuss all medications they are taking with their cardiologist. A new thienopyridine derivative, prasugrel (Effient®), is available, but early studies have demonstrated a significantly higher risk of bleeding compared to clopidogrel (Wright et al., 2011).

Patients presenting with STEMI should be evaluated for immediate reperfusion therapy with either catheter-based or pharmacologic means (see Figure 5-6). Although a catheter-based strategy (angioplasty or stenting) is preferred, if a cardiac catheterization laboratory is not immediately available, thrombolysis with thrombolytic agents such as alteplase or reteplase can be considered. Ideally, thrombolytic agents should be administered within 30 minutes of symptom onset and no longer than 12 hours after onset (Antman & Morrow, 2012). Many contraindications to thrombolytic therapy exist in patients with cancer, and the benefit of the therapy must be weighed against the risk of serious bleeding (Antman & Morrow, 2012). For example, thrombolytics are contraindicated in patients with primary or metastatic brain lesions (Ewer & Yeh, 2006). Underlying coagulopathy or bleeding disorders are relative contraindications that must be considered as well (Ewer & Yeh, 2006). Patients with NSTEMI are not candidates for thrombolysis, as thrombolytic agents have not shown to provide benefit in these patients and may actually worsen outcomes (Matulevicius et al., 2009).

Glycoprotein IIb/IIIa inhibitors, such as abciximab, eptifibatide, and tirofiban, are IV medications that prevent the final common pathway of platelet inhibition. They are used in conjunction with standard medical and invasive management in some high-risk patients with ACS. Although they carry a low (less than 2.5%) risk of major bleeding

---

Figure 5-6. Treatment of ST-Elevation Myocardial Infarction

- Initial evaluation (should be done within 10 minutes of presentation)
  - Set up continuous electrocardiogram (ECG) and automated blood pressure and heart rate monitoring.
  - Conduct focused history and physical examination.
  - Start IV (preferably two large-bore peripherial IVs).
  - Send blood for serum cardiac biomarkers, chemistry, hematology, coagulation studies, and lipid panel.
  - Obtain 12-lead ECG.
  - Obtain chest x-ray.
- Initial medical treatment
  - Aspirin 325 mg (chewed)
  - Nitroglycerin (sublingual or continuous IV infusion)
  - Supplemental O_2 to keep saturation above 92%
  - Morphine 2–4 mg IV PRN for analgesia
- Reperfusion
  - The goal timing of reperfusion therapy is door to balloon in under 90 minutes. (If giving tissue plasminogen activator, door to drug delivery in less than 30 minutes.)
  - Provide adjunctive anticoagulation and antithrombotics (heparin, aspirin, thienopyridine derivatives).
  - Provide hemodynamic support, if indicated (intra-aortic balloon pump, etc.).

Note. Based on information from Antman & Morrow, 2012.

and a very low (0.5%) risk of thrombocytopenia, these agents generally have not been studied in patients with cancer, so their use must be weighed against inherent risk depending on the patient's status (Antman & Morrow, 2012). Recent clinical trials show a decreased incidence of recurrent ischemic events with the use of glycoprotein IIb/IIIa inhibitors. However, the increased risk of major bleeding may outweigh the benefit of use in many patients with cancer (Wright et al., 2011).

Anticoagulants such as unfractionated heparin (UFH) or low-molecular-weight heparin (LMWH) have long been cornerstones of therapy for ACS. UFH has the advantage of a short half-life and monitoring parameters, which may be desirable in patients with cancer. However, the Efficacy and Safety of Subcutaneous Enoxaparin in Unstable Angina and Non-Q-Wave MI (ESSENCE) trial, which compared LMWH plus aspirin to UFH plus aspirin in patients with unstable angina and non-Q-wave MI, found LMWH to be more effective in reducing the recurrence of ischemic events (Cohen et al., 1997).

Nitrates can be useful in ACS by providing vasodilation and improved perfusion to ischemic territories, reduced preload, and relief of anginal discomfort. Available in sublingual, oral, transdermal, and IV formulations, nitroglycerin should be avoided in patients with hypotension or suspected right ventricular infarct. Nitrates are contraindicated in patients who have taken phosphodiesterase inhibitors in the previous 24 hours because of the risk of profound hypotension with concurrent administration (Matulevicius et al., 2009).

Morphine often is used for analgesia in patients with ACS. By relieving chest pain and associated anxiety, morphine reduces the metabolic demands on the heart. It also decreases the work of breathing and has shown beneficial effects, possibly due to vasodilation, in patients with acute pulmonary edema (Antman, 2012).

Intensive lipid-lowering therapy after ACS has been shown to improve outcomes (Vale et al., 2011). The PROVE-IT-TIMI 22 study demonstrated that early and intensive lipid lowering after ACS reduced the risk of death and MI 30, 90, and 180 days after ACS (Cannon et al., 2004). Furthermore, statin therapy has been shown to decrease the risk of unstable angina by 25% following ACS (Vale et al., 2011). The National Cholesterol Education Program Adult Treatment Panel III guidelines recommended an LDL goal of less than 100 mg/dl with an optional goal of less than 70 mg/dl for all patients with coronary artery disease or a coronary artery disease risk equivalent (Grundy et al., 2004).

Beta-blockers decrease myocardial oxygen demand by lowering blood pressure, heart rate, and cardiac index (Antman & Morrow, 2012). With the exception of patients in cardiogenic shock or hypotension, second- or third-degree heart block, or bradycardia, beta-blockers should be administered by mouth early in the care of patients with ACS. By decreasing myocardial oxygen demand, they relieve ischemic chest pain and decrease infarct size. They also are useful in prevention of cardiac arrhythmias associated with myocardial ischemia (Antman & Morrow, 2012).

The use of angiotensin-converting enzyme (ACE) inhibitors in patients after ACS has been shown to improve patient outcomes (Anderson et al., 2007). Along with beta-blockers and statins, ACE inhibitors are recommended as standard care in most patients who have had ACS and especially those with left ventricular systolic dysfunction (ejection fraction less than 40%), high-risk chronic coronary artery disease, or diabetes, in the absence of contraindications (Lee, Cooke, & Robertson, 2008). Clinical trials have shown the benefit of ACE inhibitors in decreasing both the occurrence and severity of clinical heart failure, ventricular remodeling after ACS, and mortality (Anderson et al., 2007). Angiotensin receptor blockers such as candesartan (Atacand®) may be useful in post-ACS patients who are intolerant to ACE inhibitors (Matulevicius et al., 2009). See Table 5-6 for more information about pharmacologic therapies.

Table 5-6. Pharmacologic Therapy in Acute Coronary Syndrome

Medication	Route	Dose
Aspirin	Oral	81–325 mg PO
Clopidogrel	Oral	75 mg PO daily, 300–600 mg PO loading dose
Unfractionated heparin	IV	Based on weight, to keep partial thrombo-plastin time 50–70
Enoxaparin	Subcutaneous	1 mg/kg every 12 hrs
Bivalirudin	IV	0.1 mg/kg bolus, followed by 0.25 mg/kg/hr infusion
Abciximab	IV	0.25 mg/kg bolus, followed by 0.125 mcg/kg/min infusion for 12–24 hrs
Eptifibatide	IV	180 mcg/kg bolus, followed by 2 mcg/kg/min infusion
Nitroglycerin	Sublingual (SL), trans-dermal, IV	0.3–0.6 mg SL, up to max of 1.5 mg 0.2–0.8 mg/hr transdermal every 12 hrs 5–200 mcg/min IV
Morphine	IV	2–4 mg IV PRN
Beta-blockers (metopro-lol, esmolol)	IV, oral (metoprolol only)	Metoprolol 25–100 mg PO BID or 5 mg IV every 4–6 hrs Esmolol 50–200 mcg/kg/min
Angiotensin-converting enzyme inhibitors (lisino-pril, captopril, ramipril)	Oral	Lisinopril 5–40 mg PO daily Captopril 25–100 mg PO BID–TID Ramipril 2.5–5 mg PO BID

Note. Based on information from Matulevicius et al., 2009.

Ventricular arrhythmias, including premature ventricular contractions, ventricular tachycardia, and even ventricular fibrillation, can occur in patients with ACS (Viswa-nathan, Rho, & Page, 2009). Prophylactic use of antiarrhythmics such as lidocaine or amiodarone is no longer advised (Antman & Morrow, 2012). However, maintain-ing adequate potassium levels (around 4.5 mEq/L) and magnesium levels (around 2–3 mEq/L) may raise the fibrillation threshold and prevent tachyarrhythmias (An-tman & Morrow, 2012).

Nursing Management

Nursing management of patients with ACS incorporates a variety of nursing diagno-ses and interventions. As mentioned previously, the triage or bedside nurse often is the first to recognize the signs and symptoms of a patient who may be experiencing ACS. This puts the nurse in a key position to ensure that the patient receives the necessary interventions and care without delay.

In taking the initial history from the patient, it is important to consider the patient's history and cardiac risk factors and to have a low threshold for reporting patient complaints of chest discomfort. All patients complaining of chest pain should be placed on a continuous telemetry monitor. Supplemental oxygen may be provided via nasal cannula, and IV access should be obtained (Urden & Stacy, 2000). Initial diagnostic testing including a 12-lead ECG, cardiac biomarkers, complete blood count, basic metabolic panel, and coagulation studies should be performed in the first 10 minutes of patient presentation. Abnormal findings should be promptly communicated to the patient's cardiology team.

Being familiar with common medications used in ACS, as outlined previously, is crucial. This includes knowing the usual dosing of each, as well as the potential side effects and adverse drug effects. Nurses should remember that patients receiving nitrates often require analgesics for nitroglycerin-induced headache. Patients receiving UFH require regular partial thromboplastin time monitoring and dose adjustments. Blood pressure and heart rate should be measured prior to the administration of beta-blockers (Hausman & Ignatavicius, 2002). When in doubt, the nurse should look up any unfamiliar drugs prior to administration.

The nurse plays a vital role in patient and family education. The patient's disease process, diagnostic tests being performed, and medications being given are all important teaching points (Hausman & Ignatavicius, 2002). A patient with ACS often is motivated to learn about lifestyle modifications, such as a healthy diet and tobacco cessation. Providing a quiet, low-stress environment can lower the patient's level of anxiety, which, in turn, reduces heart rate and myocardial oxygen demand (Urden & Stacy, 2000).

Patients who undergo diagnostic or interventional procedures in the cardiac catheterization laboratory require special nursing care. Frequent vital sign monitoring and continuous telemetry monitoring are necessary. Close monitoring of the catheterization sheath site (whether femoral, radial, or brachial), as well as the pulses of the extremity distal to the puncture site, is critical. The cardiology team should be immediately notified of any bleeding, hematoma, pain, or changes in vital signs (Hausman & Ignatavicius, 2002). Postcatheterization guidelines are institution specific and differ depending on the site of arterial access, the type and dose of any anticoagulation given, the use of a vascular closure device, and any intervention that was performed. Generally, patients who had a femoral artery access site require bed rest for a minimum of two hours with the affected leg extended straight and the head of the bed no higher than a 30° angle (Hausman & Ignatavicius, 2002) (see Figure 5-7).

Patients should be instructed on care of the access site upon discharge (Hausman & Ignatavicius, 2002). Depending on the type of stent placed (bare metal or drug-eluting), patients should be instructed on the importance of daily, uninterrupted aspirin and clopidogrel to prevent stent thrombosis (see Table 5-7).

Prevention

Primary and secondary prevention of coronary artery disease remains a crucial element of treatment and patient education. As discussed earlier, many risk factors are modifiable and should be aggressively addressed based on the patient's level of risk. Control of blood pressure (lower than 140/80 mm Hg in nondiabetic patients and lower than 130/80 in diabetic patients) is an important risk management strategy (Kahn, Robertson, Smith, & Eddy, 2008). Lipid lowering through lifestyle modification and/ or pharmaceutical therapy is also a component. Patients at high risk for coronary artery disease should achieve an LDL level of less than 130 mg/dl, and patients with known coronary disease or with diabetes should achieve an LDL level of less than 100 mg/dl and preferably less than 70 mg/dl (Amsterdam & Liebson, 2005). Patients should be encouraged to maintain a healthy weight and a body mass index of less than 30. Diabetic patients should achieve blood glucose control and a goal hemoglobin A1c level of less than 7%. Patients with the metabolic syndrome (central obesity, elevated serum triglyceride level, low high-density lipoprotein cholesterol, elevated blood pressure, and

---

Figure 5-7. Nursing Care of the Post–Cardiac Catheterization Patient

- Hemodynamic monitoring
  - Monitor and record the patient's vital signs frequently (based on hospital-specific policy).
  - Report any abnormal vital signs to the cardiology team.
  - Attach the patient to continuous telemetry monitoring.
  - Report any arrhythmias to the cardiology team.
- Vascular access site monitoring
  - Keep the patient on bed rest for the designated period of time ordered.
  - Monitor the vascular access site (femoral, radial, brachial) for signs of bleeding or hematoma frequently, and document findings.
  - In the event of bleeding or hematoma, apply manual pressure to the arterial site immediately and page the cardiology team.
  - Monitor the extremity distal to the access site frequently for signs of adequate perfusion (pulses, sensation, temperature) and document findings.
  - Notify the cardiology team of any bleeding, hematoma, or swelling at the access site, loss of distal perfusion (weak or absent pulses, cool extremity), or patient complaints of groin pain, back pain, chest pain, or leg pain.
  - If a vascular sheath needs to be discontinued, follow institutional protocol.
- Medications
  - Review and administer any post–cardiac catheterization medications.
  - See Table 5-7 for further details on common medications.
- Teaching
  - Provide patient education about the above.

Note. Based on information from Hausman & Ignatavicius, 2002; Urden & Stacy, 2000.

Table 5-7. Types of Cardiac Stents

Name of Stent/Manufacturer	Medication Released by the Stent	Recommended Duration of Antiplatelet Therapy
Cypher®, Cordis Corp. Taxus®, Boston Scientific Endeavour®, Medtronic Xience V®, Guidant, Abbott Laboratories Promus®, Boston Scientific	Sirolimus Paclitaxel Zotarolimus Everolimus Everolimus	Aspirin 81–325 mg and clopidogrel 75 mg daily for at least 12 months
VeriFLEX™, Express²®, Boston Scientific Integrity®, Medtronic	None (bare metal stent) None (bare metal stent)	Aspirin 81–325 mg and clopidogrel 75 mg for at least 4–6 weeks, and ideally for 12 months

elevated fasting glucose) should receive intensive medical therapy, ideally from a multidisciplinary team (O'Rourke, 2009). All patients should be instructed to follow a diet that is low in salt, saturated fat, and cholesterol and high in fruits and vegetables (Anderson et al., 2007). Patients should be encouraged to adopt a regular aerobic exercise program (Anderson et al., 2007). All patients who use tobacco products should be encouraged to quit, and assistance should be provided to aid them in their efforts (Anderson et al., 2007). Risk assessment tools such as the well-validated Framingham Risk Score are readily available online for both clinician and patient use and can serve as a quick and easily understood tool for patient education (Huang et al., 2009).

Conclusion

ACS is a potentially life-threatening condition that occurs fairly commonly in patients with cancer. Although interventional cardiology was once far removed from the world of oncology, it is gradually being incorporated into the care of patients with cancer. As cancer treatments advance, patients are surviving malignancies that were once considered terminal illnesses. It is important, then, for healthcare providers to recognize and aggressively treat the other leading cause of mortality in the Unites States—heart disease. With continued research and growing interest and expertise, the treatment of patients with cancer and coronary artery disease is better understood now than ever before. Many challenges remain, and ongoing investigation must continue.

References

Amsterdam, E.A., & Liebson, P.R. (2005). *Contemporary diagnosis and management of the post-MI patient* (2nd ed.). Newtown, PA: Handbooks in Health Care.

Anderson, J.L., Adams, C.D., Antman, E.M., Bridges, C.R., Califf, R.M., Casey, D.E., Jr., ... Riegel, B. (2007). ACC/AHA 2007 guidelines for the management of patients with unstable angina/non-ST-elevation myocardial infarction: A report of the American College of Cardiology/American Heart Association Task Force on Practice Guidelines. *Journal of the American College of Cardiology, 50*, e1–e157. doi:10.1016/j.jacc.2007.02.013

Antman, E.M. (2012). ST-segment elevation myocardial infarction: Pathology, pathophysiology, and clinical features. In R.O. Bonow, D.L. Mann, D.P. Zipes, & J. Libby (Eds.), *Braunwald's heart disease: A textbook of cardiovascular medicine* (9th ed., pp. 1087–1109). Philadelphia, PA: Elsevier Saunders.

Antman, E.M., & Morrow, D.A. (2012). ST-segment elevation myocardial infarction: Management. In R.O. Bonow, D.L. Mann, D.P. Zipes, & J. Libby (Eds.), *Braunwald's heart disease: A textbook of cardiovascular medicine* (9th ed., pp. 1111–1177). Philadelphia, PA: Elsevier Saunders.

Blann, A.D., & Dunmore, S. (2011). Arterial and venous thrombosis in cancer patients. *Cardiology Research and Practice, 2011*, Article ID 394740. doi:10.4061/2011/394740

Bouillon, K., Haddy, N., Delaloge, S., Garbay, J.R., Garsi, J.P., Brindel, P., ... de Vathaire, F. (2011). Long-term cardiovascular mortality after radiotherapy for breast cancer. *Journal of the American College of Cardiology, 57*, 445–452. doi:10.1016/j.jacc.2010.08.638

Brilakis, E.S., Banerjee, S., & Berger, P.B. (2007). The risk of drug-eluting stent thrombosis with noncardiac surgery. *Current Cardiology Reports, 9*, 406–411.

Cannon, C.P., & Braunwald, E. (2012). Unstable angina and non-ST segment elevation myocardial infarction. In R.O. Bonow, D.L. Mann, D.P. Zipes, & P. Libby (Eds.), *Braunwald's heart disease: A textbook of cardiovascular medicine* (9th ed., pp. 1178–1209). Philadelphia, PA: Elsevier Saunders.

Cannon, C.P., Braunwald, E., McCabe, C.H., Rader, D.J., Rouleau, J.L., Belder, R., ... Skene, A.M. (2004). Intensive versus moderate lipid lowering with statins after acute coronary syndromes. *New England Journal of Medicine, 350*, 1495–1504. doi:10.1056/NEJMoa040583

Cayley, W.E., Jr. (2005). Diagnosing the cause of chest pain. *American Family Physician, 72*, 2012–2021.

Centers for Disease Control and Prevention National Program of Cancer Registries. (2011). United States cancer statistics. Retrieved from http://www.cdc.gov/cancer/npcr/uscs/2007/technical_notes/

Clopidogrel in Unstable Angina to Prevent Recurrent Events Trial Investigators. (2001). Effects of clopidogrel in addition to aspirin in patients with acute coronary syndromes without ST-segment elevation. *New England Journal of Medicine, 345*, 494–502. doi:10.1056/NEJMoa010746

Cohen, M., Demers, C., Gurfinkel, E.P., Turpie, A.G., Fromell, G.J., Goodman, S., … Bigonzi, F. (1997). A comparison of low-molecular-weight heparin with unfractionated heparin for unstable coronary artery disease. Efficacy and Safety of Subcutaneous Enoxaparin in Non-Q-Wave Coronary Events Study Group. *New England Journal of Medicine, 337*, 447–452. doi:10.1056/NEJM199708143370702

Costa, M.A., & Jozic, J. (2009). Cardiac catheterization and coronary angiography. In R.A. O'Rourke, R.A. Walsh, & V. Fuster (Eds.), *Hurst's the heart manual of cardiology* (12th ed., pp. 82–94). New York, NY: McGraw-Hill Medical.

Cutter, D.J., Darby, S.C., & Yusuf, S.W. (2011). Risks of heart disease after radiotherapy. *Texas Heart Institute Journal, 38*, 257–258.

Davignon, J., & Ganz, P. (2004). Role of endothelial dysfunction in atherosclerosis. *Circulation, 109*(23, Suppl. 1), III27–III32. doi:10.1161/01.CIR.0000131515.03336.f8

Ewer, M.S., & Yeh, E. (2006). *Cancer and the heart.* Hamilton, Ontario, Canada: BC Decker.

Fadol, A., & Lech, T. (2011). Cardiovascular adverse events associated with cancer therapy. *Journal of the Advanced Practitioner in Oncology, 2*, 229–242.

Grundy, S.M., Cleeman, J.I., Merz, C.N., Brewer, H.B., Jr., Clark, L.T., Hunninghake, D.B., … Stone, N.J. (2004). Implications of recent clinical trials for the National Cholesterol Education Program Adult Treatment Panel III guidelines. *Circulation, 110*, 227–239. doi:10.1161/01.CIR.0000133317.49796.0E

Harrington, R.A., Becker, R.C., Cannon, C.P., Gutterman, D., Lincoff, A.M., Popma, J.J., … Goodman, S.G. (2008). Antithrombotic therapy for non-ST-segment elevation acute coronary syndromes: American College of Chest Physicians evidence-based clinical practice guidelines (8th ed.). *Chest, 133*, 607S–707S. doi:10.1378/chest.08-0691

Hausman, K.A., & Ignatavicius, D.D. (2002). *Clinical companion for medical-surgical nursing: Critical thinking for collaborative care* (4th ed.). Philadelphia, PA: Saunders.

Hoffmann, U., Brady, T.J., & Muller, J. (2003). Use of new imaging techniques to screen for coronary artery disease. *Circulation, 108*, e50–e53. doi:10.1161/01.CIR.0000085363.88377.F2

Huang, R.L., Maron, D.J., Ridker, P.M., Grundy, S.M., & Pearson, T.A. (2009). Dyslipidemia and other cardiac risk factors. In R.A. O'Rourke, R.A. Walsh, & V. Fuster (Eds.), *Hurst's the heart manual of cardiology* (12th ed., pp. 237–260). New York, NY: McGraw-Hill Medical.

Iliescu, C., Durand, J.B., & Kroll, M. (2011). Cardiovascular interventions in thrombocytopenic cancer patients. *Texas Heart Institute Journal, 38*, 259–260.

Kahn, R., Robertson, R.M., Smith, R., & Eddy, D. (2008). The impact of prevention on reducing the burden of cardiovascular disease. *Circulation, 118*, 576–585. doi:10.1161/CIRCULATIONAHA.108.190186

Khorana, A.A., Francis, C.W., Culakova, E., Fisher, R.I., Kuderer, N.M., & Lyman, G.H. (2006). Thromboembolism in hospitalized neutropenic cancer patients. *Journal of Clinical Oncology, 24*, 484–490. doi:10.1200/JCO.2005.03.8877

Lee, H.Y., Cooke, C.E., & Robertson, T.A. (2008). Use of secondary prevention drug therapy in patients with acute coronary syndrome after hospital discharge. *Journal of Managed Care Pharmacy, 14*, 271–280.

Matulevicius, S.A., Rohatgi, A., & de Lemos, J.A. (2009). Diagnosis and management of patients with unstable angina and non-ST-segment elevation myocardial infarction. In R.A. O'Rourke, R.A. Walsh, & V. Fuster (Eds.), *Hurst's the heart manual of cardiology* (12th ed., pp. 296–314). New York, NY: McGraw-Hill Medical.

Morrow, D.A., & Boden, W.E. (2012). Stable ischemic heart disease. In R.O. Bonow, D.L. Mann, D.P. Zipes, & P. Libby (Eds.), *Braunwald's heart disease: A textbook of cardiovascular medicine* (9th ed., pp. 1210–1269). Philadelphia, PA: Elsevier Saunders.

O'Rourke, R.A. (2009). Management of patients with chronic ischemic heart disease. In R.A. O'Rourke, R.A. Walsh, & V. Fuster (Eds.), *Hurst's the heart manual of cardiology* (12th ed., pp. 261–275). New York, NY: McGraw-Hill Medical.

Raggi, P., & Berman, D.S. (2005). Computed tomography coronary calcium screening and myocardial perfusion imaging. *Journal of Nuclear Cardiology, 12*, 96–103.

Roger, V.L., Go, A.S., Lloyd-Jones, D.M., Adams, R.J., Berry, J.D., Brown, T.M., … Wylie-Rosett, J. (2011). Executive summary: Heart disease and stroke statistics—2011 update. A report from the American Heart Association. *Circulation, 123*, 459–463. doi:10.1161/CIR.0b013e31820c7a50

Sabatine, M.S., & Cannon, C.P. (2012). Approach to the patient with chest pain. In R.O. Bonow, D.L. Mann, D.P. Zipes, & P. Libby (Eds.), *Braunwald's heart disease: A textbook of cardiovascular medicine* (9th ed., pp. 1076–1086). Philadelphia, PA: Elsevier Saunders.

Sarkiss, M.G., Yusuf, S.W., Warneke, C.L., Botz, G., Lakkis, N., Hirch-Ginsburg, C., ... Durand, J.B. (2007). Impact of aspirin therapy in cancer patients with thrombocytopenia and acute coronary syndromes. *Cancer, 109,* 621–627. doi:10.1002/cncr.22434

Sweeny, J.M., & Fuster, V. (2009). Definitions and pathogenesis of acute coronary syndromes. In R.A. O'Rourke, R.A. Walsh, & V. Fuster (Eds.), *Hurst's the heart manual of cardiology* (12th ed., pp. 276–284). New York, NY: McGraw-Hill Medical.

Thygesen, K., Alpert, J.S., & White, H.D. (2007). ESC/ACCF/AHA/WHF expert consensus document: Universal definition of myocardial infarction. *Journal of the American College of Cardiology, 50,* 2173–2195. doi:10.1016/j.jacc.2007.09.011

Udelson, J.E., Dilsizian, V., & Bonow, R.O. (2012). Nuclear cardiology. In R.O. Bonow, D.L. Mann, D.P. Zipes, & P. Libby (Eds.), *Braunwald's heart disease: A textbook of cardiovascular medicine* (9th ed., pp. 289–339). Philadelphia, PA: Elsevier Saunders.

Urden, L.D., & Stacy, K.M. (Eds.). (2000). *Priorities in critical care nursing* (3rd ed.). St. Louis, MO: Mosby.

Vale, N., Nordmann, A.J., Schwartz, G.G., de Lemos, J., Colivicchi, F., den Hartog, F., ... Briel, M. (2011). Statins for acute coronary syndrome. *Cochrane Database of Systematic Reviews, 2011*(6). doi:10.1002/14651858.CD006870.pub2

Viswanathan, M.N., Rho, R.W., & Page, R.L. (2009). Ventricular arrhythmias. In R.A. O'Rourke, R.A. Walsh, & V. Fuster (Eds.), *Hurst's the heart manual of cardiology* (12th ed., pp. 141–146). New York, NY: McGraw-Hill Medical.

World Heart Federation. (n.d.). Cardiovascular disease risk factors. Retrieved from http://www.world -heart-federation.org/cardiovascular-health/cardiovascular-disease-risk-factors

Wright, R.S., Anderson, J.L., Adams, C.D., Casey, D.E., Jr., Ettinger, S.M., Fesmire, F.M., ... Zidar, J.P. (2011). 2011 ACCF/AHA focused update of the guidelines for the management of patients with unstable angina/non-ST-elevation myocardial infarction (updating the 2007 guideline): A report of the American College of Cardiology Foundation/American Heart Association Task Force on Practice Guidelines developed in collaboration with the American College of Emergency Physicians, Society for Cardiovascular Angiography and Interventions, and Society of Thoracic Surgeons. *Journal of the American College of Cardiology, 57,* 1920–1959. doi:10.1016/j.jacc.2011.02.009

Yang, E.H., & Gersh, R.J. (2009). Diagnosis and management of patients with ST-segment elevation myocardial infarction. In R.A. O'Rourke, R.A. Walsh, & V. Fuster (Eds.), *Hurst's the heart manual of cardiology* (12th ed., pp. 285–295). New York, NY: McGraw-Hill Medical.

Yeh, E.T.H., & Bickford, C.L. (2009). Cardiovascular complications of cancer therapy: Incidence, pathogenesis, diagnosis and management. *Journal of the American College of Cardiology, 53,* 2231–2247. doi:10.1016/j.jacc.2009.02.050

Yusuf, S.W., Sami, S., & Daher, I.N. (2010). Radiation-induced heart disease: A clinical update. *Cardiology Research and Practice, 2011,* Article ID 317659. doi:10.4061/2011/317659

Cardiac Inflammatory Conditions and Cardiac Tamponade in Patients With Cancer

Myrshia L. Woods, MHS, PA-C

Introduction

Among all the unfortunate collateral damage and negative consequences of cancer and its therapies, patients may face several life-threatening cardiac conditions. Included in the targets of damage are the pericardium, myocardium, and endocardium. The heart appears to be extremely susceptible to damage from cancer and cancer treatment at each level of its anatomy. An inflammatory reaction can erupt and cause disease progression in each portion of the heart muscle. Resulting from a largely compromised immune system, the vulnerability of patients with cancer is significant, as it makes patients susceptible to a myriad of opportunistic infections. This chapter will focus on the diagnosis, management, and prognosis of pericarditis, myocarditis, endocarditis, and cardiac tamponade. Clinicians face special challenges in treating patients with cancer who develop these serious cardiac complications.

Specific cancers can cause insult to the heart and produce grave consequences. Some of these cancers invade the heart tissue simply by means of location or proximity. Other cancers are known to spread diffusely and can target the heart in their pathway of metastasis, such as breast cancer (Garg, Moorthy, Agrawal, Pandey, & Kumari, 2011), lung cancer, lymphoma, leukemia, melanoma, renal cell carcinoma, and nasopharyngeal carcinoma (Chen et al., 2011). Furthermore, some cancer therapies can cause inflammation directly or immunosuppression that allows for microorganism infiltration, which in turn initiates an inflammatory response.

Pericarditis

Anatomy and Pathophysiology

A close analysis of the outer protective layer of the heart is necessary in understanding how injury to it occurs. The pericardium is a thin, double-walled sac that contains the heart and the roots of the great vessels. The pericardial sac has two layers: the outermost fibrous pericardium and the inner serous pericardium. The visceral pericardium surrounds the major blood vessels, and ligaments are attached to the spinal column, diaphragm, and other parts of the mediastinum. The parietal pericardium, which is part of the epicardium, is attached to the heart muscle. In between the visceral and parietal layers is a potential space known as the pericardial cavity, which contains about 15–50 ml of clear, straw-colored fluid that lubricates as the heart beats and moves within the sac (Texas Heart Institute, 2010).

The normal pericardium has important functions, including maintaining a fixed and constant position of the heart, creating a barrier to infection, and providing lubrication between the visceral and parietal layers of the pericardium (LeWinter, 2008). When any type of injury occurs, the amount of fluid between the two layers can increase. The increase in fluid can be a gradual process over months to years, or it can occur extremely rapidly over hours in response to an acute insult. Pericardial effusions can be serous, serosanguineous, hemorrhagic, or chylous (Yarlagadda, 2011). Obviously, any tumor or malignant process that is adjacent to these areas can have an effect upon the pericardium, initiating an inflammatory reaction.

In the general population, the cause of pericarditis is often unknown. However, in patients with cancer, pericarditis often results from malignancy, chemotherapy, radiation to the chest, renal failure, or infectious processes and other conditions as listed in Figure 6-1.

It also is important to address the specific anticancer agents that can cause pericarditis, such as anthracyclines. Pericarditis should always be considered in patients with cancer who are exposed to anthracycline chemotherapy. Several other chemotherapeutic agents can cause pericarditis as listed in Table 6-1 (Fadol & Lech, 2011).

Figure 6-1. Causes of Pericarditis in Patients With Cancer

- Viral (echovirus, Coxsackie virus, adenovirus, cytomegalovirus, hepatitis B, infectious mononucleosis, HIV/AIDS)
- Bacterial (*Pneumococcus*, *Staphylococcus*, *Streptococcus*, *Mycoplasma*, Lyme disease, *Haemophilus influenzae*, *Neisseria meningitidis*)
- Fungal (histoplasmosis, coccidiomycosis)
- Myocardial infarction (heart attack)
- Tumor metastasis
- Radiation therapy to the mediastinum or left chest
- Blunt injury to the chest wall, esophagus, or heart (surgical resection, placement of mesh or devices, or post–cardiopulmonary resuscitation (CPR)
- Chemotherapy or immunosuppressant agents
- Renal failure

Note. Based on information from LeWinter, 2008.

Table 6-1. Chemotherapeutic Agents That Can Cause Pericarditis	
Drug Class	**Agents**
Antimetabolite	Cytarabine
Anthracycline	Doxorubicin, daunorubicin
Folic acid antagonist	Methotrexate
Small-molecule tyrosine kinase inhibitor	Imatinib
Antitumor antibiotic	Bleomycin
Alkylating agent	Cyclophosphamide

Note. Based on information from Fadol & Lech, 2011.

Signs and Symptoms

A typical symptom of patients experiencing pericarditis is pleuritic chest pain that is sharp and stabbing and intensified in certain positions. The reason why patients will report having worse pain when either lying down or shifting position in bed is because any movement that causes the inflamed pericardium to rub against the heart muscle will cause more friction and incite further inflammation, leading to worsening chest pain. Usually sitting up and leaning forward can help to alleviate the pain, as it allows the pericardium to tilt forward. A reporting of this specific symptom should tip off the evaluating clinician that pericarditis is the likely diagnosis. Also, on physical examination, a pericardial friction rub heard in both diastole and systole, which is auscultated over the precordium, is an audible clue that pericarditis is likely. Although pericarditis is the likely cause for the patient's symptoms, it is always imperative to rule out myocardial infarction during the evaluation as well. It is important to note that there may be a transient and slight elevation in the cardiac troponin levels; however, they should not be elevated in the high range, which may signify a true myocardial infarction (Texas Heart Institute, 2010). Other commonly reported symptoms are listed in Figure 6-2.

Diagnostic Studies

Diagnostic studies are particularly useful in confirming pericarditis because they can clearly highlight the typical features. Several studies must be ordered when

---

Figure 6-2. Symptoms of Pericarditis

- Pleuritic chest pain that may radiate into the neck, shoulder, back, or abdomen
- Fever
- Dry cough
- Painful swallowing (odynophagia)
- Dyspnea or trouble taking deep breaths
- Malaise and/or fatigue
- Anxiety
- Ankle, feet, and leg swelling

evaluating these patients, and it also is imperative to compare older studies to the new ones, as this will help to confirm progression of disease or necessitate urgency of treatment.

Specific electrocardiogram (ECG) changes are diagnostic for pericarditis. These changes can be acute, and when noted in addition to the clinical finding of a pericardial rub, coupled with the patient's symptoms of pleuritic chest pain, can be indicative of acute pericarditis. The typical ECG changes suggestive of pericarditis are diffuse ST segment elevation, with PR segment depression as shown in Figure 6-3. Another feature can be electrical alternans, which is a change in the voltage of the QRS complex based on the constant swinging and changing axis of the myocardium in the presence of an accompanying pericardial effusion (Texas Heart Institute, 2010). Other diagnostic studies that maybe helpful in the diagnosis of pericarditis are listed in Table 6-2.

Medical Management

Once pericarditis is confirmed in the patient with cancer, several viable treatment options are available. Priority is given to alleviating the patient's pain. Pain relief can be achieved with anti-inflammatory medications such as the nonsteroidal anti-inflammatory drugs ibuprofen or indomethacin. However, the use of these medications may be limited, and patients with cancer may have renal impairment (Unsworth, Sturman, Lunec, & Blake, 1987). With respect to indomethacin, oncologists may shy away from its use because of concern for potential bone marrow suppression. Therefore, another choice is steroid therapy if no other contraindications for its use are present. How-

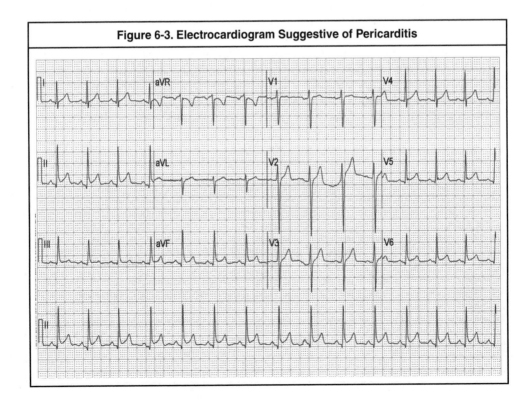

Figure 6-3. Electrocardiogram Suggestive of Pericarditis

Table 6-2. Diagnostic Studies for Pericarditis	
Test	**Findings Indicative of Pericarditis**
Chest x-ray	Cardiomegaly
Electrocardiogram	Low voltage, electrical alternans
Echocardiography	Visualization of fluid and how it is affecting contraction of the heart
Computed tomography	Visualization of fluid
Cardiac magnetic resonance imaging	Visualization of fluid and/or scarring or contracture of the pericardium
Radionuclide scanning	Visualization of fluid

Note. Based on information from LeWinter, 2008.

ever, from the cardiac standpoint, the conflicting issue with steroid use is that once the steroids are halted, pericarditis can recur. Discontinuation of steroid therapy is associated with a higher incidence of recurrent pericarditis (Imazio & Adler, 2012; Shabetai, 2005).

Another treatment choice is a type of chemotherapeutic agent named thiotepa (Maisch, Ristic, & Pankuweit, 2010). This agent has been studied in limited settings for this indication and has been approved for treatment of this condition. The only stipulation is that it must be used in the first 24–48 hours after the diagnosis, which will ensure its most effective treatment mechanism as a sclerosing agent.

If associated pericardial effusion exists in the setting of pericarditis and it becomes necessary to aspirate the fluid (in a procedure termed *pericardiocentesis*), the fluid should be analyzed for several possible pathogens; these are listed in the section under Cardiac Tamponade discussed later in this chapter.

Pericardial constriction is another pericardial complication of cancer therapy, particularly radiation to the chest. This entity is also termed *constrictive pericarditis* and is essentially a hardening or stiffening of the pericardium. Barbetakis et al. (2010) noted that 20% of patients with cancer who have undergone chest radiation therapy develop radiation-induced constrictive pericarditis. In the progression of this disease process, the pericardium can constrain the myocardium and restrict its ability to adequately fill and contract. This process can worsen over time and unfortunately carries a grim prognosis. Potential treatment options are available and have been reported in the literature. A study of six patients in Greece showed that radiation-induced constrictive pericarditis is a clinical entity that should be considered in the differential diagnosis of patients with cancer who show signs of heart failure (Barbetakis et al., 2010). Currently, surgery is the only effective treatment that will yield satisfactory results. The outcome of treatment, however, is dependent upon any associated damage to the myocardium that may permanently impair left ventricular systolic function.

It is also important to recognize that patients who receive radiation to the chest are at risk for the development of calcification, specifically of the pericardium. See Figure 6-4 for an example of calcific pericardium. Other conditions that cause this phenomenon include tuberculosis and hemorrhagic pericardial effusion.

Figure 6-4. Calcified Portion of Pericardium on Routine Chest X-Ray

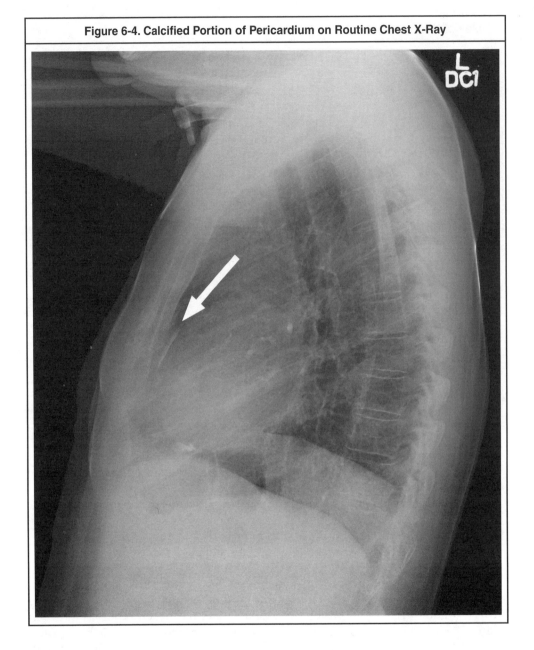

Myocarditis

The term *myocarditis* carries a broad definition involving a generalized inflammation of the heart muscle. The diagnosis of myocarditis in the patient with cancer portends a very poor prognosis if it is not immediately recognized and appropriately and aggressively treated. Oftentimes, clinicians can be misguided by other suspected conditions, especially those seen in the cancer setting. Again, if not properly identified and treated early, myocarditis can lead to severe heart failure and even death in the cancer population.

Myocarditis has various etiologies in the general population, and this is likely the case in patients with cancer as well. According to established heart failure guidelines, the potential etiologies of myocarditis include toxins, medications, physical agents, and infections (Heart Failure Society of America, 2010). Tests for all of these etiologic agents should be included in the evaluation when clinical myocarditis is suspected. The laboratory tests and viral titers listed in Figure 6-5 should be ordered to determine the specific etiology and guide therapy.

Figure 6-5. Recommended Diagnostic Tests for the Evaluation of Myocarditis

Diagnostic Tests	**Viral Titers**
• Erythrocyte sedimentation rate	• Enterovirus
• Eosinophils	• Coxsackie B
• Complement 3 and complement 4	• Echovirus
• High-sensitivity C-reactive protein	• Adenovirus
• Brain natriuretic peptide	• Epstein-Barr virus
• Creatine phosphokinase (CK) and MB	• Parvovirus
• Troponin	• Influenza
• Tuberculosis (acid-fast bacteria)	• Hepatitis C
	• Cytomegalovirus

Note. Based on information from Cooper, 2009.

Pathophysiology

In animal studies, the pathophysiology has been well established that myocardial inflammatory damage results from postinfectious and/or autoimmune-mediated processes (Heart Failure Society of America, 2010).

The pathogenesis of myocarditis in patients with cancer typically follows a classic paradigm of cardiac injury, which is usually the involvement of a multisystem injury in an immunocompromised patient. Most commonly, myocarditis ensues from an external trigger, such as a virus, in patients with cancer, causing an overwhelming degree of inflammation. Patients with cancer are generally already exposed to high levels of inflammatory markers, and this may mark their exaggerated response to the viral insult (Sumantran & Tillu, 2012).

Signs and Symptoms

Symptoms of myocarditis essentially mimic the symptoms of any patient experiencing acute decompensated heart failure. Often in patients with cancer, it is difficult to discern symptoms of cancer from symptoms of heart failure because they can overlap. The specific symptoms that can overlap include fatigue, dyspnea, and edema (Ewer, Swain, Cardinale, Fadol, & Suter, 2011). As a typical rule, however, if there is a sudden and rapid clinical decline with corresponding physical examination findings of decompensation, myocarditis should be suspected. Figure 6-6 highlights some of the common clinical symptoms of myocarditis.

Myocarditis should be considered in patients with cancer who experience an acute and rapid clinical decline with hemodynamic instability, generally from sepsis, following recent cancer therapy including various chemotherapeutic agents or stem cell transplantation. A classic example of this entity is demonstrated in a case study reported about a patient with non-Hodgkin lymphoma who was receiving lenalidomide and ex-

Figure 6-6. Clinical Symptoms of Myocarditis	
• Clinical heart failure • Fever • Viral prodrome including fever, malaise, fatigue, headache, and lack of appetite • Fatigue • Dyspnea on exertion	• Chest pain • Palpitations • Presyncope or syncope • Palpitations or abnormal heartbeat (arrhythmia)

Note. Based on information from Cooper, 2009.

perienced an acute episode of heart failure within 17 days of treatment initiation. It is postulated that the mechanism of the patient's heart failure exacerbation was a T-cell infiltration of the myocardium. This suggests that lenalidomide led to drug-induced myocarditis (Carver et al., 2010).

Various complications can arise from myocarditis, especially in the setting of cancer therapy. Patients can experience thromboembolic events even in the setting of critical thrombocytopenia with critical platelet values being below 10,000, arrhythmias, and sudden death (Heart Failure Society of America, 2010). Therefore, aggressive intervention must take place in order to lower the risk for these grave cardiovascular consequences.

Diagnostic Studies

The diagnostic studies for a patient with myocarditis include ECG, chest x-ray, cardiac magnetic resonance imaging (MRI), echocardiography, and blood tests including viral titers. Cardiac MRI may offer confirming evidence of the diagnosis because it will show delayed enhancement within the myocardial tissue. Another diagnostic study that may be indicated specifically for myocarditis is cardiac catheterization with endomyocardial biopsy. The cardiac biopsy will give definite cellular evidence of the offending agent if isolated in the collected specimens. Table 6-3 lists the recommended diagnostic tests for myocarditis.

Medical Management

These patients usually require ventilatory and hemodynamic support, which in extreme cases can include an intra-aortic balloon pump or extracorporeal membrane

Table 6-3. Recommended Diagnostic Tests for Myocarditis	
Test	**Findings Indicative of Myocarditis**
Electrocardiogram	Loss of QRS voltage, tachyarrhythmia
Chest x-ray	Cardiomegaly, pulmonary edema, or pleural effusions
Cardiac magnetic resonance imaging	Delayed enhancement of myocardium
Echocardiography	Global hypokinesis of myocardial function, dilated left ventricle with regurgitant valvular lesions
Viral titers	Cytology showing viral load or antibodies

oxygenation. It may become necessary to transfer these patients to specialized centers where more directed cardiac care can be given. In severe cases, clinicians must consider whether the patient is a suitable candidate for a potential artificial heart, left ventricular assist device, or cardiac transplantation (Heart Failure Society of America, 2010). Other treatment usually follows standard heart failure guidelines. See Chapter 10 for the management of heart failure.

Endocarditis

Patients with cancer also are susceptible to valvular lesions as they are exposed to various cancer treatments. As previously mentioned, because the immune response is compromised in this population, the risk for opportunistic infections is increased. Oftentimes this can result in infective endocarditis lesions. The full spectrum of endocarditis has been observed in the cancer population, including marantic endocarditis (Jameson et al., 2009) and isolated fungal lesions involving the heart valves.

Causes

Because the port of entry is often the mouth, it may be that the integrity of the lining of the mouth of patients with cancer may offer more of an entryway because patients frequently experience oral candidiasis or thrush following chemotherapy treatments. Figure 6-7 summarizes the common organisms causing infective endocarditis.

Less common causes of endocarditis include *Pseudomonas, Serratia,* and *Candida.* These must also be considered in the cancer population because these infections can follow immunocompromising treatments such as chemotherapy and stem cell transplantation.

Another consideration for patients with cancer that makes them susceptible is multiple blood draws, as well as foreign devices within their bodies such as port-a-caths, central lines, Ommaya devices, pain medication infusion pumps, and pacemakers. These patients constantly battle infections, including line infections, pneumonias, urinary tract infections, and cellulitis. The varying infectious exposures must certainly play a role in the introduction of pathogens into their immunocompromised systems, lending to more serious infections such as endocarditis (American Cancer Society, 2010).

Some patients with cancer have a predisposition to valvular complications because of a past history of unrelated valvular disease and have received a valve replacement. This makes this population susceptible to prosthetic valve endocarditis.

Figure 6-7. Microorganisms Typically Causing Endocarditis

- Streptococci
- Enterococci
- *Staphylococcus aureus*
- Coagulase-negative staphylococci
- Gram-negative bacteria (*Haemophilus, Actinobacillus actinomycetemcomitans, Cardiobacterium hominis*)
- Fungi
- Polymicrobial

Note. Based on information from Wilson et al., 2007; Xiong et al., 2009.

Moreover, radiation therapy plays a significant role in causing destruction of valvular tissue, which can be seen up to decades later after radiation treatment. As a result of injury to the integrity of the heart valves, patients are subject to valvular stenosis and/or regurgitation. This can lead to serious valvular complications requiring cessation of cancer therapy. Valvular disease must be addressed expediently but in the context of the priority of cancer treatment. One must consider which diagnosis carries the higher mortality—the cancer or the valvular disease—and this should direct care. Figures 6-8, 6-9, and 6-10 are echocardiogram pictures of significant valvular lesions resulting from extensive radiation therapy to the chest. Radiation damage occured to all four valves including mitral, aortic, pulmonic, and tricuspid valves.

Medical Management

In the management of each inflammatory condition, the first priority of the clinician is to provide symptom management. It is important to relieve dyspnea, fatigue, and edema by initiation of diuretic therapy as tolerated by the patient's hemodynamics and renal function. Next, it is necessary to treat the underlying etiology for the inflammatory condition with agents such as antibiotics, antivirals, or antifungal medications. With respect to myocarditis and endocarditis, if heart failure ensues, it is important to initiate standard heart failure treatment as outlined in Chapter 10.

Cardiac Tamponade

Cardiac tamponade is a life-threatening situation when a large amount of blood or fluid is inside the pericardial sac causing hemodynamic compromise resulting in severe hypotension, shock, and death if not intervened in a timely manner. Cardiac tamponade occurs in up to 15% of patients with cancer and can develop as a result of malignant involvement of the pericardium under metastatic disease conditions, contiguous extension of neighboring tumors, or primary involvement (Oida et al., 2010). Cardiac tamponade can occur in any type of pericarditis case, but it is more commonly observed in neoplastic, tuberculous, and purulent pericarditis cases than in viral or idiopathic cases (Oida et al., 2010). Pericardial effusion is a known complication in many advanced cancers and unfortunately has a strong impact on both quality of life and overall prognosis (Oida et al., 2010).

Pathophysiology

The pathophysiology of this emergent condition can be divided into three distinct phases. Phase I includes the accumulation of pericardial fluid that causes increased stiffness of the ventricle, requiring a higher filling pressure. It is in this phase that the filling pressures of the right and left ventricles are higher than the intrapericardial pressures. During phase II, further accumulation of fluid occurs, and the pericardial pressure increases above the ventricular filling pressure, which causes a reduced cardiac output. Lastly, in phase III the cardiac output decreases further, which is due to the equilibration of pericardial and left ventricular filling pressure.

The main pathologic process in cardiac tamponade is the markedly diminished diastolic filling from the heart being compressed by the increasing intrapericardial fluid or pericardial effusion (see Figure 6-11). As the pericardial effusion increases,

Figure 6-8. Radiation-Induced Mitral Valvular Stenosis and Regurgitation

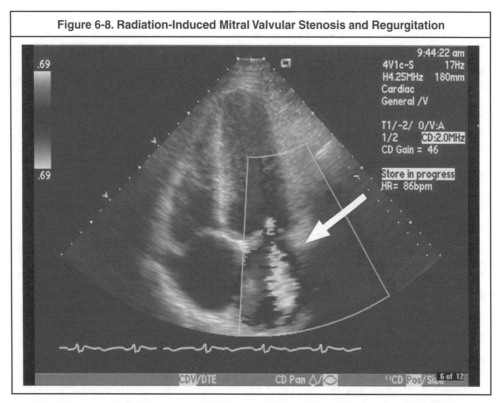

Figure 6-9. Radiation-Induced Tricuspid and Mitral Stenosis and Regurgitation

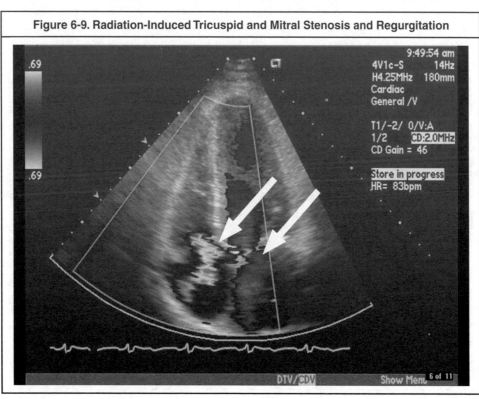

Figure 6-10. Radiation-Induced Valvular Stenosis

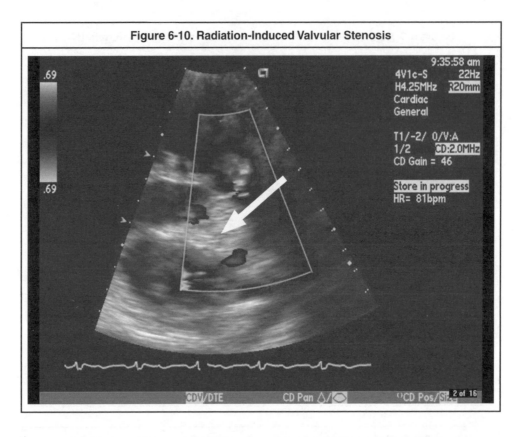

Figure 6-11. Large Pericardial Perfusion Surrounding the Myocardium

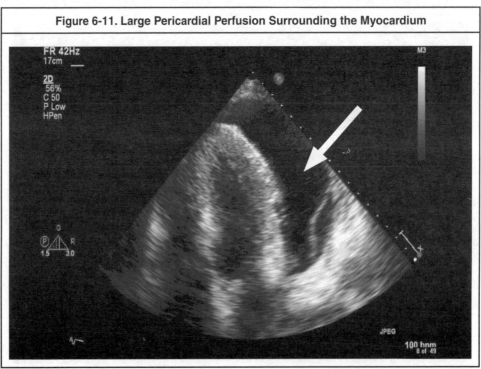

systemic venous return is altered because of the heart being compressed resulting in cardiac tamponade. Figure 6-12 shows an example of right ventricular collapse during cardiac tamponade. Figure 6-13 shows a mass within a large pericardial effusion causing cardiac tamponade. Moreover, occasionally the pericardium can become calcified as shown previously in Figure 6-4, which may contribute to the development of increased pressure in the pericardium (Gautam, Gautam, Sogunuru, & Subramanyam, 2012).

Signs and Symptoms and Diagnostic Studies

Patients with cancer with cardiac tamponade are no different from the general population in their symptomatology, which includes acute shortness of breath or tachypnea, chest discomfort, and/or palpitations or rapid heartbeat. Concurrently, patients can be severely hypotensive on the verge of experiencing a cardiac arrest. This occurs as the pericardial effusion causes collapse of the right-sided cardiac chambers, including the right atrium and right ventricle, preventing filling of the chambers. With inadequate filling of the right side of the heart, consequently there is no forward flow to the pulmonary system and the left side of the heart is depleted of volume, which significantly lowers the cardiac output to the body. In this scenario, the cardiac output can fatally drop, leading to death. This signifies the emergency of this condition (Heart Failure Society of America, 2010).

Emergent attention must be given to these patients and usually involves pericardiocentesis. Using sterile technique with echocardiographic guidance, a cardiologist or

Figure 6-12. Right Ventricular Collapse During Diastole With Large Surrounding Pericardial Effusion Seen in Cardiac Tamponade

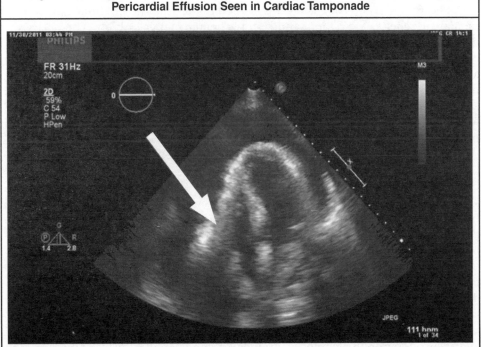

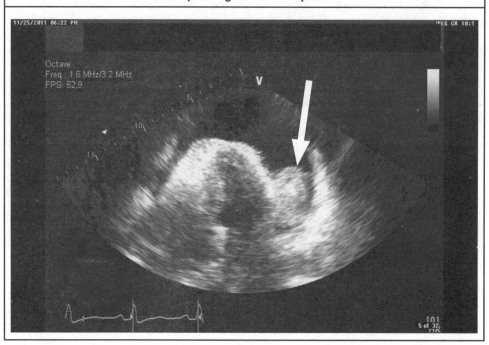

Figure 6-13. Mass Adjacent to Left Ventricle With Surrounding Pericardial Effusion, With Impending Cardiac Tamponade

trained clinician can introduce a needle into the pericardium, and the pericardial fluid can be aspirated and collected with a catheter. The aspiration of fluid usually offers immediate relief to the patient and restores hemodynamic stability. The pericardial drain is not recommended to be left longer than five to seven days because infection can ensue, as there is a direct pathway for entrance into the pericardium. It is imperative to be aware that fungal infections can possibly develop in persistent indwelling intrapericardial catheters and can lead to development of a pericardial empyema, as noted in an actual patient case at the University of Texas MD Anderson Cancer Center by the cardiology department. This outcome should be avoided at all costs if possible.

The amount of pericardial fluid aspirated is variable. In the MD Anderson experience, the yield of pericardial fluid has been observed to range from a few hundred milliliters up to a maximum of 1.5 L. When more than a liter of fluid is drained at one time, usually the patient's pericardial effusion has been chronically developing over time ranging from months to a year. It is unlikely that any patient could tolerate an acute amount of fluid this large. Rather, this amount of fluid would likely cause right-sided heart chamber collapse and subsequent death (Heart Failure Society of America, 2010).

The pericardial drain and collection bag may be emptied as it fills, usually once daily, and if the amount of drainage does not exceed more than 50 ml/day, then the drain can be pulled. If the drainage is excessive, then a pericardial window should be considered for the patient. A pericardial window is a surgical procedure where a thin incision is placed within the pericardium to allow drainage of the effusion and absorption into the lymphatic drainage system (Mueller, 2011). The cardiothoracic surgeon must be consulted to evaluate the suitability of the patient to undergo this procedure.

The collected fluid should also be analyzed for pathogens, including cancer cells and other microorganisms. The color and consistency of the pericardial fluid can portend certain prognoses. The range of color of the pericardial fluid can be from serous to serosanguineous to frank bloody. Unfortunately, a bloody effusion often signifies a malignant pericardial effusion. Table 6-4 lists the diagnostic tests for the evaluation for pericardial effusion. Incidentally, sometimes myopericarditis can occur simultaneously. Myopericarditis is an inflammatory condition of the heart involving both the myocardium and the pericardium that can be marked by pronounced heart failure symptoms and sequelae (Broder, Gottlieb, & Lepor, 2008).

Often, the pericardial effusion may test positive for malignant cells. The presence of malignant pericardial effusion in advanced cancer can portend a poor prognosis. Cardiac tamponade due to malignant pericardial effusion is thus a rare clinical entity and often acutely life threatening (Hsi, Krishnamurthy, Ryan, Luo, & Woodlock, 2010). Furthermore, in patients presenting with cardiac tamponade, malignancy accounts for 65% of primary etiology, and one-year mortality was 76.5% in patients with malignant disease and 13.3% in those without malignant disease (Cornily et al., 2008).

Medical and Nursing Management

Once the emergent condition of cardiac tamponade is resolved, the next priority is to prevent recurrence. Effective management in this regard can be achieved by instillation in the pericardial sac of varying agents with sclerosing or cytostatic activity such as tetracyclines, bleomycin, thiotepa, or radionuclides (Martinoni et al., 2000). Intrapericardial sclerotherapy is associated with good results in terms of prevention of recurrence and improvement in survival (Martinoni et al., 2000).

Oida et al. (2010) studied a series of these patients who underwent pericardiocentesis followed by intrapericardial cisplatin for treatment of malignant pericardial effusion secondary to esophageal cancer. The authors concluded that this method of treatment successfully prevented recurrence.

Table 6-4. Diagnostic Tests for the Evaluation for Pericardial Effusion	
Pericardial Effusion Evaluation	**Findings Indicative of Pericarditis**
Acid-fast bacteria	*Mycobacterium* tuberculosis
Complete blood count	Elevated white blood cell count
Cytology	Presence of malignant or immature cells
Culture	Bacteria or fungi
Brain natriuretic peptide (BNP)	Elevated BNP indicates myocardial strain
Flow cytometry (in patients with leukemia and lymphoma)	Malignant cells and/or chromosomes
Note. Based on information from Liff et al., 2011.	

Conclusion

The heart is a vulnerable organ susceptible to various insults and attacks from offending agents that are used frequently in cancer therapy. Careful attention must be given to these special considerations of patients with cancer to properly diagnose acute problems and to aggressively treat these grave conditions. This should be the ultimate goal of clinicians who practice in the cancer setting in order to improve patient outcomes and enhance the quality of life of patients undergoing cancer therapy.

References

American Cancer Society. (2010). Infections in people with cancer. Retrieved from http://www.cancer.org/acs/groups/cid/documents/webcontent/002871-pdf.pdf

Barbetakis, N., Xenikakis, T., Paliouras, D., Asteriou, C., Samanidis, G., Kleontas, A., ... Tsilikas, C. (2010). Pericardiectomy for radiation-induced constrictive pericarditis. *Hellenic Journal of Cardiology, 51*, 214–218.

Broder, H., Gottlieb, R.A., & Lepor, N.E. (2008). Chemotherapy and cardiotoxicity. *Reviews in Cardiovascular Medicine, 9*, 75–83.

Carver, J.R., Nasta, S., Chong, E.A., Stonecypher, M., Wheeler, J.E., Ahmadi, T., & Schuster, S.J. (2010). Myocarditis during lenalidomide therapy. *Annals of Pharmacotherapy, 44*, 1840–1843. doi:10.1345/aph.1P044

Chen, F., Mo, Y., Ding, H., Xiao, X., Wang, S.Y., Huang, G., ... Wang, S.Z. (2011). Frequent epigenetic inactivation of Myocardin in human nasopharyngeal carcinoma. *Head and Neck, 33*, 54–59. doi:10.1002/hed.21396

Cooper, L.T., Jr. (2009). Myocarditis. *New England Journal of Medicine, 360*, 1526–1538. doi:10.1056/NEJMra0800028

Cornily, J.C., Pennec, P.Y., Castellant, P., Bezon, E., Le Gal, G., Gilard, M., ... Blanc, J.J. (2008). Cardiac tamponade in medical patients: A 10-year follow-up survey. *Cardiology, 111*, 197–201. doi:10.1159/000121604

Ewer, M.S., Swain, S.M., Cardinale, D., Fadol, A., & Suter, T.M. (2011). Cardiac dysfunction after cancer treatment. *Texas Heart Institute Journal, 38*, 248–252.

Fadol, A., & Lech, T. (2011). Cardiovascular adverse events associated with cancer therapy. *Journal of the Advanced Practitioner in Oncology, 2*, 229–242.

Garg, N., Moorthy, N., Agrawal, S.K., Pandey, S., & Kumari, N. (2011). Delayed cardiac metastasis from phyllodes breast tumor presenting as cardiogenic shock. *Texas Heart Institute Journal, 38*, 441–444.

Gautam, M.P., Gautam, S., Sogunuru, G., & Subramanyam, G. (2012). Constrictive pericarditis with a calcified pericardial band at the level of left ventricle causing mid-ventricular obstruction. *BMJ Case Reports*. doi:10.1136/bcr.09.2011.4743

Heart Failure Society of America. (2010). Section 16: Myocarditis: Current treatment. *Journal of Cardiac Failure, 16*, e176–e179. doi:10.1016/j.cardfail.2010.05.025

Hsi, D.H., Krishnamurthy, M., Ryan, G.F., Luo, P., & Woodlock, T.J. (2010). Successful management of hemopericardium and cardiac tamponade secondary to occult malignancy and anticoagulation. *Experimental and Clinical Cardiology, 15*(2), e33–e35.

Imazio, M., & Adler, Y. (2012). Treatment with aspirin, NSAID, corticosteroids, and colchicine in acute and recurrent pericarditis. *Heart Failure Reviews*. Advance online publication. doi:10.1007/s10741-012-9328-9

Jameson, G.S., Ramanathan, R.K., Borad, M.J., Downhour, M., Korn, R., & Von Hoff, D. (2009). Marantic endocarditis associated with pancreatic cancer: A case series. *Case Reports in Gastroenterology, 3*, 67–71. doi:10.1159/000207195

LeWinter, M.M. (2008). Pericardial diseases. In P. Libby, R.O. Bonow, D.L. Mann, & D.P. Zipes (Eds.), *Braunwald's heart disease: A textbook of cardiovascular medicine* (8th ed., pp. 1829–1854). Philadelphia, PA: Elsevier Saunders.

Liff, D., Babaliaros, V., & Khattar, R. (2011, July 18). Evaluation of pericardial effusion. Retrieved from https://online.epocrates.com/u/2911458/Evaluation+of+pericardial+effusion/Differential/Overview

Maisch, B., Ristic, A., & Pankuweit, S. (2010). Evaluation and management of pericardial effusion in patients with neoplastic disease. *Progress in Cardiovascular Diseases, 53,* 157–163. doi:10.1016/j.pcad.2010.06.003

Martinoni, A., Cipolla, C.M., Civelli, M., Cardinale, D., Lamantia, G., Colleoni, M., ... Fiorentini, C. (2000). Intrapericardial treatment of neoplastic pericardial effusions. *Herz, 25,* 787–793. doi:10.1007/PL00001998

Mueller, D.K. (2011, August 3). Pericardial window. Retrieved from http://emedicine.medscape.com/article/1829679-overview

Oida, T., Mimatsu, K., Kano, H., Kawasaki, A., Kuboi, Y., Fukino, N., & Amano, S. (2010). Pericardiocentesis with cisplatin for malignant pericardial effusion and tamponade. *World Journal of Gastroenterology, 16,* 740–744. doi:10.3748/wjg.v16.i6.740

Shabetai, R. (2005). Recurrent pericarditis: Recent advances and remaining questions. *Circulation, 112,* 1921–1923. doi:10.1161/CIRCULATIONAHA.105.569244

Sumantran, V.N., & Tillu, G. (2012). Cancer, inflammation, and insights from Ayurveda. *Evidence-Based Complementary and Alternative Medicine, 2012,* 306346. doi:10.1155/2012/306346

Texas Heart Institute. (2010). Pericarditis. Retrieved from http://www.texasheartinstitute.org/HIC/Topics/cond/pericard.cfm

Unsworth, J., Sturman, S., Lunec, J., & Blake, D.R. (1987). Renal impairment associated with nonsteroidal anti-inflammatory drugs. *Annals of the Rheumatic Diseases, 46,* 233–236.

Wilson, W., Taubert, K.A., Gewitz, M., Lockhart, P.B., Baddour, L.M., Levison, M., ... Durack, D.T. (2007). Prevention of infective endocarditis: Guidelines from the American Heart Association: A guideline from the American Heart Association Rheumatic Fever, Endocarditis, and Kawasaki Disease Committee, Council on Cardiovascular Disease in the Young, and the Council on Clinical Cardiology, Council on Cardiovascular Surgery and Anesthesia, and the Quality of Care and Outcomes Research Interdisciplinary Working Group. *Circulation, 116,* 1736–1754. doi:10.1161/CIRCULATIONAHA.106.183095

Xiong, Y.Q., Fowler, V.G., Yeaman, M.R., Perdreau-Remington, F., Kreiswirth, B.N., & Bayer, A.S. (2009). Phenotypic and genotypic characteristics of persistent methicillin-resistant *Staphylococcus aureus* bacteremia in vitro and in an experimental endocarditis model. *Journal of Infectious Diseases, 199,* 201–208. doi:10.1086/595738

Yarlagadda, C. (2011, August 11). Cardiac tamponade. Retrieved from http://emedicine.medscape.com/article/152083-overview

CHAPTER 7

Hypertension in Patients With Cancer

*Myrshia L. Woods, MHS, PA-C, Tara Lech, PharmD, BCPS,
and Anecita P. Fadol, PhD, RN, FNP-BC, FAANP*

Introduction

Hypertension (HTN) is a progressive cardiovascular syndrome associated with functional and structural cardiac and vascular abnormalities that can damage the heart, brain, kidneys, and other organs and lead to premature morbidity and death (Ram, 2007). Approximately 76.4 million adults in the United States have been diagnosed with HTN (Roger et al., 2012), and as many as 29% of patients with cancer have pretreatment elevated blood pressure (BP) (Chu et al., 2007). Certain cancer treatments may provoke or exacerbate existing HTN. Antiangiogenic therapies targeting the vascular endothelial growth factor signaling pathway (VSP) are notably associated with hypertensive cardiotoxic adverse effects (Launay-Vacher & Deray, 2009). Other cancer treatments that may cause HTN include calcineurin inhibitors, steroids, radiation, and surgical intervention involving the head and neck area.

Calcineurin inhibitors (i.e., cyclosporine and tacrolimus) are frequently used for immunosuppression following hematopoietic stem cell transplantation (HSCT). These agents can cause de novo HTN or acceleration of preexisting HTN. The concomitant use of steroids in many drug protocols, radiation therapy, and extensive surgery involving the head and neck also may result in HTN.

As the diagnosis and treatment of cancer continue to improve, resulting in increased survivorship, management of HTN becomes increasingly important to prevent end-organ damage. In fact, the risk of mortality from ischemic heart disease and stroke begins at BP levels as low as 115/75 mm Hg, and the risk doubles with each incremental increase of 20 mm Hg systolic or 10 mm Hg diastolic (Lewington, Clarke, Qizilbash, Peto, & Collins, 2002). Thus, adequate management of HTN in patients with cancer is critical to prevent cardiovascular complications while receiving cancer treatment. This chapter will discuss the most common causes of HTN in patients with cancer and identify recommended diagnostic workup, pharmacologic management, and monitoring of patients while on antineoplastic therapies that may induce or exacerbate HTN.

Definition

The Joint National Committee on Prevention, Evaluation, and Treatment of High Blood Pressure 7th Edition (JNC 7) guidelines define HTN as a systolic blood pressure (SBP) of 140–159 mm Hg or a diastolic blood pressure (DBP) of 90–99 mm Hg (Chobanian et al., 2003). The JNC 7 classification of HTN is listed in Table 7-1. This definition is widely adhered to by general healthcare practitioners, whereas oncologists tend to apply the HTN classification as defined by the National Cancer Institute (NCI) Cancer Therapy Evaluation Program's *Common Terminology Criteria for Adverse Events* (CTCAE) to report adverse effects in chemotherapy clinical trials. The older CTCAE (versions 2 and 3) did not include reporting of SBP less than 150 mm Hg or DBP less than 100 mm Hg. However, the latest CTCAE (version 4.03) updated the grading system to be in agreement with the JNC7 criteria (NCI Cancer Therapy Evaluation Program, 2006, 2010). A summary of the CTCAE classification of HTN is shown in Table 7-2.

Table 7-1. Classification of Blood Pressure

Category	Systolic and Diastolic Pressure (mm Hg)
Normal	< 120 and < 80
Prehypertension	120–139 or 80–99
Hypertension, stage 1	140–159 or 90–99
Hypertension, stage 2	≥ 160 or ≥ 100

Note. Based on information from Chobanian et al., 2003.

Table 7-2. Hypertension as Defined by *Common Terminology Criteria for Adverse Events* (CTCAE)

Grade	CTCAE Version 3.0	CTCAE Version 4.03
1	Asymptomatic, transient (< 24 hours) increase by > 20 mm Hg (diastolic) or to > 150/100 if previously within normal limits; no treatment required	Prehypertension (120–139/80–89 mm Hg)
2	Recurrent or persistent (≥ 24 hours) or symptomatic increase by > 20 mm Hg (diastolic) or to > 150/100 mm Hg if previously within normal limits; monotherapy may be indicated	Stage 1 hypertension (140–159/90–99 mm Hg)
3	Requiring more than one drug or more intensive therapy than previously	Stage 2 hypertension (≥ 160/100 mm Hg)
4	Life-threatening consequences	Life-threatening consequences; > 180/120 mm Hg with impending or progressive target organ damage
5	Death	Death

Note. Based on information from National Cancer Institute Cancer Therapy Evaluation Program, 2006, 2010.

Pathophysiology

The exact mechanism of antineoplastic agent–induced HTN remains unclear. It is postulated that different pathophysiologic processes exist for the different types of anticancer agents.

Vascular Endothelial Growth Factor Signaling Pathway Inhibitors

The term *VSP inhibitors* includes a subclass of antiangiogenesis inhibitors that blocks signaling of vascular endothelial growth factor (VEGF) and its primary cognate receptor on endothelial cells, VEGF receptor-2 (referred to as VEGFR2) (Bhargava, 2009; Maitland et al., 2010). Table 7-3 lists the VSP inhibitors approved by the U.S. Food and Drug Administration for cancer treatment and new agents in development (Escudier et al., 2007; Meinardi et al., 2000; Rossi, Seccia, Maniero, & Pessina, 2011).

VEGF has been associated with decreases in blood pressure because it enhances the production of the vasodilator nitric oxide (NO) and decreases vascular resistance through the generation of new blood vessels (Henry et al., 2003; Hood, Meininger, Ziche, & Granger, 1998). VSP inhibitor–induced HTN is postulated to result from the antagonism of the normal effect of VEGF on endothelial cells to stimulate NO synthase to produce NO (Zachary, 2001). NO promotes vasodilation, and reducing NO will cause vasoconstriction and therefore increased blood pressure (Brunner et al., 2005). Moreover, lower levels of NO have been linked with sodium and water retention, which can lead to development of HTN (Granger & Alexander, 2000). The VSP inhibitor mechanism for inducing HTN is shown in Figure 7-1.

Table 7-3. Incidence of Hypertension With VSP Inhibitors		
VSP Inhibitors	**Total Incidence of Hypertension (%)**	**Incidence of CTCAE Grade ≥ 3 Hypertension (%)**
FDA-approved agents		
Bevacizumab	22	11
Pazopanib	37	8
Sorafenib	17	4
Sunitinib	24	8
Vandetanib	21	2
New agents in development		
Aflibercept	46	18
Axitinib	30	5
Cediranib	72	33
Motesanib	56	25

CTCAE—National Cancer Institute *Common Terminology Criteria for Adverse Events*; FDA—U.S. Food and Drug Administration; VSP—vascular endothelial growth factor signaling pathway

Note. Based on information from Escudier et al., 2007; Meinardi et al., 2000; Rossi et al., 2011.

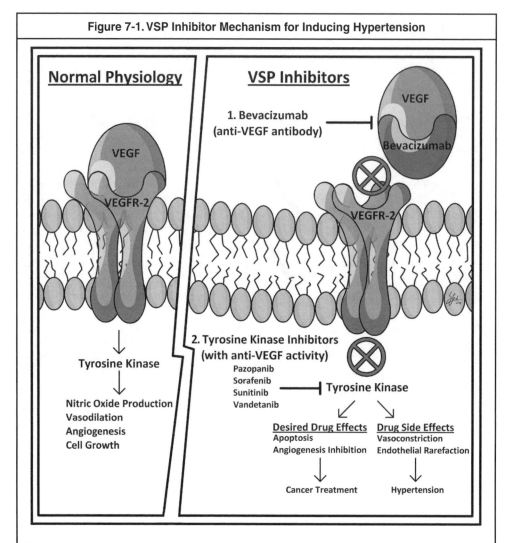

Figure 7-1. VSP Inhibitor Mechanism for Inducing Hypertension

(A) Normal physiology: Binding of vascular endothelial growth factor (VEGF) to its receptor triggers intracellular signaling pathways including tyrosine kinase leading to nitric oxide production, vasodilation, angiogenesis, and cell growth. (B) Vascular signaling pathway inhibitors work through various mechanisms: Bevacizumab binds to VEGF and prevents activation of the VEGF receptor while tyrosine kinase inhibitors prevent the activation of tyrosine kinase. The desired anti-cancer effect of these medications is to promote apoptosis and angiogenesis inhibition leading to treatment of the cancer. The undesired effect of hypotension is a result of the decreased nitric oxide bioavailability with secondary vasoconstriction and increased peripheral resistance.

VEGFR-2—vascular endothelial growth factor receptor-2; VSP—vascular endothelial growth factor signaling pathway

Note. Artwork created and copyrighted by Mr. Zbigniew Lech. Used with permission.

Calcineurin Inhibitors

This classification of medications is routinely used in immunosuppressive regimens following organ transplantation and HSCT. Since the widespread use of cyclosporine and tacrolimus in patients following kidney transplantation, the prevalence of HTN has increased from 40%–50% to up to 90%–100% (Curtis, 2002). The proposed mechanism underlying HTN caused by calcineurin inhibitors is believed to be the result of the sympathetic activation and an increase in the endothelin-1 synthesis leading to vasoconstriction and a decrease in water, sodium, and potassium excretion (Rossi et al., 2011). HTN usually develops within the first six weeks of therapy.

Corticosteroids

HTN secondary to steroid use is dose dependent and occurs in at least 20% of patients treated with synthetic corticosteroids (Rossi et al., 2011). Long-term use of steroid preparations such as topical ointments or nasal drops also can induce HTN. The physiologic mechanism of steroid-induced HTN is complex and includes increased angiotensinogen synthesis and activation of the sympathetic nervous system (Rickard, Funder, Morgan, Fuller, & Young, 2007). Increased production of angiotensinogen induces salt and fluid retention and greater patient sensitivity to vasoactive substances.

Radiation Therapy and Head and Neck Surgery

These treatment regimens may cause HTN when the baroreceptors are involved. The mechanism of HTN includes alteration in the autonomic pathways connecting the baroreceptors and the carotid bodies to the brain stem, resulting in an imbalance in the sympathetic and parasympathetic systems. This leads to labile, volatile HTN or severe hypertensive crisis (Ketch, Biaggioni, Robertson, & Robertson, 2002).

Risk Factors

A baseline evaluation of the underlying hypertensive risk prior to initiation of cancer therapies associated with HTN is critical. Uncontrolled HTN may result in adverse cardiovascular events. Understanding the causes of HTN is important, as some of these risk factors are similar for the development of cancer. Risk factors for the development of HTN are classified as modifiable or nonmodifiable. Modifiable risk factors include obesity, tobacco and alcohol abuse, physical inactivity, diabetes mellitus, renal insufficiency/failure, thyroid and parathyroid abnormalities, and hyperlipidemia (Whitworth, 2003) and the use of antineoplastic agents with hypertensive adverse effects (Bhargava, 2009; Chu et al., 2007; Curtis, 2002). It is conceivable that many of the risk factors associated with an increased risk of malignancy also play a significant role in the pathophysiology of HTN (Kurtin, 2009).

Nonmodifiable risk factors include increasing age, family history, and certain ethnic groups in which HTN is most often genetically based. The specific ethnic groups that are disproportionately affected are Afro-Caribbean, Native American, and Asian/Pacific Islander in comparison to lower rates of HTN observed in Caucasian and Hispanic populations (Roger et al., 2012). Given that this specific risk factor is inherited, clinicians should recognize the importance of individualizing care of these patients based on certain genetic predispositions. It is well established that certain ethnicities respond to specific classes of antihypertensive treatment that prove to have a mortality benefit. This important aspect of treatment is highlighted in the JNC 7 guidelines as well. A summary of the risk factors for assessment of HTN appears in Figure 7-2. The interplay of these risk factors in the development of HTN in patients with cancer is illustrated in Figure 7-3.

Figure 7-2. Risk Factors for Hypertension

Modifiable Risk Factors
- Obesity (body mass index > 30)
- Dyslipidemia
- Diabetes mellitus
- Cigarette smoking
- Physical inactivity
- Antineoplastic agents (VSP inhibitors)

Nonmodifiable Risk Factors
- Increasing age
- Family history
- Ethnic background

Note. Based on information from Maitland et al., 2010.

Figure 7-3. Risk Factors for Hypertension in Patients With Cancer

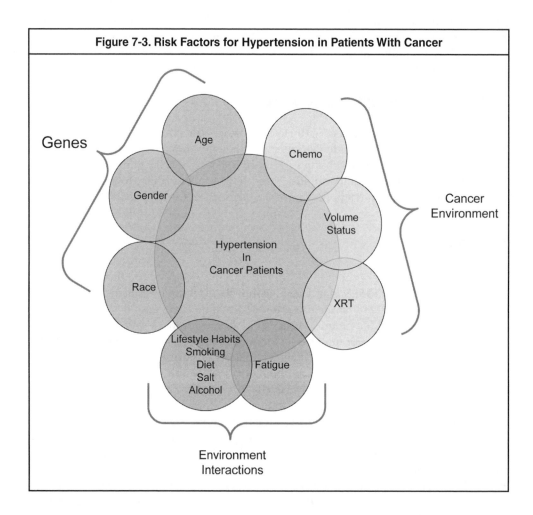

Diagnostic Workup

A comprehensive evaluation is recommended when considering cancer treatments associated with HTN. The JNC 7 guidelines recommend that the diagnostic workup for HTN should include the following goals: (a) detection and confirmation of HTN, (b) detection of target organ disease (e.g., renal damage, congestive heart failure), (c) identification of other risk factors for cardiovascular disease (e.g., diabetes mellitus, hyperlipidemia), and (d) detection of secondary causes of HTN (Chobanian et al., 2003). For patients with a complex cardiovascular history, a cardiology consult may be necessary. A baseline evaluation should include a complete physical examination with particular attention to the cardiopulmonary system and laboratory analysis (hepatic and renal profile, lipid panel, thyroid function tests). Patients with preexisting HTN may undergo a baseline electrocardiogram and echocardiogram to evaluate for left ventricular hypertrophy. Patients with a high risk profile for the presence of coronary artery disease may benefit from a baseline myocardial perfusion stress test.

Management of Hypertension

The primary goal in HTN management is to reduce morbidity and mortality and lower the risk of target organ damage, such as cardiovascular and cerebrovascular events and renal failure. Successful HTN treatment is associated with a 30%–40% reduction in stroke, 20%–25% reduction in myocardial infarction, and greater than 50% reduction in congestive heart failure (Neal, MacMahon, & Chapman, 2000). The target BP goal for treatment should be based on the JNC 7 classification of the patient. All patients should be treated to a goal of lower than 140/90 mm Hg, except for those with preexisting coronary artery disease, diabetes, or chronic kidney disease, in which the goal should be lower than 130/80 mm Hg. If the patient is already receiving antihypertensive medication and the BP target goal is still not achieved, adherence should be verified. If the dose is already at the maximum, a second agent may be added to achieve the target BP goal. Generally, two or more antihypertensive agents will be required to achieve the goal BP, especially in patients on VSP inhibitor agents. Before starting VSP inhibitor therapy, adequate BP control is recommended (Maitland et al., 2010). If the patient is not receiving antihypertensive therapy, the patient should be monitored closely after initiation of VSP therapy. The pace of titration of the medications to achieve the target goal is dependent on the patient's response to the medication.

According to the JNC 7 guidelines, the first-line treatment for uncomplicated HTN without compelling indications includes a thiazide-type diuretic either alone or in combination with an agent from another class (Chobanian et al., 2003). If a thiazide-type diuretic is not the first drug selected, it should be the second drug in the regimen if no contraindications exist. The major classes of antihypertensive agents are diuretics, beta-blockers, angiotensin-converting enzyme inhibitors, angiotensin receptor blockers, and calcium channel blockers (see Table 7-4). All of these agents have been shown to reduce cardiovascular events such as stroke, acute coronary syndromes, and heart failure (Neal et al., 2000). In cases with compelling indications, the JNC 7 recommendations for initial treatment are outlined in Table 7-5.

Blood Pressure Monitoring

It is important to monitor patients' BP closely while they are on VSP inhibitor therapy. The NCI clinical trial protocols recommend monitoring BP weekly during the first cycle of VSP inhibitor therapy and then at least every two to three weeks for the duration of treatment (Maitland et al., 2010). In clinical trials, initial elevations of BP were noted during the first week of treatment with sorafenib and sunitinib, the most com-

Table 7-4. Major Classes of Antihypertensive Agents

Antihypertensive Agent	Indications	Contraindications
Thiazide diuretics	Isolated HTN, HF	Gout, glucose intolerance, and pregnancy
ACE inhibitors	LVD, HF, post-MI, diabetic nephropathy, LVH, metabolic syndrome	Hyperkalemia, bilateral renal artery stenosis, peripheral vascular disease, angioedema, pregnancy
Angiotensin receptor antagonists	Intolerance to ACE inhibitors, HF, post-MI, diabetic nephropathy, LVH	Hyperkalemia, bilateral renal artery stenosis, peripheral vascular disease, angioedema, pregnancy
Beta-blockers	HF, post-MI, tachyarrhythmias, atrial fibrillation	Asthma, COPD, atrioventricular block (second and third degree)
Calcium channel blockers (dihydropyridine)	Elderly patients, isolated systolic HTN, SVT, angina pectoris	Preexisting edema, HF

ACE—angiotensin-converting enzyme; COPD—chronic obstructive pulmonary disease; HF—heart failure; HTN—hypertension; LVD—left ventricular dysfunction; LVH—left ventricular hypertrophy; MI—myocardial infarction; SVT—supraventricular tachycardia

Note. Based on information from Maitland et al., 2010; Mancia et al., 2007.

Table 7-5. Compelling Indications for Individual Drug Classes

Condition	Drug Therapy	Comments
Chronic kidney disease	ACE inhibitor, ARB	–
Diabetes	Diuretic, beta-blocker, ACE inhibitor, ARB, CCB	Avoid CCB as single therapy.
Heart failure	Diuretic, beta-blocker, ACE inhibitor, ARB, aldosterone antagonist	FDA-approved beta-blockers include carvedilol and metoprolol succinate. Avoid alpha-blockers and CCBs, except amlodipine.
High coronary disease risk	Diuretic, beta-blocker, ACE inhibitor, CCB	–
Post–myocardial infarction	Beta-blocker, ACE inhibitor, aldosterone antagonist	Avoid dihydropyridine CCBs, except amlodipine or felodipine.
Recurrent stroke prevention	Diuretic, ACE inhibitor	–

ACE—angiotensin-converting enzyme; ARB—angiotensin receptor blocker; CCB—calcium channel blocker; FDA—U.S. Food and Drug Administration

Note. Based on information from Chobanian et al., 2003.

monly used VSP inhibitors (Azizi, Chedid, & Oudard, 2008; Maitland et al., 2010). Early detection and management of HTN might prevent some of the complications of VSP inhibitor therapy. This can be achieved with weekly office visits and ambulatory BP monitoring. Patients are encouraged to maintain BP diaries, recording the readings at least once daily. They should be instructed to report to the clinician any BP readings above the recommended parameters. Clinicians must provide adequate education to patients regarding BP measurement techniques (e.g., using the right cuff size, using brachial cuff measurement instead of wrist or finger devices), when to hold BP medications, and when to report for clinical follow-up in the event of persistently uncontrolled blood pressure despite full compliance to prescribed antihypertensive therapy. Different BP measurement techniques are listed in Table 7-6.

Patients who are on chronic pain management should be monitored closely. Baseline BP measurement should be reassessed after adequate pain control is achieved. Pain medications such as opioids and narcotics can lower the BP significantly, whereas nonsteroidal anti-inflammatory agents can potentially increase BP. If patients are continued on antihypertensive agents while taking high-dose opioids or narcotics for pain control, they are at risk to experience symptomatic hypotension, possibly potentiating presyncope or syncope. Close monitoring is necessary when the patient with cancer is on antihypertensive regimens as pain management becomes a higher priority in the patient's overall care.

Table 7-6. Blood Pressure Measurement Techniques	
Method	**Comments**
In-office	Two readings, 5 minutes apart, sitting in chair, legs uncrossed, with arm at level of heart. Confirm elevated reading in the contralateral arm.
Ambulatory blood pressure monitoring	Indicated for evaluation of white-coat hypertension. Absence of 10%–20% blood pressure decrease during sleep may indicate increased cardiovascular risk.
Patient self-check	Provides information on response to therapy. May help to improve adherence to therapy and is useful for evaluating white-coat hypertension.

Note. Based on information from Chobanian et al., 2003.

Resistant Hypertension

Resistant or refractory HTN is defined as a blood pressure of 140/90 mm Hg or higher (or at least 130/80 mm Hg in patients with diabetes or renal disease) despite adherence to treatment with full doses of at least three antihypertensive medications including a diuretic (Chobanian et al., 2003). When resistant HTN is encountered, the clinician must begin investigating for potential secondary causes of HTN (see Table 7-7). It is possible to unveil secondary disease processes in the background of cancer that may be exacerbating HTN. Referral to a specialist should be considered in patients whose HTN is difficult to control despite an assessment of adherence and dose of antihypertensive agents and other factors that may exacerbate the condition (Moser & Setaro, 2006).

Table 7-7. Secondary Causes of Resistant Hypertension

Findings	Disorder Suspected	Further Diagnostic Studies
Snoring, daytime somnolence, obesity	Obstructive sleep apnea	Sleep study
Hypernatremia, hypokalemia	Primary aldosteronism	Ratio of plasma aldosterone to plasma renin activity, CT scan of adrenal glands
Renal insufficiency, atherosclerosis, edema, elevated BUN/Cr, proteinuria	Renal parenchymal disease	Creatinine clearance, renal ultrasound
Systolic/diastolic abdominal bruit	Renovascular disease	Magnetic resonance angiography, captopril-augmented radioisotopic renography, renal arteriography
Use of sympathomimetics, perioperative setting, acute stress, tachycardia	Excess catecholamines	Confirm patient is normotensive in absence of high catecholamines.
Decreased or delayed femoral pulses, abnormal chest radiograph	Coarctation of aorta	Doppler or CT imaging or aorta
Weight gain, fatigue, weakness, hirsutism, amenorrhea, moon facies, dorsal hump, purple striae, truncal obesity, hypokalemia	Cushing syndrome	Dexamethasone-suppression test
High salt intake, excessive alcohol intake, obesity	Diet side effects	Trial of dietary modification
Erythropoietin use in renal disease, polycythemia in COPD	Erythropoietin side effect	Trial off drug
Paroxysmal hypertension, headaches, diaphoresis, palpitations, tachycardia	Pheochromocytoma	Urinary catecholamine metabolites (vanillylmandelic acid, metanephrines, normetanephrines, plasma-free metanephrines
Fatigue, weight loss, hair loss, diastolic hypertension, muscle weakness	Hypothyroidism	TSH levels
Heat intolerance, weight loss, palpitations, systolic hypertension, exophthalmos, tremor, tachycardia	Hyperthyroidism	TSH levels
Kidney stones, osteoporosis, depression, lethargy, muscle weakness	Hyperparathyroidism	Serum calcium, parathyroid hormone levels
Headaches, fatigue, visual problems, enlargement of hands, feet, and tongue	Acromegaly	Growth hormone level

BUN/Cr—blood urea nitrogen/creatinine; COPD—chronic obstructive pulmonary disease; CT—computed tomography; TSH—thyroid-stimulating hormone

Note. Based on information from Onusko, 2003.

Withdrawal of Hypertensive Medications

The appropriate discontinuation of antihypertensive agents from a patient's regimen should be considered when HTN-causing cancer therapy ceases. If patients begin to notice a steady drop in BP after completion of cancer therapy, especially the VSP inhibitors, and become symptomatic with hypotensive episodes, then antihypertensive medications should be discontinued. Frequent BP monitoring should continue despite being off antihypertensive treatment to confirm that normal pressure is being maintained.

Another important aspect in BP monitoring while patients are on VSP inhibitor therapy is *white-coat HTN*, which consists of a sustained difference between arterial BP measurements obtained within and outside the medical office setting. Sometimes, patients may claim that their BP at home is much lower than the BP measured in the clinic. The exact pathophysiology is not well defined; however, several authors have proposed that environmental, anthropometric, and autonomic factors are contributory in white-coat HTN (Gualdiero, Niebauer, Addison, Clark, & Coats, 2000; Mansoor, McCabe, & White, 1996). This can be true in patients with cancer, who are exposed to psychological and emotional trauma as they undergo complicated protocols of treatments and battle multiple side effects. In a study of 69 women with breast cancer undergoing chemotherapy, the mean white-coat effect was 7.8 mm Hg (standard deviation [SD] 16.5) for systolic BP and 8.8 mm Hg (SD 11.0) for diastolic BP (Costa, Varella, & Del Giglio, 2003). The clinician must recognize this phenomenon and be willing to alter medications accordingly, being careful not to overmedicate these patients because of higher readings observed in the clinical setting.

Nursing Implications

Recognizing all the important aspects regarding HTN, it is imperative for the clinician to dedicate time in educating patients. This also is a unique opportunity for the nurse to provide education that will likely increase patient adherence to the prescribed medical regimen. There is a need to increase patients' awareness of the problem, as well as their knowledge about the consequences of poor control. Patients need to be educated on which cancer therapies cause HTN, the side effects of elevated BP, the negative consequences of poor control, and the available treatment options for effective control.

Patient education should outline the importance of effective HTN management to allow continuation of therapy, discussing reportable signs and symptoms and demonstrating home BP monitoring and periodic calibration of the home BP-monitoring equipment (Kurtin, 2009). Using patient education materials specifically designed for this patient population will be most helpful. The Department of Cardiology at MD Anderson developed a patient educational booklet, *High Blood Pressure and You: Treating High Blood Pressure During and After Cancer Treatment,* specifically for this unique patient population.

Conclusion

HTN remains a highly prevalent comorbid condition in patients with cancer and is associated with increased risk for adverse cardiovascular outcomes and potential deleterious consequences. Identifying the underlying cause of HTN is critical to guide treatment and avoid unnecessary changes in cancer therapy. It is imperative for oncologists and cardiologists to work in collaboration to prevent and manage HTN so that these potentially life-sustaining anticancer agents can benefit the greatest number of patients and prevent morbidity and mortality secondary to end-organ damage, improve overall outcomes, and enhance the quality of life of these patients.

References

Azizi, M., Chedid, A., & Oudard, S. (2008). Home blood-pressure monitoring in patients receiving sunitinib [Letter to the editor]. *New England Journal of Medicine, 358,* 95–97. doi:10.1056/NEJMc072330

Bhargava, P. (2009). VEGF kinase inhibitors: How do they cause hypertension? *American Journal of Physiology: Regulatory, Integrative and Comparative Physiology, 297,* R1–R5. doi:10.1152/ajpregu.90502.2008

Brunner, H., Cockcroft, J.R., Deanfield, J., Donald, A., Ferrannini, E., Halcox, J., ... Webb, D.J. (2005). Endothelial function and dysfunction. Part II: Association with cardiovascular risk factors and diseases. A statement by the Working Group on Endothelins and Endothelial Factors of the European Society of Hypertension. *Journal of Hypertension, 23,* 233–246. doi:10.1097/00004872-200502000-00001

Chobanian, A.V., Bakris, G.L., Black, H.R., Cushman, W.C., Green, L.A., Izzo, J.L., Jr., & Roccella, E.J. (2003). JNC 7: Complete report: Seventh report of the Joint National Committee on Prevention, Detection, Evaluation, and Treatment of High Blood Pressure. *Hypertension, 42,* 1206–1252. doi:10.1161/01.HYP.0000107251.49515.c2

Chu, T.F., Rupnick, M.A., Kerkela, R., Dallabrida, S.M., Zurakowski, D., Nguyen, L., ... Chen, M.H. (2007). Cardiotoxicity associated with tyrosine kinase inhibitor sunitinib. *Lancet, 370,* 2011–2019. doi:10.1016/S0140-6736(07)61865-0

Costa, L.J., Varella, P.C., & Del Giglio, A. (2003). White coat effect in breast cancer patients undergoing chemotherapy. *European Journal of Cancer Care, 12,* 372–373. doi:10.1046/j.1365-2354.2003.00416.x

Curtis, J.J. (2002). Hypertensinogenic mechanism of the calcineurin inhibitors. *Current Hypertension Reports, 4,* 377–380. doi:10.1007/s11906-002-0067-5

Escudier, B., Eisen, T., Stadler, W.M., Szczylik, C., Oudard, S., Siebels, M., ... Bukowski, R.M. (2007). Sorafenib in advanced clear-cell renal-cell carcinoma. *New England Journal of Medicine, 356,* 125–134. doi:10.1056/NEJMoa060655

Granger, J.P., & Alexander, B.T. (2000). Abnormal pressure–natriuresis in hypertension: Role of nitric oxide. *Acta Physiologica Scandinavica, 168,* 161–168. doi:10.1046/j.1365-201x.2000.00655.x

Gualdiero, P., Niebauer, J., Addison, C., Clark, S.J., & Coats, A.J. (2000). Clinical features, anthropometric characteristics, and racial influences on the 'white-coat effect' in a single-centre cohort of 1553 consecutive subjects undergoing routine ambulatory blood pressure monitoring. *Blood Pressure Monitoring, 5,* 53–57.

Henry, T.D., Annex, B.H., McKendall, G.R., Azrin, M.A., Lopez, J.J., Giordano, F.J., ... McCluskey, E.R. (2003). The VIVA trial: Vascular endothelial growth factor in ischemia for vascular angiogenesis. *Circulation, 107,* 1359–1365. doi:10.1161/01.CIR.0000061911.47710.8A

Hood, J.D., Meininger, C.J., Ziche, M., & Granger, H.J. (1998). VEGF upregulates ecNOS message, protein, and NO production in human endothelial cells. *American Journal of Physiology, 274,* H1054–H1058.

Ketch, T., Biaggioni, I., Robertson, R., & Robertson, D. (2002). Four faces of baroreflex failure: Hypertensive crisis, volatile hypertension, orthostatic tachycardia, and malignant vagotonia. *Circulation, 105,* 2518–2523. doi:10.1161/01.CIR.0000017186.52382.F4

Kurtin, S.E. (2009). Hypertension management in the era of targeted therapies for cancer. *Oncology, 23*(4, Suppl. Nurse Ed.), 41–45.

Launay-Vacher, V., & Deray, G. (2009). Hypertension and proteinuria: A class-effect of antiangiogenic therapies. *Anti-Cancer Drugs, 20,* 81–82. doi:10.1097/CAD.0b013e3283161012

Lewington, S., Clarke, R., Qizilbash, N., Peto, R., & Collins, R. (2002). Age-specific relevance of usual blood pressure to vascular mortality: A meta-analysis of individual data for one million adults in 61 prospective studies. *Lancet, 360,* 1903–1913. doi:10.1016/S0140-6736(02)11911-8

Maitland, M.L., Bakris, G.L., Black, H.R., Chen, H.X., Durand, J.-B., Elliott, W.J., ... Tang, W.H.W. (2010). Initial assessment, surveillance, and management of blood pressure in patients receiving vascular endothelial growth factor signaling pathway inhibitors. *Journal of the National Cancer Institute, 102,* 596–604. doi:10.1093/jnci/djq091

Mancia, G., De Backer, G., Dominiczak, A., Cifkova, R., Fagard, R., Germano, G., ... Zamorano, J.L. (2007). 2007 guidelines for the management of arterial hypertension: The Task Force for the Management of Arterial Hypertension of the European Society of Hypertension (ESH) and of the European Society of Cardiology (ESC). *European Heart Journal, 28*, 1462–1536. doi:10.1093/eurheartj/ehm236

Mansoor, G.A., McCabe, E.J., & White, W.B. (1996). Determinants of the white-coat effect in hypertensive subjects. *Journal of Human Hypertension, 10*, 87–92.

Meinardi, M.T., Gietema, J.A., van der Graaf, W.T., van Veldhuisen, D.J., Runne, M.A., Sluiter, W.J., ... Sleijfer, D.T. (2000). Cardiovascular morbidity in long-term survivors of metastatic testicular cancer. *Journal of Clinical Oncology, 18*, 1725–1732.

Moser, M., & Setaro, J.F. (2006). Clinical practice. Resistant or difficult-to-control hypertension. *New England Journal of Medicine, 355*, 385–392. doi:10.1056/NEJMcp041698

National Cancer Institute Cancer Therapy Evaluation Program. (2006). *Common terminology criteria for adverse events* [v.3.0]. Retrieved from http://ctep.cancer.gov/protocolDevelopment/electronic_applications/docs/ctcaev3.pdf

National Cancer Institute Cancer Therapy Evaluation Program. (2010). *Common terminology criteria for adverse events* [v.4.03]. Retrieved from http://evs.nci.nih.gov/ftp1/CTCAE/CTCAE_4.03_2010-06-14_QuickReference_5x7.pdf

Neal, B., MacMahon, S., & Chapman, N. (2000). Effects of ACE inhibitors, calcium antagonists, and other blood-pressure-lowering drugs: Results of prospectively designed overviews of randomised trials. Blood Pressure Lowering Treatment Trialists' Collaboration. *Lancet, 356*, 1955–1964. doi:10.1016/S0140-6736(00)03307-9

Onusko, E. (2003). Diagnosing secondary hypertension. *American Family Physician, 67*, 67–74.

Ram, C.V. (2007). The evolving definition of systemic hypertension. *American Journal of Cardiology, 99*, 1168–1170. doi:10.1016/j.amjcard.2006.11.046

Rickard, A.J., Funder, J.W., Morgan, J., Fuller, P.J., & Young, M.J. (2007). Does glucocorticoid receptor blockade exacerbate tissue damage after mineralocorticoid/salt administration? *Endocrinology, 148*, 4829–4835. doi:10.1210/en.2007-0209

Roger, V.L., Go, A.S., Lloyd-Jones, D.M., Benjamin, E.J., Berry, J.D., Borden, W.B., ... Turner, M.B.. (2012). Heart disease and stroke statistics—2012 update: A report from the American Heart Association. *Circulation, 125*, e2–e220. doi:10.1161/CIR.0b013e31823ac046

Rossi, G.P., Seccia, T.M., Maniero, C., & Pessina, A.C. (2011). Drug-related hypertension and resistance to antihypertensive treatment: A call for action. *Journal of Hypertension, 29*, 2295–2309. doi:10.1097/HJH.0b013e32834c465d

Whitworth, J.A. (2003). 2003 World Health Organization (WHO)/International Society of Hypertension (ISH) statement on management of hypertension. *Journal of Hypertension, 21*, 1983–1992. doi:10.1097/00004872-200311000-00002

Zachary, I. (2001). Signaling mechanisms mediating vascular protective actions of vascular endothelial growth factor. *American Journal of Physiology: Cell Physiology, 280*, C1375–C1386.

CHAPTER 8

Venous Thromboembolism

Edgar C. Salire, RN, MSN, NP-C

Introduction

Venous thromboembolism (VTE) is a serious and life-threatening disorder that represents the second leading cause of death in hospitalized patients with cancer (Lyman & Khorana, 2009). VTE consists of deep vein thrombosis (DVT), which typically involves deep veins of the legs or pelvis, and its complication, pulmonary embolism (PE). VTE may indicate an occult cancer, represent a complication of a known malignancy, or complicate hospitalization, surgery, or various systemic cancer treatments (Prandoni et al., 2002; Varki, 2007).

The incidence of VTE in the cancer population is estimated at approximately 1 in 200, a fivefold increase compared to the general population (Lee et al., 2003). A recent retrospective study of about two million patients hospitalized in the United States reported an overall VTE rate of 4.1% among patients with cancer (Khorana, Francis, Culakova, Kuderer, & Lyman, 2007). Approximately 10% of all patients with a noncancer diagnosis who have VTE will be diagnosed with malignancy in two years with a worse prognosis (Yeh, Lenihan, & Ewer, 2008). The link between venous thrombosis and hypercoagulability, known as *Trousseau sign of malignancy*, was first described in 1865 by French internist Armand Trousseau, which he later found in himself when he was diagnosed with gastric cancer (Lyman & Khorana, 2009).

With the aging population, sedentary lifestyles, and the increasing incidence of cancer, VTE will become an increasing healthcare issue that will be an added strain to the overburdened and underfunded healthcare system unless we develop more cost-efficient management strategies. This chapter will discuss the pathogenesis of VTE, signs and symptoms, differential diagnoses, diagnostic tests, medical and surgical management, preventive measures, and the nursing implications in the management of patients with cancer who are at higher risk for this life-threatening complication.

Pathogenesis

VTE in patients with cancer is best explained by the Virchow triad: stasis or alteration in the normal blood flow, vessel damage, and alteration in the blood components (see Table 8-1). The underlying factor associated with increased risk of thrombosis in patients with cancer includes the activation of thrombin and fibrin formation, both directly by the release of procoagulants in tumor cells and indirectly by the activation of the endothelial cells, leukocytes, and platelets by cytokines and the production of factor X–activating cysteine protease, mucinous glycoproteins, and circulating tissue factor–bearing microparticles (Furie & Furie, 2008) (see Figure 8-1). Patients with cancer have an increased risk of VTE in the first few months after diagnosis and when distant metastases are present. Multiple risk factors predispose patients to the development of VTE (see Figure 8-2). The types of cancers with higher risk are cancers of the pancreas, stomach, brain, kidney, uterus, lung, and ovary (Wun & White, 2009). Those with hematologic malignancies, lymphoma and myeloma, have the highest rate (Khorana et al., 2007). The risk of VTE is increased further among patients with cancer receiving systemic chemotherapy, as listed in Table 8-2. The use of antiangiogenic agents such as bevacizumab can increase the risk of both arterial and venous thrombosis (Lyman & Khorana, 2009).

Signs and Symptoms

Deep Vein Thrombosis

Many cases are completely asymptomatic and are diagnosed after embolization. Physical examination alone is often unreliable for diagnosing DVT; hence, clinical decisions should be based on the patient's signs and symptoms and risk factors, and the diagnosis should be confirmed with imaging studies. The most common signs and symptoms are pain, swelling, increase in temperature, and increase in respiratory and heart rate. Homan sign is an unreliable test for DVT and is only 50% sensitive. Massive edema with cyanosis and ischemia (phlegmasia cerulea dolens) is a rare medical emergency (Tiller, 2007).

Table 8-1. Pathogenesis of Venous Thromboembolism	
Component of Virchow Triad	**Predisposing Factors**
Stasis	Bed rest and immobility, extrinsic compression of vessels by mass
Blood components	Tumors and macrophages produce procoagulants, inflammatory cytokines increase blood viscosity and thrombopoietin, causing spontaneous platelet aggregation.
Vessel damage	Direct tumor invasion, indwelling catheters, chemotherapy, erythropoietin, antiangiogenic agents
Note. Based on information from Lyman & Khorana, 2009; Shannon, 2006.	

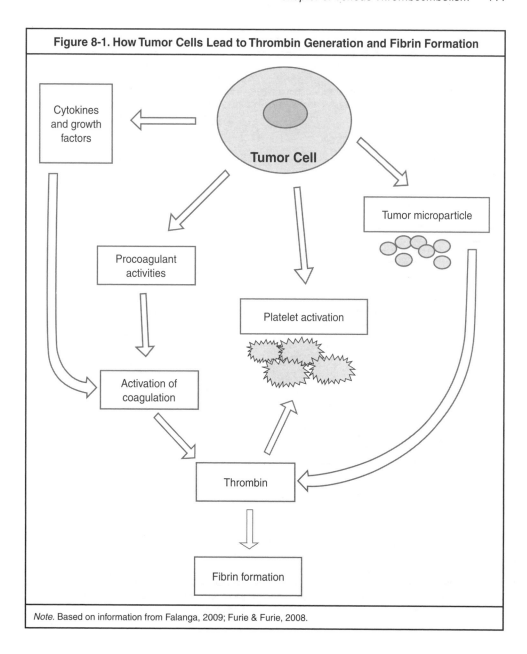

Figure 8-1. How Tumor Cells Lead to Thrombin Generation and Fibrin Formation

Note. Based on information from Falanga, 2009; Furie & Furie, 2008.

Pulmonary Embolism

When unexplained dyspnea in patients with cancer is present, PE should always be considered. Pleuritic chest pain and hemoptysis also are common in patients with PE. Tachypnea and tachycardia are the most common signs, but they are also nonspecific. The most common finding on physical examination is jugular venous distention, pleural friction rub, wheezes or rales, and an accentuated (P2) pulmonic component of the second heart sound (Fedullo, 2008). Figure 8-3 summarizes the signs and symptoms of DVT and PE.

Figure 8-2. Risk Factors for Thromboembolic Events in Patients With Cancer

- Immobilization/paralysis
- Genetic
  - Inherited coagulopathy (factor V Leiden mutation, antithrombin III deficiency)
  - Polymorphism causing risk for thrombosis
- Surgery
- Trauma
- Heart failure
- Estrogen therapy
- Prior history of thrombosis
- Indwelling catheters, cardiovascular access catheters
- Permanent pacemakers, automatic implantable cardioverter defibrillator

- Chemotherapy or other agents
  - Tamoxifen
  - Thalidomide
  - Bevacizumab
  - Cyclooxygenase-2 inhibitor (rofecoxib)
- Mechanical effects of cancer (i.e., compression tumors)
- Erythropoiesis-stimulating agents: epoetin alfa, darbepoetin alfa
- Obesity

Note. Based on information from Streiff, 2011; Yeh et al., 2008.

Table 8-2. Oncologic Agents That Cause Venous Thromboembolism

Drug	Incidence
Alkylating agent: Cisplatin	8.5%
Angiogenesis inhibitors[a]	
• Thalidomide	1%–58%
• Lenalidomide	3%–75%
Histone deacetylase inhibitor: Vorinostat	4.7%–8%
Small-molecule tyrosine kinase inhibitor (TKI): Erlotinib	2.9%–11%
Monoclonal antibody-based TKI: Bevacizumab	8.5%
Selective estrogen receptor modulator: Tamoxifen	6.8%
Antimetabolite: 5-fluorouracil	4%–16%

[a] The incidence of venous thromboembolism for angiogenesis inhibitors reported in the literature varies considerably depending on the patient's disease status, concomitant use of high- or low-dose steroids, erythropoietin, or other chemotherapeutic agents and whether or not proper thromboprophylaxis was employed during the study period.

Note. Based on information from Fadol & Lech, 2011; Falanga & Zacharski, 2005; Orlando et al., 2000.

Differential Diagnosis

The variability of presentation for PE sets up the clinician for potentially missing the correct diagnosis. The typical "classic" presentation of PE, which includes sudden onset of pleuritic chest pain, shortness of breath, and hypoxia, is rarely seen. Forty percent of patients had been seen by a physician in weeks prior to their demise. Some patients complained of nagging symptoms for weeks before dying. Multiple conditions have presenting symptoms similar to PE and DVT and should be ruled out in the differential diagnoses listed in Figure 8-4. These patients should have a working diagnosis confirmed before ruling out PE and discontinuing the workup (Kline & Runyon, 2006).

Figure 8-3. Signs and Symptoms of Pulmonary Embolism and Deep Vein Thrombosis

Pulmonary Embolism
- Sudden onset of shortness of breath
- Dyspnea
- Pleuritic chest pain
- Tachypnea
- Hemoptysis
- Tachycardia
- Syncope (massive pulmonary embolism)
- Hypotension
- Sudden cardiac death
- Cyanosis
- Pleural rub
- Jugular venous distention
- Increased P_2 sound
- S_3 gallop

Deep Vein Thrombosis (depending on location)
- Pain
- Unilateral or bilateral swelling in arm or leg (hallmark of venous thromboembolism)
- Erythema
- Bluish discoloration
- Pallor
- Pulselessness
- Positive Homan sign (leg pain on dorsal flexion of foot)

Note. Based on information from Barreiro, 2007; Tiller, 2007.

Figure 8-4. Differential Diagnoses

Pulmonary Embolism
- Pneumonia
- Bronchitis
- Myocardial infarction
- Congestive heart failure
- Viral pleuritis
- Asthma
- Chronic obstructive pulmonary disease exacerbation
- Pulmonary edema
- Aortic dissection
- Rib fracture(s)
- Pneumothorax
- Musculoskeletal chest wall pain
- Pericarditis
- Anxiety states
- Costochondritis

Deep Vein Thrombosis
- Cellulitis
- Lymphedema
- Extrinsic compression of vein by tumor or enlarged lymph nodes
- Pulled, strained, or torn muscle
- Compartment syndrome
- Localized allergic reaction
- Filariasis

Note. Based on information from Barreiro, 2007; Fedullo, 2008; Tiller, 2007.

Diagnostic Tests

Laboratory Examinations

D-dimer helps to rule out the presence of a thrombus, DVT, PE, stroke, and disseminated intravascular coagulation (DIC). D-dimers are small protein particles not normally present in the blood, except when the coagulation system has been activated (Fischbach, 2009). Normal D-dimer values are less than or equal to 250 ng/ml D-dimer units (DDU) or less than or equal to 0.50 mcg/ml fibrinogen equivalent units (FEU). Within the reportable normal range (110–250 ng/mL DDU; 0.22–0.50 mcg/ml FEU), measured values may reflect the activation state of the procoagulant and fibrinolytic systems, but the clinical utility of such quantitation is not established (Mayo Clinic Mayo Medical Laboratories, n.d.). The sensitivity and negative predictive value of D-dimer assays are high, and their specificity is low (Wells, Owen, Doucette, Ferguson, & Tran, 2006). Other factors causing elevated levels of D-dimer include recent surgery, trauma, infection, heart disease, cancer, and liver diseases. Conditions that can cause false-positive results include rheumatoid arthritis, increased triglycerides, hyperlipidemia, and hemolysis. The likelihood of finding a normal D-dimer level in a patient with cancer is less than 30%, which significantly decreases the utility of this examination in a cancer setting (ten Wolde, Kraaijenhagen, Prins, & Büller, 2002) (see Figure 8-5).

Imaging Studies

Imaging studies used to diagnose thromboembolism include pulmonary angiography, ventilation/perfusion (V/Q) scan, computed tomography (CT), magnetic resonance imaging (MRI), and electrocardiogram (ECG). The choice of diagnostic modality is determined for each clinical situation.

Pulmonary angiography: The current gold standard of diagnosing PE is pulmonary angiography; however, it is rarely used as a first-line diagnostic tool because it is more invasive than either the V/Q scan or helical CT. It involves injecting contrast media into the main pulmonary artery and looking for intraluminal filling defects of arterial branches (Fedullo, 2008).

V/Q scan: V/Q scan is a medical imaging technique using scintigraphy and medical isotopes to evaluate the circulation of air and blood in the lungs. A defect in the perfusion image requires a mismatched ventilation defect to be indicative of PE. This usually is ordered when radio contrast media cannot be used because of renal failure (Linkins & Kearon, 2009).

CT scan: CT scans produce x-rays similar to those used in conventional radiography, but they are taken with a special scanning system. A computer provides rapid, complex calculations that determine the extent to which tissues absorb multiple x-ray beams. This is unique because it produces cross-sectional images (i.e., "slices") of anatomic structures without superimposing tissues on each other. The helical (spiral) scan is the initial imaging study of choice for patients suspected of having PE because of its high sensitivity (53%–100%) and spec-

---

Figure 8-5. Laboratory Examinations

Pulmonary Embolism	Deep Vein Thrombosis
• D-dimer > 500 ng/ml • Arterial blood gases: normal or decreased PO_2, decreased PCO_2	• D-dimer (sensitive but not specific) • Baseline laboratory tests: complete blood count, platelet count, activated partial thromboplastin time, prothrombin time/international normalized ratio • Factor V Leiden, factor VIII level, serum homocysteine, lupus anticoagulant • Protein C and S antigen levels, antithrombin activity, anticardiolipin antibodies

Note. Based on information from Barreiro, 2007; Tiller, 2007.

ificity (67%–100%). It has superseded the V/Q scan in many institutions and is only reserved to patients with contraindications for IV contrast media (Fischbach, 2009).

MRI: MRI is a diagnostic modality that employs a superconducting magnet and radiofrequency signals to cause hydrogen nuclei to emit their own signals. The computer uses this signal to construct detailed, sectional images of the body (Fischbach, 2009). Although MRI produces high tissue contrast without ionizing radiation, this technique is less popular than CT because of technical limitations, higher costs, limited availability, and other logistical considerations (Kanne & Lalani, 2004) (see Figures 8-6, 8-7, and 8-8).

ECG: The most common ECG finding in PE is sinus tachycardia. Other tachydysrhythmias (usually atrial) are rarely seen and usually denote a large PE (Ferrari et al., 2007). The typical ECG changes known as the $S_1Q_3T_3$ pattern described by McGinn and White in 1935 show the classic triad of a tall S wave in lead I, Q wave in lead III, and a T-wave inversion in lead III. This pattern is considered pathognomonic of PE and is present in 10%–50% of patients (Ferrari et al., 2007) (see Figure 8-9). The other ECG changes that are seen are usually due to right-sided heart dilation. These include T-wave changes on V_2-V_3 (massive PE), ST segment abnormalities, incomplete or complete right bundle branch block, and right axis deviation in the limb leads (Fedullo, 2008).

Figure 8-6. Imaging Studies

Pulmonary Embolism (PE)

- Computed tomography (CT) angiogram (spiral CT)—becoming test of choice (see Figure 8-7)
- Pulmonary angiogram—gold standard, intraluminal filling defects and/or arterial cutoffs
- Echocardiogram—may reveal a thrombus in the right ventricle (RV) or pulmonary outflow tract, septal flattening with paradoxical septal motion or dilated RV (see Figure 8-8)
- Ultrasound of the lower and upper extremities
- Gadolinium-enhanced magnetic resonance angiography
- Ventilation/perfusion (V/Q) (showing multiple segmental or lobar perfusion defects with normal ventilation)
  - Normal V/Q = no PE
  - Intermediate probability = need another test
  - High probability = positive PE
- Chest x-ray—nonspecific
  - Enlargement of the pulmonary artery with focal oligemia distal to the PE (Westermark sign)
  - Parenchymal infiltrates
  - Atelectasis
  - Can be used to exclude other pathology

Deep Vein Thrombosis (DVT)

- Duplex ultrasonography—preferred diagnostic modality for symptomatic proximal DVT
  - Noninvasive, highly sensitive (90%) for popliteal and femoral thrombi
  - Does not identify in pelvic vein or vena cava
- Contrast venography
  - Gold standard, but should not be initial screening tool
  - Costly and invasive. May cause superficial phlebitis or hypersensitivity reactions, but generally safe and accurate.
  - Disadvantages include discomfort and technical difficulty.
- Impedance plethysmography
  - Accurate as duplex ultrasound
  - Less operator dependency, but poor at detecting calf thrombi
  - Rarely used due to availability of duplex ultrasound
- Magnetic resonance imaging
  - As accurate as contrast venography
  - Accurate, noninvasive alternative to venography especially for patient with contraindication for contrast material
  - Excellent resolution of inferior vena cava and pelvic vein

Note. Based on information from Barreiro, 2007; Fedullo, 2008; Meaney et al., 1997; Shannon, 2006; Tapson, 1997.

Figure 8-7. Spiral Computed Tomography Showing Saddle Pulmonary Embolism

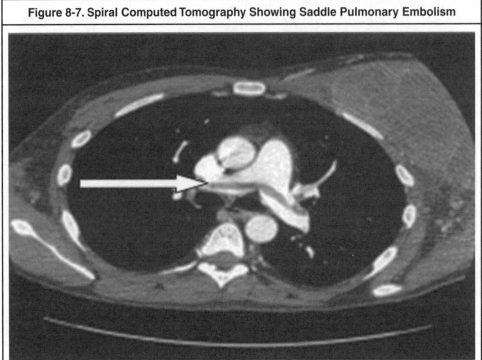

Figure 8-8. Transthoracic Echocardiogram Showing Right Ventricular Thrombus in Transit

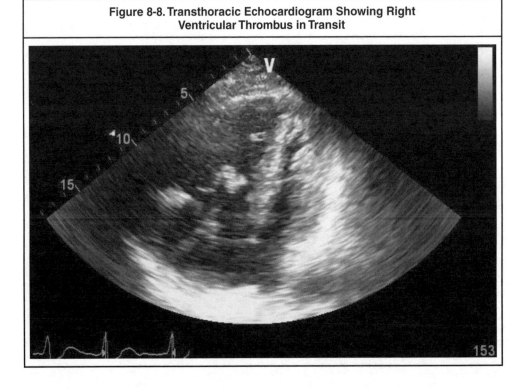

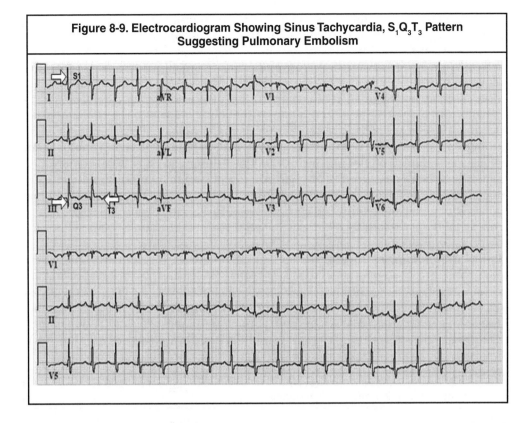

Figure 8-9. Electrocardiogram Showing Sinus Tachycardia, $S_1Q_3T_3$ Pattern Suggesting Pulmonary Embolism

Treatment

The mainstay in the management of acute massive PE is the stabilization of cardio-vascular hemodynamics and attempting to prevent secondary complications related to the clot. Hemodynamically unstable patients should be monitored closely, preferably in the intensive care unit (ICU) setting. Judicious fluid resuscitation can improve cardiac output and systemic hypotension.

Inotropic Agents

Drugs such as dobutamine (starting at 0.5–2.0 mcg/kg/min) are favored because of their inotropic and vasodilatory properties. The beneficial effect is usually attained around 15–20 mcg/kg/min. Norepinephrine with its alpha- and beta-adrenergic properties can improve blood pressure, cardiac output, and peripheral vascular resistance. It is administered in a continuous infusion (2–4 mcg/min) and titrated to achieve hemodynamic stability (Shannon, 2006).

Thrombolytics

These agents are used to dissolve clots or induce thrombolysis. In the absence of contraindications, thrombolytics such as urokinase, streptokinase, and tissue plasminogen activators (TPAs) usually are the established therapy for hemodynamically unstable patients with massive PE, phlegmasia cerulea dolens, and upper extremity DVT in patients with a central venous catheter that must be kept patent. Urokinase and streptokinase are rarely used because of the risk of anaphylactic reaction. TPA is a serine protease, the major enzyme that catalyzes the conversion of plasminogen to plasmin, resulting in clot breakdown (Rivera-Bou, Cabañas, & Villanueva, 2012). At the time of this writing, no large clinical trial existed that demonstrated increased survival in patients with massive PE who were given thrombolytics versus conventional heparin therapy. The efficacy of these thrombolytic agents is almost the same, although TPA infused at a shorter time with a loading dose of 10 mg followed by an IV infusion of 90 mg in two hours, or 100 mg over two hours without a loading dose, achieves the same results compared to a 12–24-hour infusion of streptokinase or urokinase. During the infusion of TPA or soon after discontinuation, heparin treatment should be initiated (Goldhaber, 2009). These drugs can be given directly into selected pulmonary arteries or systemically.

Initial Anticoagulant Therapy

Anticoagulants are agents that prevent the formation of clots. Several factors exist in selecting the initial anticoagulant, whether it is unfractionated heparin (UFH), low-molecular-weight heparin (LMWH), or fondaparinux (see Table 8-3). The National Com-

Table 8-3. Recommended Anticoagulants for the Initial Treatment of Venous Thromboembolism in Patients With Cancer	
Drug	**Dosage**
Dalteparin[a]	200 IU/kg SC q 24 hrs or 100 units/kg SC q 12 hrs (maximum single dose: 18,000 IU)
Enoxaparin[b]	1 mg/kg SC q 12 h or 1.5 mg/kg SC q 24 hrs (start warfarin on day 1 of enoxaparin treatment per ACCP guidelines)
Tinzaparin[a]	175 IU/kg SC q 24 hrs for at least 6 days and until adequately anticoagulated with warfarin (INR of at least 2 for 2 consecutive days)
Fondaparinux[c]	Weight < 50 kg = 5 mg SC q 24 hrs Weight 50–100 kg = 7.5 mg SC q 24 hrs Weight > 100 kg = 10 mg SC q 24 hrs
Unfractionated heparin	Weight-based dosing: 80 IU/kg bolus followed by 18 IU/kg/hr continuous infusion adjusted to therapeutic aPTT[d]

ACCP—American College of Chest Physicians; aPTT—activated partial thromboplastin time; INR—international normalized ratio; SC—subcutaneous

[a] U.S. Food and Drug Administration (FDA)-approved severe renal insufficiency dosage guidelines are not available for dalteparin or tinzaparin.

[b] The FDA-approved enoxaparin regimen for patients with severe renal insufficiency (creatinine clearance < 30 ml/min) is 1 mg/kg q 24 hrs. *Note:* There is limited information on the use of this dose regimen in patients requiring renal replacement therapy.

[c] Fondaparinux should not be used in patients with severe renal insufficiency (creatinine clearance < 30 ml/min).

[d] aPTT therapeutic range should be based upon heparin levels measured by chromogenic factor Xa inhibition or protamine titration, not an arbitrarily selected aPTT control range of 1.5–2.5

Note. Based on information from Clinical Pharmacology, 2010; Geerts et al., 2008; Streiff, 2011.

prehensive Cancer Network (NCCN) VTE guidelines recommend that all of these anti-coagulants can be used in patients with cancer depending on renal function, financial status, inpatient versus outpatient treatment, laboratory monitoring, ease of administration, and reversibility (Wagman et al., 2008).

Unfractionated Heparin

UFH is a naturally occurring anticoagulant produced by basophils and mast cells. It binds to antithrombin III, causing the inactivation of thrombin and clotting factors, most notably factor Xa. The advantages of UFH are its short half-life of 1.5 hours, making it preferable for patients at high risk for bleeding and in need of invasive procedures; its nonrenal clearance, making it a good choice for patients with renal impairment; its low cost; and that it is completely reversible by protamine sulfate at a dose of 1–1.5 mg per 100 units of heparin. Disadvantages include a higher risk for heparin-induced thrombocytopenia (HIT), the need for close laboratory monitoring, and significant intra- and interindividual dose variability (Clinical Pharmacology, 2010).

Low-Molecular-Weight Heparin

LMWH consists of heparin salts having an average molecular weight of less than 8,000 Da (Dalton) compared to UFH, which has an average molecular weight of 12,000 Da. Unlike heparin, where partial thromboplastin time or activated clotting time can be measured, LMWH is monitored by anti–factor Xa assay measuring its activity. LMWH has a more predictable pharmacologic profile and is dosed on weight without close laboratory monitoring, making therapy simpler and allowing for outpatient treatment; therefore, it is a more popular option. It also is associated with a lower risk of HIT. Disadvantages include partial reversibility with protamine (60%–80%), longer half-life averaging 3.5–7 hours, and, because it is renally cleared, a reduced dose is given to patients with renal insufficiency (Clinical Pharmacology, 2010).

Fondaparinux

Fondaparinux is a factor Xa inhibitor with the same advantages as LMWH: weight-based dosing, longer half-life (17–21 hours), rare incidence of HIT, and use with patients who have a history of HIT. Because it is primarily cleared renally, it cannot be given if the patient's creatinine clearance is less than 30 ml/min. It is also protamine irreversible (Clinical Pharmacology, 2010).

A meta-analysis of randomized controlled trials (RCTs) including patients with cancer found that LMWH was associated with lower mortality than UFH (RR = 0.71; 95% CI [0.52, 0.98]) and equivalent frequency of recurrent VTE (RR = 0.78; 95% CI [0.29, 2.08]) (Akl, Rohilla, et al., 2008). Equivalent mortality was also seen in studies comparing UFH and fondaparinux (Büller et al., 2003).

Chronic Anticoagulant Therapy

LMWH and vitamin K antagonists (VKAs), such as warfarin, are the principal chronic anticoagulants in VTE in patients with cancer, although fondaparinux has been used in some patients (Shetty et al., 2007) (see Table 8-4).

Table 8-4. Recommended Anticoagulants for the Chronic Treatment of Venous Thromboembolism in Patients With Cancer	
Drug	**Dosage**
Dalteparin	200 IU/kg SC q 24 h for the first month followed by 150 units/kg SC q 24 hrs (max single dose of 18,000 IU)
Enoxaparin	1.5 mg/kg SC q 24 hrs or 1 mg/kg SC q 12 hrs or at least 3–6 months or until cancer is resolved
Tinzaparin	175 IU/kg SC q 24 hrs or at least 3–6 months or until cancer is resolved
Warfarin	Start with 2.5–5 mg daily and adjust to INR of 2–3. Continue parenteral anticoagulation (e.g., UFH, LMWH, fondaparinux) for at least 5–7 days until INR is 2 or more before warfarin monotherapy. Treat for ≥ 12 months.

INR—international normalized ratio; LMWH—low-molecular-weight heparin; SC—subcutaneous; UFH—unfractionated heparin

Note. Based on information from Clinical Pharmacology, 2010; Streiff, 2011.

Low-Molecular-Weight Heparin

Several RCTs compared LMWH and VKAs, including the largest and most definitive study of anticoagulation in patients with cancer, the CLOT trial (Comparison of LMWH vs. Oral Anticoagulation Therapy for the Prevention of Recurrent VTE in Patients With Cancer), which compared dalteparin and VKAs for six months. Dalteparin showed a 50% reduction in VTE recurrence and an equivalent risk of major bleeding compared with VKAs (Lee et al., 2003). The superiority of LMWH was confirmed by a recent meta-analysis of RCTs comparing LMWH and VKAs for long-term treatment of VTE (Akl, Barba, et al., 2008). This prompted NCCN and other guideline committees such as American Society of Clinical Oncology and American College of Chest Physicians to recommend LMWH as the first-line drug for long-term therapy in patients with cancer (Wagman et al., 2008).

Warfarin

Warfarin is an anticoagulant that acts by inhibiting vitamin K–dependent coagulation factors. Choosing the right dose of warfarin is very important, as most patients with cancer are older, use several medications, and have poor nutritional intake and impaired organ function. Warfarin is initially started at a dose of 2.5–5 mg PO daily to maintain an international normalized ratio (INR) of 2–3 and after an overlap of at least five days of parenteral anticoagulation to avoid recurrent episodes of VTE. Maintaining a therapeutic INR in patients with cancer is a challenge, and failure to attain the therapeutic level results in frequent visits to the clinic or the emergency room while adding discomfort to the patient and support system (Kearon et al., 2008). The duration of anticoagulation therapy is generally at least three months or as long as the cancer is active or under treatment, provided that no contraindication occurs (Streiff, 2010).

New Oral Anticoagulants

Rivaroxaban: Recently, the U.S. Food and Drug Administration approved rivaroxaban, a direct factor Xa inhibitor, for the prophylaxis of DVT, which may lead to PE in adults undergoing hip and knee surgery. It also is used for nonvalvular atrial fibrillation. The EINSTEIN-DVT (Oral Rivaroxaban Versus Standard Therapy in the Initial Treatment of Symptomatic DVT and Long-Term Prevention of Recurrent VTE) evaluation study found that rivaroxaban can be a single-drug approach to short-term and continued treatment of venous thrombosis without laboratory monitoring and also can improve the risk-benefit profile of anticoagulation. It was found to be of comparable efficacy compared with enoxaparin followed by VKA in patients with acute, symptomatic DVT (Bauersachs et al., 2010). The dose for hip replacement is 10 mg PO every day for 35 days starting 6–10 hours postoperatively once hemostasis is established. The dose for knee replacement is 10 mg PO for 12 days starting 6–10 hours postoperatively once hemostasis is established. For patients with nonvalvular atrial fibrillation and creatinine clearance greater than 50 ml/min, the dose is 20 mg PO daily with evening meals. Those with creatinine clearance of 15–50 ml/min will be given a dose of 15 mg daily, also with the evening meal.

Apixaban: Another factor Xa inhibitor that has been approved in Europe and soon in the United States, apixaban, at a dose of 2.5 mg twice daily for 35 days showed superiority compared to enoxaparin at a dose of 40 mg subcutaneously daily for VTE prophylaxis following hip surgery (Lassen et al., 2010).

Dabigatran etexilate: Dabigatran etexilate is a direct thrombin inhibitor used to reduce the risk of stroke and systemic embolism in nonvalvular atrial fibrillation. The dose is usually 150 mg PO twice daily, but for patients with renal impairment with a creatinine clearance of 15–20 ml/min, the dose is 75 mg PO twice daily. Prior to invasive and surgical procedures, the drug is discontinued one to two days if creatinine clearance is 50 ml/min or greater or three to five days if the creatinine clearance is 50 ml/min or less. Longer times should be considered for major surgery, spinal puncture, or placement of a spinal or epidural catheter or port. This should be restarted as soon as possible after the procedure (Boehringer Ingelheim Pharmaceuticals, Inc., 2012) (see Table 8-5).

Table 8-5. New Oral Anticoagulants		
Drug	**Indications**	**Dosage**
Dabigatran etexilate (Pradaxa®)	Reduces the risk of stroke and systemic embolism in nonvalvular atrial fibrillation	Creatinine clearance (CrCl) > 30 ml/min; 150 mg PO BID with or without food CrCl 15–30 ml/min; 75 mg PO BID with or without food
Rivaroxiban (Xarelto®)	Reduces the risk of stroke and systemic embolism in nonvalvular atrial fibrillation	CrCl > 50 ml/min 20 mg PO daily with evening meals CrCl 15–50 ml/min 15 mg PO daily with evening meals
	Deep vein thrombosis prophylaxis • Hip replacement • Knee replacement	10 mg PO daily with or without food Duration is 35 days for hip replacement, 12 days for knee replacement. The initial dose should be given at least 6–10 hours after surgery once hemostasis has been established.

Note. Based on information from Clinical Pharmacology, 2010.

Management of Venous Thromboembolism Recurrence in Patients With Cancer

The recurrence of VTE in patients with cancer is approximately 20.7% compared to 6.8% in patients with a noncancer diagnosis (Prandoni et al., 2002). Female patients, patients with lung cancer, and patients with prior episodes of VTE are at higher risk for recurrent thromboembolism, whereas patients with breast cancer and stage I disease are at lower risk (Louzada et al., 2012). Causes of recurrent VTE include subtherapeutic anticoagulation, intrinsic compression/venous stasis by tumor, nodal mass, Trousseau syndrome, HIT, and rarely, antiphospholipid syndrome (see Table 8-6). Subtherapeutic anticoagulation is not uncommon among patients with cancer on VKAs. The different factors that cause subtherapeutic anticoagulation include chemotherapy-induced thrombocytopenia and nausea and vomiting, resulting in withholding the anticoagulants and invasive procedures that require discontinuation of therapy. Management includes increasing the target INR to 2.5–3.5, although there are no data to support this practice. Using parenteral anticoagulation with LMWH showed a low recurrence rate in VTE (Luk, Wells, Anderson, & Kovacs, 2001). An empiric dose escalation of 25% of LMWH has also proved to be a useful strategy (Carrier et al., 2009).

Trousseau syndrome is a hypercoagulable disorder in patients with cancer characterized by warfarin resistance, recurrent superficial thrombophlebitis, arterial thrombosis and/or VTE, disseminated intravascular coagulation, and nonbacterial thrombotic endocarditis. This is usually controlled with UFH or LMWH (Varki, 2007).

HIT is usually seen in patients who have recently received UFH or LMWH and presents with recurrent VTE in the presence of thrombocytopenia. Heparin should be eliminated, and a direct thrombin inhibitor, such as argatroban or lepirudin, should be used (see Table 8-6).

Table 8-6. Recommended Management for Recurrent Venous Thromboembolism in Patients With Cancer

Clinical Scenario	Management
Subtherapeutic anticoagulation	If on VKA, transition to therapeutic INR with parenteral agent, consider higher INR target (2.3–3.5).
Therapeutic anticoagulation	If on VKA, switch to LMWH or fondaparinux; if on parenteral agent, consider dose escalation or alternative parenteral agent.
Anatomic vascular compression (nodal, tumor masses, etc.)	Reduce/relieve vascular compression; reinstitute anticoagulation.
Trousseau syndrome	Switch to UFH or LMWH.
Heparin-induced thrombocytopenia	Eliminate heparin; start direct thrombin inhibitor (argatroban, lepirudin, bivalirudin) and selective factor Xa inhibitor fondaparinux.
Antiphospholipid syndrome	Increase INR target or switch to alternative anticoagulant (e.g., LMWH).

INR—international normalized ratio; LMWH—low-molecular-weight heparin; UFH—unfractionated heparin; VKA—vitamin K antagonist

Note. Based on information from Streiff, 2011; Warkentin et al., 2008.

Pulmonary Embolectomy

This is a thoracic surgical procedure that involves the removal of thrombus from the pulmonary artery. Pulmonary embolectomy is a life-saving procedure in patients with massive PE and persistent hypotension despite a mortality rate of approximately 30% (Barreiro, 2007). A good alternative to this is thrombolytic therapy if not contraindicated.

Inferior Vena Cava Filter

The inferior vena cava (IVC) filter is a vascular filter that vascular surgeons or interventional radiologists place in the IVC to prevent PE. Vena cava interruption using IVC filters is indicated in patients with permanent contraindication for anticoagulation, failed anticoagulation, massive PE, severe cardiopulmonary disease with DVT, or free-floating iliofemoral or IVC thrombus to prevent lower extremity thrombi from embolizing to the lungs (Zalpour, Hanzelka, Patlan, Rozner, & Yusuf, 2011). An RCT on permanent IVC filters showed that they were associated with reduced risk of PE but increased risk of DVT and no overall effect on mortality (PREPIC Study Group, 2005). Therefore, in cases where anticoagulation is only temporarily not feasible, retrievable filters should be used (Coleman & MacCallum, 2010).

Preventive Measures

Patients with cancer are essentially at high risk for VTE, so pharmacologic and mechanical prophylaxis should be a mainstay in their management (see Table 8-7). In a

---

Table 8-7. Chemical and Mechanical Venous Thromboembolism Prophylaxis in Patients With Cancer

Agent	Dosage	Duration
Unfractionated heparin	5,000 units SC q 8 hrs or 7,500 units SC q 12 hrs	10–14 days or duration of hospitalization, whichever is longer[a]
Dalteparin	5,000 units SC q 24 hrs	10–14 days or duration of hospitalization, whichever is longer[a]
Enoxaparin	40 mg SC q 24 hrs or 30 mg SC q 12 hrs	10–14 days or duration of hospitalization, whichever is longer[a]
Tinzaparin	4,500 units (or 75 units/kg) SC q 24 hrs	10–14 days or duration of hospitalization, whichever is longer[a]
Fondaparinux	2.5 mg SC q 24 hrs if weight is > 50 kg	10–14 days or duration of hospitalization, whichever is longer[a]
Sequential (pneumatic) compression devices ± graduated compression stockings[b]	Continuous use unless ambulating	Duration of hospitalization

[a] Extended outpatient VTE prophylaxis should be considered for high-risk cancer surgery patients (up to 4 weeks) or patients receiving thalidomide- or lenalidomide-based combination chemotherapy.

[b] Only use as sole prophylaxis modality when contraindications to pharmacologic prophylaxis present.

Note. Based on information from Clinical Pharmacology, 2010; Streiff, 2011.

multinational survey (Impact of Managed Pharmaceutical Care on Resource Utilization and Outcomes in the Veterans Affairs Medical Centers [IMPROVE]), only 45% of patients with cancer were given VTE prophylaxis compared to 77% of ICU patients. Results of the study suggested suboptimal physician practices in providing VTE prophylaxis to acutely ill hospitalized medical patients and the need for improved implementation of existing evidence-based guidelines in hospitals (Tapson et al., 2007).

Pharmacologic Prophylaxis

Bleeding is a main concern of the surgical oncologist when patients are on pharmacologic VTE prophylaxis prior to surgery. However, in a prospective observational study of 2,373 surgical patients followed for about one month, only 7% died of hemorrhagic complications, while 45% died of VTE (Agnelli et al., 2006). This confirmed that in surgical oncology patients, thromboembolism is a greater risk than bleeding. Multiple studies—MEDENOX (Medical Patients with Enoxaparin), PREVENT (Prevention of Recurrent Venous Thromboembolism), and ARTEMIS (ARixtra for Thromboembolism Prevention in Medical Indications Study)—have shown that LMWH, UFH, and fondaparinux are all effective in medical and surgical patients (Leizorovicz & Mismetti, 2004).

NCCN guidelines recommend that all patients with cancer receive pharmacologic VTE prophylaxis in the absence of contraindications and that mechanical prophylaxis alone should be used until contraindications are no longer present (see Figure 8-10).

Anticoagulants should be administered up to four weeks for patients following cancer surgery (Streiff, 2010). Thrombocytopenia does not preclude the use of mechanical prophylaxis. Studies have shown, particularly in hematopoietic stem cell transplant recipients, that VTE occurred in 34% of patients with a platelet count of less than 50,000 and in 13% of patients with a platelet count less than 20,000; 14% of PE and 12.5% of all lower extremity DVT occurred in patients with platelet counts of less than 20,000 (Gerber et al., 2008).

Mechanical Prophylaxis

Antiembolic stockings, intermittent pneumatic compression devices, and mechanical foot pumps are mechanical ways of preventing DVT.

Figure 8-10. Contraindications to Pharmacologic Thrombophylaxis

- Active bleeding (cerebral, gastrointestinal, genitourinary)
- Neurosurgery within 24–48 hours
- Brain metastases conferring risk of bleeding (renal, choriocarcinoma, melanoma, thyroid cancer)
- Spinal procedure and/or epidural placement
- Major abdominal surgery within 48 hours
- Severe hypertension (systolic blood pressure > 200 mm Hg, diastolic blood pressure > 120 mm Hg)
- Endocarditis, pericarditis
- Preexisting coagulopathy
- Thrombocytopenia (primary team to evaluate)
- Hypersensitivity to heparin or heparin-induced thrombocytopenia
- Patient on active protocol that prohibits use of anticoagulation

Note. Based on information from Lyman et al., 2007; Streiff et al., 2011.

Antiembolic Stockings

Antiembolic stockings are graduated compression stockings (high pressure at the ankle and low pressure at the knee or thigh) that increase venous flow velocity and prevent venous stasis. Antiembolic stockings that exert a graduated pressure range of 18 mm Hg at the ankle, 14 mm Hg at the mid-calf, and 8 mm Hg at the upper thigh achieve maximum femoral venous blood flow velocity of 138.4% of baseline and thus increase venous return. Used alone, they reduce the incidence of DVT by more than 60%, and when used in conjunction with other mechanical and pharmacologic methods of prophylaxis, they reduce the incidence up to 85% (Autar, 2009). Based on the available evidence favoring the use of thigh-length antiembolic stockings, the National Institute for Health and Clinical Excellence (2007) recommends that all patients having surgery should be offered thigh-length antiembolic stockings upon admission unless contraindicated.

Intermittent Pneumatic Compression

Sequential compression devices (SCDs) deliver pressure in a sequential fashion up the legs, producing a wave-like milking effect to evacuate the leg veins. The compression is set to cycle regularly, for example, every 60 seconds. They are available for the feet (Auguste, Quiñones-Hinojosa, & Berger, 2004). Like the SCDs, intermittent pneumatic compression includes an inflatable compression sleeve and a characteristic pressure modulation to reduce the risk of DVT. In a study comparing two intermittent pneumatic compression systems, the SCD showed hemodynamic superiority compared to a rapid flow device (Kakkos, Nicolaides, Griffin, & Geroulakos, 2005).

Mechanical Foot Pumps

Unlike the SCD, which compresses the ankle, calves, and thigh, the mechanical foot pump uses a foot sleeve with rigid base that fills with air and then deflates. The pressure from the inflated balloon activates the plantar venous plexus, which in turn sends blood back to the heart. The major advantage is that it only requires access to the foot (Roger, Cipolle, Velmahos, & Rozycki, 2002).

Recent analysis of studies of all three mechanical methods of thrombophylaxis indicated that when used alone (i.e., without pharmacologic measures), mechanical thrombophylaxis reduces the frequency of DVT by 66% and PE by 31% (Lyman et al., 2007). They could be used alone in cases where contraindication to pharmacologic prophylaxis is present or used in combination with pharmacologic prophylaxis in high-risk patients. These methods of mechanical VTE prophylaxis usually are attractive to clinicians because they are not associated with bleeding risk, but they also have harmful consequences such as skin irritation and breakdown.

It is important to carefully assess patients prior to initiating mechanical VTE prophylaxis, particularly antiembolic stockings, as they are contraindicated in some patients (see Figure 8-11). Careful selection of appropriate size of the stockings/device, proper application, and patient compliance should be considered (Geerts et al., 2008).

Nursing Implications

Prevention of VTE should be a major nursing priority. Constant monitoring is paramount given that 50% of the patients with VTE and 90% with lower-extremity DVT

Figure 8-11. Contraindications to Antiembolic Stockings

- Arterial insufficiency (peripheral arterial disease including symptoms of claudication and lower-extremity pain with elevation)
- Absent peripheral pulse
- Cellulitis
- Allergy to material
- Any vascular intervention to the lower extremity
- Severe peripheral neuropathy
- Dermatitis, including stasis dermatitis
- Anatomic deformity associated with rheumatoid arthritis
- Loss of skin integrity
- Massive edema of legs or pulmonary edema from congestive heart failure
- Suspected or actual acute deep vein thrombosis
- Lower-extremity ischemia or gangrene
- Vein ligation or saphenous vein harvest within six months
- Skin graft within six months

Note. Based on information from Institute for Clinical Systems Improvement, 2008; National Institute for Health and Clinical Excellence, 2010.

---

are asymptomatic (Crowther & McCourt, 2005). Prophylaxis is the most cost-effective and clinically appropriate measure to avert this problem. Nurses can have a significant impact on VTE prophylaxis by meticulous assessment, identification of risk factors, education of patients regarding ambulation and range-of-motion exercise, and early intervention with pharmacologic and mechanical prophylaxis such as antiembolic stockings and SCDs (Dunn, 2004).

Conclusion

Venous thromboembolism, which includes PE and DVT, is one of the major causes of mortality and morbidity in patients with cancer, and its treatment poses a major challenge. However, early identification, thorough assessment, and prompt implementation of appropriate mechanical or pharmacologic prophylaxis can improve overall patient outcome.

References

Agnelli, G., Bolis, G., Capussotti, L., Scarpa, R.M., Tonelli, F., Bonizzoni, E., … Gussoni, G. (2006). A clinical outcome-based prospective study on venous thromboembolism after cancer surgery: The @RISTOS project. *Annals of Surgery, 243,* 89–95. doi:10.1097/01.sla.0000193959.44677.48

Akl, E.A., Barba, M., Rohilla, S., Terrenato, I., Sperati, F., Muti, P., & Schünemann, H.J. (2008). Low-molecular-weight heparins are superior to vitamin K antagonists for long term treatment of venous thromboembolism in patients with cancer: A Cochrane systematic review. *Journal of Experimental Clinical Cancer Research, 27,* 21. doi:10.1186/1756-9966-27-21

Akl, E.A., Rohilla, S., Barba, M., Sperati, F., Terrenato, I., Muti, P., … Schünemann, H.J. (2008). Anticoagulation for the initial treatment of venous thromboembolism in patients with cancer: A systematic review. *Cancer, 113,* 1685–1694. doi:10.1002/cncr.23814

Autar, R. (2009). A review of the evidence for the efficacy of anti-embolism stockings (AES) in venous thromboembolism prevention. *Journal of Orthopedic Nursing, 13,* 41–49. doi:10.1016/j.joon.2009.01.003

Auguste, K.I., Quiñones-Hinojosa, A., & Berger, M.S. (2004). Efficacy of mechanical prophylaxis for venous thromboembolism in patients with brain tumors. *Neurosurgical Focus, 17*(4), E3. doi:10.3171/foc.2004.17.4.3

Barreiro, T.J. (2007). Pulmonary embolism. In F.J. Domino (Ed.), *The 5-minute clinical consult 2007* (pp. 1030–1031). Philadelphia, PA: Lippincott Williams & Wilkins.

Bauersachs, R., Berkowitz, S.D., Brenner, B., Buller, H.R., Decousus, H., Gallus, A.S., … Schellong, S. (2010). Oral rivaroxaban for symptomatic venous thromboembolism. *New England Journal of Medicine, 363*, 2499–2510. doi:10.1056/NEJMoa1007903

Boehringer Ingelheim Pharmaceuticals, Inc. (2012). *Pradaxa*® (dabigatran) [Prescribing information]. Ridgefield, CT: Author.

Büller, H.R., Davidson, B.L., Decousus, H., Gallus, A., Gent, F., Piovella, M.H., … Lensing, A.W. (2003). Subcutaneous fondaparinux versus intravenous unfractionated heparin in the initial treatment of pulmonary embolism. *New England Journal of Medicine, 349*, 1695–1702. doi:10.1056/NEJMoa035451

Carrier, M.B., Le Gal, G., Cho, R., Tierney, S., Rodger, M., & Lee, A.Y. (2009). Dose escalation of low molecular heparin to manage recurrent venous thromboembolic events despite systemic anticoagulation in cancer patients. *Journal of Thrombosis and Haemostasis, 7*, 760–765. doi:10.1111/j.1538-7836.2009.03326.x

Clinical Pharmacology. (2010). Online database. Retrieved from http://www.clinicalpharmacology-ip.com

Coleman, R., & MacCallum, P. (2010). Treatment and secondary prevention of venous thromboembolism in cancer. *British Journal of Cancer, 102*(Suppl. 11), S17–S23. doi:10.1038/sj.bjc.6605601

Crowther, M., & McCourt, K. (2005). Venous thromboembolism: A guide to prevention and treatment. *Nurse Practitioner, 30*(8), 26–43. doi:10.1097/00006205-200508000-00006

Dunn, D. (2004). Preventing perioperative complications in an older adult. *Nursing, 34*(11), 36–41.

Fadol, A., & Lech, T. (2011). Cardiovascular adverse events associated with cancer therapy. *Journal of the Advanced Practitioner in Oncology, 2*, 229–242.

Falanga, A. (2009). The incidence and risk of venous thromboembolism associated with cancer and nonsurgical cancer treatment. *Cancer Investigation, 27*, 105–115. doi:10.1080/07357900802563028

Falanga, A., & Zacharski, L. (2005). Deep vein thrombosis in cancer: The scale of the problem and approaches to management. *Annals of Oncology, 16*, 696–701. doi:10.1093/annonc/mdi165

Fedullo, P. (2008). Pulmonary embolism. In V. Fuster, R. Walsh, R. O'Rourke, & P. Poole-Wilson (Eds.), *Hurst's the heart* (pp. 1649–1672). New York, NY: McGraw-Hill.

Ferrari, E., Imbert, A., Chevalier, T., Mihoubi, A., Morand, M., & Baudouy, M. (2007). The ECG in pulmonary embolism. Predictive value of negative T waves in precordial leads—80 case reports. *Chest, 111*, 537–543. doi:10.1378/chest.111.3.537

Fischbach, F. (2009). *A manual of laboratory and diagnostic tests* (8th ed.). New York, NY: Lippincott Williams & Wilkins.

Furie, B., & Furie, B.C. (2008). Mechanisms of thrombus formation. *New England Journal of Medicine, 359*, 938–949. doi:10.1056/NEJMra0801082

Geerts, W.H., Bergqvist, D., Pineo, G.F., Heit, J.A., Samama, C.M., Lassen, M.R., & Colwell, C.W. (2008). Prevention of venous thromboembolism: American College of Chest Physicians evidence-based clinical practice guidelines (8th edition). *Chest, 133*(6, Suppl.), 381S–453S. doi:10.1378/chest.08-0656

Gerber, D.E., Segal, J.B., Levy, M.Y., Kane, J., Jones, R.J., & Streiff, M.B. (2008). The incidence of and risk factors for venous thromboembolism (VTE) and bleeding among 1514 patients undergoing hematopoietic stem cell transplantation: Implications for VTE prevention. *Blood, 112*, 504–510. doi:10.1182/blood-2007-10-117051

Goldhaber, S.Z. (2009). Advanced treatment strategies for acute pulmonary embolism, including thrombolysis and embolectomy. *Journal of Thrombosis and Haemostasis, 7*(Suppl. S1), 322–327. doi:10.1111/j.1538-7836.2009.03415.x

Institute for Clinical Systems Improvement (2008, October). *Health care guideline: Venous thromboembolism prophylaxis* (5th ed.). Retrieved from http://www.icsi.org/venous_thromboembolism_prophylaxis/venous_thromboembolism_prophylaxis_4.html

Kakkos, S.K., Nicolaides, A.N., Griffin, M., & Geroulakos, G. (2005). Comparison of two intermittent pneumatic compression systems: A hemodynamic study. *International Angiology, 24*, 330–335.

Kanne, J.P., & Lalani, T.A. (2004). Role of computed tomography and magnetic resonance imaging for DVT and PE. *Circulation, 109*, I-15–I-21. doi:10.1161/01.CIR.0000122871.86662.72

Kearon, C., Kahn, S.R., Agnelli, G., Goldhaber, S., Raskob, G.E., & Comerota, A.J. (2008). Antithrombotic therapy for venous thromboembolic disease: American College of Chest Physicians evidence-based clinical practice guidelines (8th edition). *Chest, 133*(6, Suppl.), 454S–545S.

Khorana, A.A., Francis, C.W., Culakova, E., Kuderer, N.M., & Lyman, G.H. (2007). Frequency, risk factors, and trends for venous thromboembolism among hospitalized cancer patients. *Cancer, 110*, 2339–2346. doi:10.1002/cncr.23062

Kline, J.A., & Runyon, M.S. (2006). Pulmonary embolism and deep venous thrombosis. In J.A. Marx, R.S. Hockberger, & R.M. Walls (Eds.), *Rosen's emergency medicine: Concepts and clinical practice* (6th ed., pp. 1368–1382). Philadelphia, PA: Elsevier Mosby.

Lassen, M.R., Gallus, A., Raskob, G.E., Pineo, G., Chen, D., & Ramirez, L.M. (2010). Apixaban versus enoxaparin for thromboprophylaxis after hip replacement. *New England Journal of Medicine, 363*, 2487–2498. doi:10.1056/NEJMoa1006885

Lee, A.Y.Y., Levine, M.N., Baker, R.I., Bowden, C., Kakkar, A.K., Prins, M., ... Gent, M. (2003). Low-molecular-weight heparin versus a coumarin for the prevention of recurrent venous thromboembolism in patients with cancer. *New England Journal of Medicine, 349*, 146–153. doi:10.1056/NEJMoa025313

Leizorovicz, A., & Mismetti, P. (2004). Preventing venous thromboembolism in medical patients. *Circulation, 110*, 13–19. doi:10.1161/01.CIR.0000150640.98772.af

Linkins, L.-A., & Kearon, C. (2009). Venous thromboembolism In N. Key, M. Makris, D. Shaughnessy, & D. Lillicrap (Eds.), *Practical hemostasis and thrombosis* (2nd ed., pp. 135–146). Hoboken, NJ: Wiley.

Louzada, M.L., Carrier, M., Lazo-Langner, A., Dao, V., Kovacs, M.J., Ramsay, T.O., ...Wells, P.S. (2012). Development of a clinical prediction rule for risk stratification of recurrent venous thromboembolism in patients with cancer: Associated venous thromboembolism. *Circulation.* Advance online publication. doi:10.1161/CIRCULATIONAHA.111.051920

Luk, C., Wells, P.S., Anderson, D., & Kovacs, M.J. (2001). Extended outpatient therapy with low molecular weight heparin for the treatment of recurrent venous thromboembolism despite warfarin therapy. *American Journal of Medicine, 111*, 270–273. doi:10.1016/S0002-9343(01)00840-3

Lyman, G.H., & Khorana, A.A. (2009). Cancer, clots and consensus: New understanding of an old problem. *Journal of Clinical Oncology, 27*, 4821–4826. doi:10.1200/JCO.2009.22.3032

Lyman, G.H., Khorana, A.A., Falanga, A., Clarke-Pearson, D., Flowers, C., Jahanzeb, M., ... Francis, C.W. (2007). American Society of Clinical Oncology guideline: Recommendations for venous thromboembolism prophylaxis and treatment in patients with cancer. *Journal of Clinical Oncology, 25*, 5490–5505. doi:10.1200/JCO.2007.14.1283

Mayo Clinic Mayo Medical Laboratories. (n.d.). Test ID: RIAS 9292 ristocetin inhibitor assay screen, plasma. Retrieved from http://mayomedicallaboratories.com/test-catalog/print/9292

Meaney, J.F., Weg, J.G., Chenevert, T.L., Stafford-Johnson, D., Hamilton, B.H., & Prince M.R. (1997). Diagnosis of pulmonary embolism with magnetic resonance angiography. *New England Journal of Medicine, 336*, 1422–1427. doi:10.1056/NEJM199705153362004

National Institute for Health and Clinical Excellence. (2007). Reducing the risk of deep venous thrombosis and pulmonary embolism in patients undergoing surgery. Retrieved from http://www.guideline.gov/content.aspx?id=24106v

National Institute for Health and Clinical Excellence. (2010). Reducing the risk of venous thromboembolism (deep vein thrombosis and pulmonary embolism) in patients admitted to hospital (CG92). Retrieved from http://guidance.nice.org.uk/CG92

Orlando, L., Colleoni, M., Nolè, F., Biffi, R., Rocca, G., Curigliano, G., ... Goldhirsch, A. (2000). Incidence of venous thromboembolism in breast cancer patients during chemotherapy with vinorelbine, cisplatin, 5-fluorouracil as continuous infusion (ViFuP regimen): Is prophylaxis required? [Letter to the editor]. *Annals of Oncology, 11*, 117–118. doi:10.1023/A:1008364801718

Prandoni, P., Lensing, A.W., Piccioli, A., Bernardi, E., Simoni, P., Girolami, B., ... Girolami, A. (2002). Recurring venous thromboembolism and bleeding complications during anticoagulant treatment in patients with cancer and venous thrombosis. *Blood, 100*, 3484–3488. doi:10.1182/blood-2002-01-0108

PREPIC Study Group. (2005). Eight-year follow-up of patients with permanent vena cava filters in the prevention of pulmonary embolism. *Circulation, 112*, 416–422. doi:10.1161/CIRCULATIONAHA.104.512834

Rivera-Bou, W.L., Cabañas, J.G., & Villanueva, S.E. (2012). Thrombolytic therapy in emergency medicine. Retrieved from http://emedicine.medscape.com/article/811234-overview

Roger, F., Cipolle, M., Velmahos, G., & Rozycki, G. (2002). Practice management guidelines for the prevention of venous thromboembolism in trauma patients: The EAST Practice Management Guidelines Work Group. *Journal of Trauma, 53*, 142–164.

Shannon, V.R. (2006). Heart-lung interactions in the cancer patient. In M.S. Ewer (Ed.), *Cancer and the heart* (pp. 298–324). Hamilton, Ontario, Canada: BC Decker.

Shetty, R., Seddighzadeh, A., Parasuraman, S., Vallurupalli, N.G., Gerhard-Herman, M., & Goldhaber, S.Z. (2007). Once-daily fondaparinux monotherapy without warfarin for long term treatment of venous thromboembolism. *Thrombosis and Haemostasis, 98,* 1384–1386. doi:10.1160/TH07-06-0394

Streiff, M.B. (2010). The National Comprehensive Cancer Network guidelines on the management of venous thromboembolism in cancer patients. *Thrombosis Research, 125,* S128–S133. doi:10.1016/S0049-3848(10)70030-X

Streiff, M.B. (2011). Anticoagulation in the management of venous thromboembolism in the cancer patient. *Journal of Thrombosis and Thrombolysis, 31,* 282–294. doi:10.1007/s11239-011-0562-0

Streiff, M.B., Bockenstedt, P.L., Cataland, S.R., Chesney, C., Eby, C., Fanikos, J., ... Zakarija, A. (2011). Venous thromboembolic disease. *Journal of the National Comprehensive Cancer Network, 9,* 714–777.

Tapson, V.F. (1997). Pulmonary embolism: New diagnostic approaches. *New England Journal of Medicine, 336,* 1449–1451. doi:10.1056/NEJM199705153362010

Tapson, V.F., Decousus, H., Pini, M., Chong, B.H., Froehlich, J.B., Monreal, M., ... Anderson, F.A., Jr. (2007). Venous thromboembolism prophylaxis in acutely ill hospitalized medical patients: Findings from the International Medical Prevention Registry on Venous Thromboembolism. *Chest, 132,* 936–945. doi:10.1378/chest.06-2993

ten Wolde, M., Kraaijenhagen, R.A., Prins, M.H., & Büller, H.R. (2002). The clinical usefulness of D-dimer testing in cancer patients with suspected deep venous thrombosis. *Archives of Internal Medicine, 162,* 1880–1884. doi:10.1001/archinte.162.16.1880

Tiller, R. (2007). Deep vein thrombophlebitis. In F. Domino (Ed.), *The 5-minute clinical consult 2007* (pp. 338–341). Philadelphia, PA: Lippincott Williams & Wilkins.

Varki, A. (2007). Trousseau's syndrome: Multiple definitions and multiple mechanisms. *Blood, 110,* 1723–1729. doi:10.1182/blood-2006-10-053736

Wagman, L.D., Baird, M.F., Bennett, C.L., Bockenstedt, P.L., Cataland, S.R., Fanikos, J., ... Vedantham, S. (2008). Venous thromboembolic disease. NCCN Clinical Practice Guidelines in Oncology. *Journal of the National Comprehensive Cancer Network, 6,* 716–753.

Warkentin, T.E., Geinacher, A., Koster, A., & Lincoff, A.M. (2008). Treatment and prevention of heparin-induced thrombocytopenia: American College of Chest Physicians Evidence-Based Clinical Practice Guidelines (8th edition). *Chest, 133*(6, Suppl.), 340S–380S. doi:10.1378/chest.08-0677

Wells, P.S., Owen, C., Doucette, S., Ferguson, D., & Tran, H. (2006). Does your patient have deep vein thrombosis? *JAMA, 295,* 199–207. doi:10.1001/jama.295.2.199

Wun, T., & White, R.H. (2009). Epidemiology of cancer-related venous thromboembolism. *Best Practice and Research: Clinical Hematology, 22,* 9–23. doi:10.1016/j.beha.2008.12.001

Yeh, E.T., Lenihan, D., & Ewer, M. (2008). Thromboembolism. In V. Fuster, R. Walsh, R. O'Rourke, & P. Poole-Wilson (Eds.), *Hurst's the heart* (pp. 2060–2062). New York, NY: McGraw-Hill.

Zalpour, A., Hanzelka, K., Patlan, J.T., Rozner, M.A., & Yusuf, S.W. (2011). Saddle pulmonary embolism in a cancer patient with thrombocytopenia: A treatment dilemma. *Cardiology Research and Practice, 2011,* Article ID 835750. doi:10.4061/2011/835750

Stem Cell Transplantation and Cardiovascular Adverse Events

Tara Reilly-Donovan, RN, MSN, ACNP-BC

Introduction

Hematopoietic stem cell transplantation (HSCT) is an effective treatment for hematologic malignancies and some nonmalignant diseases. Approximately 15,000–20,000 patients undergo HSCT annually throughout the world (Griffith, Savani, & Boord, 2010). HSCT was initiated from the 1950s through the 1970s. The first patients were identical twins, so the recipient's immune system would believe the stem cells were its own. This is known as human leukocyte antigen (HLA) compatibility. In the late 1960s, non-twin sibling transplants were conducted (Buckner, 1999). Through the 1970s, autologous transplantation began to be performed, and work continued with HLA matching in an attempt to prevent rejection. In the 1980s, the National Marrow Donor Program was established to create a system of finding marrow from donors who were unrelated to the potential recipients (St. Jude Children's Research Hospital, 2011). One of the more serious complications of HSCT is therapy-related cardiovascular disease. This chapter will discuss the adverse cardiovascular effects of HSCT including risk factors, cardiotoxic treatments, management of cardiovascular adverse events, and HSCT in patients with preexisting cardiac conditions.

Diseases Treated With Hematopoietic Stem Cell Transplantation

HSCT is used to treat a number of conditions, both malignant and nonmalignant. This review will focus on malignancies that are treated using HSCT (see Table 9-1). Leukemia is an acute or chronic disease in humans characterized by an abnormal increase in the number of white blood cells in the tissues and often in the blood. Cer-

Table 9-1. Diseases Treated With Hematopoietic Transplantation	
Disease	**Description**
Leukemias	
• Acute leukemia	Condition usually affecting children, is distinguished by rapid increase in the numbers of immature blood cells, within the marrow and circulating blood
• Chronic myeloid leukemia	Slowly progressive disease affecting mostly adults, is characterized by the excessive production of granulocytes
• Chronic lymphocytic leukemia	Mostly affecting adults, is distinguished by the excessive production of lymphocytes
• Acute myeloid leukemia	Production of abnormal myeloblasts, which then causes the production of abnormal white blood cells. It can also interfere with the production of red blood cells and platelets.
Lymphomas	
• Non-Hodgkin: Diffuse large B-cell lymphoma	Most common subtype of non-Hodgkin lymphoma followed by diffuse large T-cell lymphoma. Large cell lymphomas may develop in the lymph system tissue in the neck, chest, throat, or abdomen.
• Hodgkin: Hodgkin lymphoma	Characterized by a specific cell type, specifically the presence of the Reed-Sternberg cell on pathologic evaluation. Hodgkin lymphoma is spread from one lymph node group to another, is notable for the development of systemic symptoms with advanced disease.
Myelodysplastic syndrome	Compilation of hematologic disorders that are characterized by dysplasia or unsuccessful production of myeloid cells within the bone marrow. This leads to anemia and cytopenias secondary to bone marrow function. It can transform to acute myeloid leukemia.
Multiple myeloma	Disorder of the plasma cells within the blood. With time, myeloma cells collect in the bone marrow. As a result of the myeloma cells, the body is unable to produce normal antibodies and produces an increased amount of abnormal antibodies.

Note. Based on information from National Cancer Institute, 2011a, 2011b.

tain types of leukemias may be treated with HSCT. Lymphomas classified as Hodgkin or non-Hodgkin type are malignant conditions of the lymphatic cells of the immune system. It is important to note that some types of non-Hodgkin lymphomas are considered to be unclassifiable. Large-cell lymphomas may develop in the lymph tissue in the neck, chest, throat, or abdomen. Both myelodysplastic syndrome and multiple myeloma are described later in this chapter.

Types of Hematopoietic Stem Cell Transplantation

In general, two types of HSCT are performed: autologous and allogeneic. *Autologous* HSCT is a type of transplant that uses the patient's own cells. The patient is usually given chemotherapy, and sometimes radiation, to debulk the malignant disease. Prior to receiving high-dose chemotherapy, the patient's cells are collected (harvested) and stored. The patient is then treated for the malignancy per protocol. The purpose of the chemotherapy and/or radiation is to eliminate the malignant cells. This, however, depletes the patient's bone marrow and thus the ability to produce new blood cells. After chemotherapy, the patient's stored cells are then returned to the patient to replace the destroyed cells and allow production of new blood cells. One of the drawbacks of autologous transplants is the risk of contamination of the graft with malignant cells (Leger & Nevill, 2004).

Allogeneic transplants use cells from another person, the donor. Ideally, if available, the donor is someone with a similar genetic makeup. Allogeneic transplant donors may be a closely HLA-matched sibling. An unrelated donor may be used if an individual with a similar HLA makeup can be identified. Unrelated donors may be found through a registry of bone marrow donors. Satisfactory unrelated donors can be identified for 80% of Caucasian patients (Leger & Nevill, 2004). The figure is lower for patients from other ethnic groups. The ideal donor is an HLA-identical sibling, as transplants with only partial matching for HLA antigens are associated with a higher risk of post-transplant complications. One drawback of an imperfect match is that the graft of donor cells is more likely to die or be destroyed by the patient's body before settling in the bone marrow. That is known as the graft not "taking." Graft-versus-host disease (GVHD), a post-transplant complication in which functional immune cells in the graft attack the host, is probably the most common complication of allogeneic transplants (Leger & Nevill, 2004).

Methods of Harvesting Cells

Harvesting refers to the collection of cells for transplantation. Stem cells have the unique ability to divide, when needed, and give rise to mature differentiated cells. Hematopoietic stem cells give rise to all types of blood cells (National Institutes of Health, 2009). Most stem cells remain in the marrow until they have matured into specialized cells and then are released into the circulating bloodstream. The methods of harvesting cells are described in Table 9-2. Stem cells as described previously are located in the bone marrow. However, stem cells also circulate in the peripheral blood and in umbilical cord blood.

Patient Selection

Patient eligibility is multifactorial but generally is based on risk versus benefit. Factors that contribute to the analysis include the type of transplant (allogeneic or autologous) and the proposed conditioning therapy or treatment used to ablate the patient's marrow. Eligibility criteria vary institutionally and throughout different countries. Most institutions look at similar criteria such as laboratory data, performance status, and organ function, including renal and cardiac function. Factors influencing survival after conditioning treatment in preparation for an allogeneic transplant include disease stage, performance status, stem cell source, HLA matching, and timing of transplant. These factors should all be considered when planning treatment (Giralt et al., 2007). Patient diagnosis alone should not determine treatment. It should instead be the result of a decision-making process including assessment of patient age, performance status,

Table 9-2. Methods of Harvesting Cells			
Method	**Procedure**	**Pros**	**Cons**
Bone marrow aspiration	Performed under general anesthesia. Using a long needle that can reach the center of the bone, the stem cells are retrieved from a long bone, usually the hip or pelvis.	Peripheral leukocyte counts do not significantly decrease.	Painful; risk with general anesthesia
Peripheral stem cell collection	Stem cell growth factor is administered, which causes stem cell reproduction and stimulates cells to leave the bone marrow and enter the peripheral blood. Venipuncture is used to obtain 10–20 L of peripheral blood, which undergoes leukapheresis. Stem cells are separated and cryopreserved.	Less painful than bone marrow aspiration	May need to repeat procedure multiple times Side effects from stimulating factor: bone marrow pains, malaise, headaches, chills, fever
Umbilical cord (cord blood has a higher concentration of stem cells than adult blood)	Cells are obtained through donation of an infant's umbilical cord and placenta after birth.	Less painful than bone marrow aspiration or peripheral collection	Adequate-sized single cord blood units are not available for full-size adults and high-weight children.

Note. Based on information from Broxmeyer, 2011; Ledger & Nevill, 2004.

medical comorbidities, family support, socioeconomic viability, and motivation to participate in self-care (Hamadani, Craig, Awan, & Devine, 2010).

Because of the rigors of transplantation, performance status is always evaluated prior to the procedure using a performance score. Many centers use the Karnofsky performance score, the Eastern Cooperative Oncology Group (ECOG) grading scale, or the Zubrod performance score.

The *Karnofsky score* is used to quantify the state of health in a patient with cancer. It is based on the patient's ability to continue normal daily activity with no evidence of disease, minor evidence of disease, or some evidence of disease. The ability to care for oneself ranges from complete independence; needing occasional assistance; often needing assistance; disabled and needing specialized care; severely disabled and hospitalized; hospitalized, very ill, and requiring supportive measures but not actively dying; to moribund with fatality and imminent death. Patients who are able to carry on normal activity with no evidence of disease obtain a score of 100, whereas death confers a score of 0, and the score is in increments of 10 (Schag, Heinrich, & Ganz, 1984).

The *ECOG performance score* is also used to quantify a patient's state of health using similar criteria: asymptomatic, meaning fully active and not restricted by disease; symptomatic but ambulatory; symptomatic, less than 50% time in bed, and able to perform self-care but unable to work; symptomatic, greater than 50% time in bed but not bedbound, and limited self-care; bedbound and unable to perform self-care; and death. The score is in increments of 1; asymptomatic patients would obtain a score of 0, and death would be a score of 5 (Buccheri, Ferrigno, & Tamburini, 1996).

The patient's current disease state is an important factor when considering HSCT. According to Hamadani et al. (2010),

> The histological type and remission status of the underlying disorder are the key determinants of whether HSCT is indicated in any given patient and which type of transplant offers the best risk/benefit ratio. . . . Autologous (and perhaps allogeneic) transplantation in patients with chemotherapy-refractory lymphomas offer[s] little prospect of cure. Similarly, outcomes of leukemia patients undergoing allografting while in complete remission are clearly superior to those with refractory disease. (p. 1260)

Based on these findings, patients with chemotherapy-refractory disease often are not eligible, whereas patients who are in remission may be ideal candidates. A previously failed HSCT is also a factor to consider when evaluating a patient because toxicities increase with repeat exposure to conditioning agents.

Age alone does not determine eligibility. Historically, younger patients have been referred for transplantation. As a result of improvements in supportive care and the advent of peripheral blood stem cell transplantation with earlier engraftment, older patients are now frequently referred for transplant. In addition, reduced-intensity conditioning (RIC) has allowed transplantation in older patients who would not have been candidates with traditional conditioning. These conditioning methods will be discussed later in the chapter. Traditionally, age 55 was considered the maximum age for conventional allografting. Although older people tend to have more comorbidities, it has been found that age older than 55 is not a prognostic indicator with RIC (Corradini et al., 2005). In the study by Giralt et al. (2007), the mean age for RIC was 55 while the mean age for conventional conditioning was 33. Furthermore, with current screening practices, age is not an absolute exclusion criterion for autologous HSCT, but rather the presence of significant medical comorbidities may result in exclusion (Reece et al., 2003).

To evaluate comorbidities prior to transplant, a full evaluation of specific organ function is performed. The National Marrow Donor Program recommends a battery of screening tests: Dental x-rays and oral examination are recommended to evaluate the oral cavity. Lung function is evaluated through pulmonary function tests and diffusing capacity for carbon monoxide, with a recommended forced vital capacity greater than 60%. A cardiac evaluation is recommended with an electrocardiogram (ECG) to evaluate for arrhythmias and echocardiogram or multigated acquisition (MUGA) scan for ejection fraction (EF) evaluation, with EF greater than 50% as the usual cutoff. Kidney function should be evaluated, with recommended serum creatinine less than 1.5 mg/dl and creatinine clearance greater than 60 ml/min. Liver function is evaluated with serum bilirubin less than 2 mg/dl. Liver function tests also evaluate for veno-occlusive disease, with serum glutamic-oxaloacetic transaminase, or SGOT, less than two times of normal and serum glutamic pyruvic transaminase, or SGPT, less than two times of normal. A neurologic evaluation is performed, as parenchymal central nervous system disease may be a contraindication to transplant because of the risk of cerebral bleeding (National Marrow Donor Program, 2011).

Pretransplant Cardiac Evaluation

Prior to undergoing HSCT, patients should receive a cardiac risk assessment to identify possible cardiovascular complications. Normal cardiac function is necessary to handle the physiologic stress of transplantation, including the rigors of chemotherapy, radiation, and volume depletion combined with prolonged bone marrow suppression, in addition to the potential hypotension that often accompanies life-threatening infections. Diagnostic testing used to assess cardiac function is described in Table 9-3. Although case reports have been published on cardiac toxicity following bone marrow transplantation (BMT), the actual risk of developing this complication has not been

Table 9-3. Pretransplant Evaluation

Test	Description	Procedure	Purpose
Electrocardiogram	Transcription of the heart's electrical activity over a period of time	Noninvasive test that uses electrodes to look at the electrical activity through the heart from different angles	To identify arrhythmias, ischemia, conduction abnormalities, atrial and ventricular enlargement, and hypertrophy
Echocardiogram	Ultrasound waves to make two- and three-dimensional images of the heart	Noninvasive procedure that uses gel and an ultrasound probe. Probe sends ultrasound beams into chest; reflections are detected and used to generate images of the heart.	To evaluate chamber size and function, cardiac valve morphology, and abnormalities of flow. Also used to assess for abnormal communication between the right and left sides of the heart, to detect wall motion abnormalities, and to determine the ejection fraction or pump function.
Multigated acquisition scan	Radioactive marker to create an image of the beating heart	Radioactive substance is added to red blood cells and then injected into patient. Outline of chambers is defined through gamma camera.	An alternative test used to evaluate ejection fraction
Stress testing	Compare left ventricular function and wall motion or left ventricular myocardial perfusion at rest and during maximum physical exertion. Stress is induced by exercise or chemical stimulation with electrocardiogram monitoring.	Nuclear tests use a radiotracer, and photos are taken with a gamma camera to capture images of the blood flow before and after exercise. Photos assess the state of perfusion of the myocardium as a surrogate for the state of the coronary arteries of the patient.	To evaluate for ischemia. Poor perfusion with stress represents ischemia, whereas absence of circulation represents infarction. Test also evaluates ejection fraction.

Note. Based on information from Givertz & Colucci, 2001; Lilly, 2001; Martin, 2001; Zangari et al., 1999.

defined (Hertenstein et al., 1994). The diagnostic cardiovascular testing that has been used for pretransplant assessment includes ECG, stress testing, MUGA scan (also known as radionuclide scan), and echocardiogram.

The usefulness of pretransplant echocardiograms to evaluate EF has been controversial. Sakata-Yanagimoto et al. (2004), in comparing studies looking at the effectiveness of echocardiograms in the pretransplant evaluation, noted conflicting results. For example, Braverman, Antin, Plappert, Cook, and Lee (1991) showed that the incidence of severe cardiac complications was higher among patients with a low EF, whereas Hertenstein et al. (1994) found no correlation between pretransplant cardiac function and the development of life-threatening cardiac events. Sakata-Yanagimoto et al. (2004) then conducted a retrospective review of 164 patients with normal left ventricular function (EF greater than 55%) who had ECG and echocardiogram within three months before HSCT and evaluated cardiac complications within 28 days following transplantation. Study results showed an increased incidence of severe cardiac toxicity in the reduced-EF group, but the difference was not statistically significant. The cumulative dose of anthracyclines was a more potent predictor of cardiac complications than the pretransplant EF.

Measuring EF through MUGA scans has also been contested. Zangari et al. (1999) evaluated the predictive value on transplantation mortality of left ventricular ejection fraction (LVEF) measured with MUGA (rest and exercise) scans for 174 patients who underwent HSCT. All patients with normal baseline LVEF were followed for at least three months after the transplant. Results showed that resting EF was a predictor for peritransplant mortality in younger patients (younger than 43 years); however, it was not a discriminating factor for early death in other subgroups. No significant difference in mortality was observed between patients with normal or decreased resting EF and appropriate cardiac reserve or in patients with normal resting EF and decreased cardiac reserve. However, presence of decreased resting EF and poor cardiac reserve defined a patient group with extremely high early mortality (n = 18, 56%). Among younger patients, none of those with a high mean LVEF (n = 26, 52%) died of congestive heart failure. They found that inadequate cardiac reserve had a worse prognosis regardless of baseline normal EF (Zangari et al., 1999). Bearman et al. (1990) found that the incidence of grade III or IV cardiac toxicity was not statistically different between patients with normal EF and mildly reduced EF. It should be noted that the prognostic value of stress testing has not been evaluated in this patient population.

Pretransplant Conditioning

Conditioning is the process prior to HSCT when the transplant recipient receives high-dose chemotherapy and, in some cases, radiation to eradicate the underlying malignant disease. In allogeneic transplants, conditioning also suppresses the recipient's immune system to prevent rejection of the donor's stem cells. In general, conditioning has been broken down into three classes: myeloablative (MA) conditioning, nonmyeloablative (NMA) conditioning, and RIC. Pretransplant days until the transplant are represented as a countdown with the conditioning days numbered as negative (e.g., –6) and the actual day of transplant being day 0 (Leger & Nevill, 2004).

Myeloablative Conditioning

Myeloablation refers to the administration of total body irradiation (TBI) and/or alkylating agents at doses that will not allow autologous hematologic recovery (Giralt et al., 2007). The agents used for myeloablation prior to BMT vary significantly but include TBI, cyclophosphamide (Cy), and busulfan (Bu). The combinations of Bu-Cy or Cy-TBI are considered to be MA regimens. Other agents have been introduced in the conditioning regimen at high doses and in different combinations with Cy or TBI, usually with the intention of further intensification. These include melphalan, thiotepa, etoposide, and dimethylbusulfan (Giralt et al., 2007). A frequently used MA for young patients with leukemia or lymphoma is either Cy 120 mg/kg and TBI 10–15 gray (Gy) (referred to as Cy-TBI) or Bu 16 mg/kg and Cy 120 mg/kg (referred to as Bu-Cy) (Bacigalupo et al., 2009). An important note is that MA can cause profound pancytopenia and myeloablation within one to three weeks from administration. Pancytopenia is long lasting, usually irreversible, and in most instances fatal unless hematopoiesis is restored by hemopoietic stem cell infusion (Giralt et al., 2007).

MA conditioning agents are considered to be cardiotoxic. Cy, Bu, and melphalan are alkylating agents that are well tolerated at lower doses; however, high-dose regimens such as those given with BMT cause a variety of adverse effects related to the total dose of an individual course received and prior treatment with anthracyclines and mediastinal radiation. The cause of cardiotoxicity is thought to be endothelial and myocyte injury mediated through a toxic metabolite. Autopsies have found increased left ventricular wall thickness with hemorrhagic myocardial necrosis (Yeh et al., 2004). Life-threatening and often fatal, cardiac toxicity as a complication of BMT was first described in patients treated with high-dose Cy. The occurrence of cardiotoxicity is characterized by the clinical manifestations of dyspnea, fluid retention, and pericardial effusion. Tissue examination shows evidence of endothelial damage and small vessel microthrombosis (Hertenstein et al., 1994). Bu, which often is used with Cy, is less cardiotoxic but has been associated with endomyocardial fibrosis and cardiac tamponade (Yeh et al., 2004).

Long-term effects of TBI are also dose dependent. With transplantation, the total dose often would be lethal if administered in one dose; therefore, the doses are fractionated. The effects on the heart, both acute and delayed, are correlated with the dose. Acute complications are rare. It can be difficult to determine whether radiation is the sole cause of the acute effects, as compared to radiation in combination with other conditioning agents. Potential effects include pericarditis, cardiac tamponade, and acute cardiomyopathy. These may be long-term risks from TBI exposure or, too frequently, may also be risks resulting from treatment of prior malignancies in patients facing a second or third malignancy and who now must be evaluated and managed through transplantation. In addition to increasing the risk of coronary artery disease (CAD), TBI is an important risk factor for consequent diabetes, dyslipidemia, and overall accumulation of factors that predispose patients to cardiovascular disease compared to patients exposed to other cancer therapies (Chow et al., 2011). The effect of radiation therapy on the cardiovascular system is discussed in further detail in Chapter 4.

Nonmyeloablative Conditioning

NMA conditioning regimens were developed to reduce toxicity, thus making transplantation available in the older patient population. Although NMA conditioning is immunosuppressive, it generally causes minimal cytopenia and little early toxicity and does not require stem cell support. When an NMA regimen is followed by peripheral blood stem cells mobilized with granulocyte–colony-stimulating factor, complete engraftment of donor stem cells usually results. To encourage engraftment, numerous donor T lymphocytes, cluster of differentiation 34+ (CD34+) cells, are required. NMA regimens involve the combination of immunoablation and large numbers of donor cells (Bacigalupo et al., 2009). NMA regimens can include fludarabine and Cy, TBI 2 Gy, TBI 1 Gy, total lymphoid irradiation, and antithymocyte globulin (ATG) (Bacigalupo et al., 2009). These regimens seem to be better tolerated than MA regimens and do not appear to be cardiotoxic. In a study looking at 26 patients undergoing allogeneic NMA HSCT, all of whom were given a combination of fludarabine and ATG, no grade 3 or 4 toxicity (World Health Organization criteria) was observed in any of the recipients (Slavin et al., 1998). There was no mention of cardiac toxicities in the study.

Reduced-Intensity Conditioning

RIC is an intermediate category of regimens that do not fit the definition for MA or NMA. RIC regimens differ from MA conditioning because the dose of alkylating agents or TBI is reduced by at least 30%. These regimens cause cytopenia and therefore require stem cell support. Although autologous recovery can occur, high morbidity and mortality exist because of the duration of pancytopenia. RIC regimens have used a wide selection of agents given at a wide range of doses. They often include a combination of fludarabine with either reduced doses of alkylating agents, such as melphalan, busulfan, or thiotepa, or reduced TBI (Bacigalupo et al., 2009). Although the doses of treatment agents have been reduced, cardiotoxicity has been associated with RIC regimens.

Melphalan, at doses of 140 mg/m^2, a frequent component of RIC regimens, has recently been associated with atrial fibrillation (A-fib). This is further supported by Olivieri et al. (1998) in a small case report of 76 patients treated with high-dose melphalan who were considered to be at risk for conduction abnormalities. Five out of the 76 patients (6.6%) developed A-fib. It is important to note that arrhythmias occurred in the absence of detectable structural heart disease. Lower doses of TBI are used to limit TBI-associated complications.

Fludarabine has rarely been associated with cardiac effects, but other purine analogs have shown evidence of cardiotoxicity. The proposed mechanism for the cardiotoxicity of these drugs is uncertain; however, related drugs can undergo phosphorylation by the mitochondrial deoxyguanosine kinase, causing impaired cellular energy metabolism. The development of severe acute left ventricular failure in 3 of 21 patients conditioned with fludarabine and melphalan conditioning contrasts with the reported rarity of cardiotoxicity with either agent individually. It is possible that the interaction of both agents is required for the toxic effect (Ritchie, Seymour, Roberts, Szer, & Grigg, 2001).

Engraftment and Cardiac Complications During Engraftment

As mentioned previously, the transplant occurs on day 0. The transplant itself is not complex; it consists of IV infusion of liquid stem cells. The process usually occurs over one to two hours. After transplant, the patient waits for the stem cells to engraft, with the transplant team providing life-saving supportive care. During this time, the patient is neutropenic, with reduced immunity leaving the patient vulnerable to infection. Patients often are put on prophylactic antibiotics including antifungals and antivirals. Patient safety is a concern during this time, and patients are placed in positive-pressure isolation rooms (Leger & Nevill, 2004).

Engraftment is the progression by which the infused stem cells migrate into the recipient's marrow and produce new blood products within the marrow. While waiting for engraftment, the patient is supported with blood products and the neutrophil count is monitored as a measure of reconstitution of the patient's immune system. Usually the absolute neutrophil count reaches greater than $0.5 \times 10^9/L$ between day +10 and +20. This is then followed by platelet and red blood cell engraftment. Engraftment occurs sooner with autografting and when stem cells are used rather than bone marrow cells (Leger & Nevill, 2004).

Cardiac complications can occur during the engraftment period. Patients who will develop cardiac adverse effects (such as heart failure) from conditioning treatments may begin to show clinical signs during this time.

Volume Overload

Volume overload should be considered in all patients, even those without heart failure, during the engraftment period. Patients with neutropenia are more susceptible to bacterial infections and may require antibiotics to combat infection. Neutropenic sepsis can be fatal in this population and requires large volumes of hydration and antibiotics. Patients are also anemic and thrombocytopenic during this period and are often supported with blood and blood products. It is important to monitor for signs of volume overload and heart failure during this time. This is discussed further in the heart failure section of this chapter.

Acute Graft-Versus-Host Disease

During the engraftment period, patients are at risk for the development of acute GVHD (aGVHD), which usually occurs before day 100 post-transplant. To prevent aGVHD, patients often are given prophylaxis with immunosuppressive drugs, including cyclosporine, tacrolimus, methotrexate, mycophenolate mofetil, corticosteroids, or ATG. If GVHD develops, patients are treated with corticosteroids along with cyclosporine or tacrolimus. Other drugs that may be included in treatment are monoclonal antibodies (e.g., anti-CD3, anti-CD5, and anti-interleukin-2 antibodies), mycophenolate mofetil, alemtuzumab, ATG, and sirolimus. Although prevention and treatment of aGVHD is critical because of subsequent post-transplant morbidity and mortality, it comes with cardiac risks.

Corticosteroids, which are used in both the prevention and treatment of acute GVHD, have cardiac adverse effects. The major adverse effects of glucocorticoids on the cardiovascular system include dyslipidemia and hypertension. The mechanisms of glucocorticoid-mediated hypertension appear to be related to increased peripheral vascular resistance (Ng & Celermajer, 2004). Dyslipidemia is more common in long-term glucocorticoid use and is characterized by increased total cholesterol, low-density lipoprotein (LDL) cholesterol, and triglycerides. Glucocorticoid activation of the mineralocorticoid receptor also may exert clinically relevant cardiovascular effects. Mineralocorticoid activation has been suggested to exacerbate heart failure by increasing sodium and fluid retention and also by promoting remodeling through fibrosis of the atria and ventricles (Ng & Celermajer, 2004). Oral glucocorticoids appear to be associated with increased risk of heart failure (odds ratio of 2.66, 95% CI [2.46, 2.87]), which appears to be dose dependent (Souverein et al., 2004).

Cyclosporine is commonly used as an immunosuppressive agent to enable tolerance and for prevention of aGVHD in BMT. Cyclosporine can be nephrotoxic and is known to cause hypertension. The specific mechanism is unknown, although there are several theories such as activation of the sympathetic nervous system, endothelin-mediated systemic vasoconstriction, impaired vasodilatation secondary to reduction in prostaglandin and nitric oxide, altered cytosolic calcium translocation, and activation of the renin-angiotensin system (Niehof & Borlak, 2011).

Alemtuzumab is a humanized monoclonal antibody shown to be effective in the prevention and treatment of aGVHD (Carella, Beltrami, Scalzulli, Carella, & Corsetti, 2004). Although not common, pulmonary and cardiac events also may occur in patients treated with alemtuzumab. It has been associated with left ventricular dysfunction, vasospasm, and myocarditis. The association among cardiac adverse events, alemtuzumab, and T-cell malignancies may be explained by a cytokine-release syndrome, defined as an increased level of serum tumor necrosis factor-alpha, interferon gamma, and interleukin-6 after alemtuzumab infusion. The cytokine release can lead to coronary vasospasm, potentially cytomegalovirus-related myocarditis, or myocardial "stunning." In general, the left ventricular dysfunction or stunning is mostly reversible, but it may be permanent if the damage is severe enough. It has also been proposed that alemtuzumab could kill T cells that infiltrate the heart, causing myocyte dysfunction or electrical disturbances. The cardiac events associated with alemtuzumab have been associated with T-cell malignancies. Cardiac adverse events developed after a median of 10 full doses of alemtuzumab (range of 1–18 doses), approximately four weeks of therapy, and a median cumulative dose of 223 mg (range of 43–553 mg). It is important to note that this was a small study of eight patients, six of whom developed cardiac adverse events, and did not include the use of alemtuzumab for the treatment or prevention of aGVHD (Lenihan et al., 2004). This was supported by another small study, which concluded that the use of in vivo alemtuzumab along with MA conditioning may increase the incidence of reversible cardiac complications. The toxicity was not solely from alemtuzumab but from conditioning and increased cytokine secretion associated with engraftment (Oshima et al., 2005).

Cardiac Complications With Stem Cell Transplantation

Cardiomyopathy

Pathophysiology: Cardiomyopathy can be caused by agents the patient was exposed to prior to HSCT such as anthracyclines and trastuzumab as discussed in Chapter 2. *Stress-induced cardiomyopathy* (SICM), also widely called *takotsubo cardiomyopathy, apical ballooning syndrome,* or *broken-heart syndrome,* is a reversible cardiomyopathy usually precipitated by a stressful event. The number of patients who experience this syndrome after HSCT is unknown, as no data examining this type of cardiomyopathy in this population have been published. The pathophysiology of this disorder is not entirely clear, but it is believed to result from myocardial stunning secondary to high levels of circulating catecholamines and stress-related neuropeptides. Catecholamines are released during the stressful event, which can lead to impaired perfusion, myocyte injury, or left ventricular outflow tract obstruction (Huffman, Wagman, Fudim, Zolty, & Vittorio, 2010). SICM in this population may be secondary to the emotional and physiologic stress of the transplant. Physiologic stressors can include conditioning chemotherapies, volume management including volume depletion and volume overload, pancytopenia, GVHD, infection, and sepsis. Emotional stressors often are present, including uncertainty about treatment without the guarantee of success and depression. Patients are in isolation during the engraftment period. Plants and fresh fruits and vegetables are not permitted because of the risk of infection, and if patients leave the room, they must wear a gown, gloves, and mask, which can cause emotional distress. Visitors are often limited, causing patients to feel isolated during a time when support is most needed.

Clinical features: Patients may have an abrupt onset of dyspnea, chest pain, or fatigue. Patients are often asymptomatic. On laboratory evaluation, cardiac enzyme levels may be increased; however, the level is usually inappropriately low relative to contractile dysfunction seen on echocardiogram (Nussinovitch, Goitein, Nussinovitch, & Altman, 2011). The incidence of SICM is higher in postmenopausal women (Nussinovitch et al., 2011).

Diagnostic tests: Echocardiogram of SICM will show hypokinesis or akinesis of the middle and apical segments of the left ventricle, which results in ballooning of the apical wall with sparing of basal systolic function, and the ejection fraction decreases 20%–49% (Huffman et al., 2010). Transient left ventricular outflow tract obstruction has also been seen on echocardiogram (Pilgrim & Wyss, 2008). ECG may have different presentations. For example, ST segment elevation is usually higher in leads V_4–V_6 rather than in V_1–V_3, with the absence of Q waves and lack of reciprocal changes, which is indicative of SICM as opposed to a myocardial infarction. T-wave abnormalities such as deep T-wave inversions and QTc prolongation usually are present in SICM as compared with myocardial infarction (Nussinovitch et al., 2011). Cardiac enzymes such as troponin may be mildly elevated (Huffman et al., 2010). Cardiac catheterization or coronary angiography is often necessary to assess for obstructive CAD and evaluate for acute coronary syndrome.

Differential diagnoses: Signs and symptoms of SICM may be interpreted as acute coronary syndrome. New-onset dyspnea is often assumed to be pneumonia or other pulmonary diagnoses. Fatigue in this population is often presumed to be secondary to the physical demands of the transplant. The sudden onset of chest pain with ECG changes in the absence of known CAD may also be confused with pericarditis or myocarditis.

Medical and nursing management: The first step in the treatment of SICM is accurate diagnosis. SICM should be considered when evaluating the patient with chest pain and ECG changes in the absence of CAD. It is equally important to investigate the possibility of acute coronary syndrome in the post-HSCT patient. An attempt should be made at identifying the cause with an attempt at resolution, although in this population there may be multiple causes. The goal of treatment in SICM is restoration of heart muscle function. Fortunately, with timely recognition, SICM is usually reversible, and recovery of left ventricular EF can occur quickly (Sharkey, Lesser, & Maron, 2011). Treatment of SICM is largely supportive. Commonly used medications include beta-blockers and angiotensin-converting enzyme inhibitors, both of which promote recovery of heart muscle. The use of these medications in the treatment of cardiomyopathy is discussed in Chapters 2 and 3. It is important to note that due to the large proportion of the heart muscle injured, heart failure may occur, which may require aggressive diuresis (Sharkey et al., 2011). The treatment of SICM in HCST recipients is more complicated. Patients may be hypotensive in the setting of neutropenic sepsis or volume depletion. In this case, hypotension should be treated first. When the patient is normotensive and can tolerate beta-blockers or angiotensin-converting enzyme inhibitors, therapy should then be initiated at low doses and titrated up with careful observation. The patient may not be a candidate for coronary angiography because of low platelet count, but if the suspicion for acute coronary syndrome is high, the patient should be treated medically until the proper diagnosis can be made. Medical and nursing management of acute coronary syndrome is discussed in Chapter 5.

Heart Failure

Pathophysiology: The etiology of heart failure in transplant recipients may differ from that in nontransplant patients. Volume overload in a transplant patient may be due to an acute decrease in left ventricular function as a result of cardiotoxic effects of chemotherapy, stress, fluid overload resulting from multiple transfusions, worsening acute renal failure, or even ischemia in the setting of sepsis or anemia. Clinical signs of heart failure occur more rapidly with Cy therapy. Cardiotoxicity can occur during treatment or within three weeks of administration (Morandi, Ruffini, Benvenuto, Raimondi, & Fosser, 2005). Left ventricular systolic function, evaluated by the fractional shortening on echocardiogram, declined substantially 5–16 days after the initiation of Cy therapy (Gottdiener, Appelbaum, Ferrans, Deisseroth, & Ziegler, 1981). For further discussion about the pathophysiology of heart failure, refer to Chapter 10.

Clinical features: In congestive heart failure (CHF), cardiac output does not match venous return. The heart cannot keep up with the normal demands placed on it; rising capillary pressure pushes sodium and water into the interstitial space, causing pulmonary edema, lower-extremity edema, weight gain, or increasing abdominal girth due to ascites (Anderson et al., 2010). The cardinal symptoms the patient may complain of include dyspnea, fatigue with declining functional capacity, and paroxysmal nocturnal dyspnea (McMurray, 2010). Patients may experience dyspnea on exertion or when lying flat (orthopnea), dizziness, orthostatic hypotension, and coughing or wheezing. Some patients may be unable to sleep unless sitting upright. Other signs noted on physical examination include jugular venous distention, cardiac enlargement with displaced apical impulse, and a third heart sound (McMurray, 2010). Commonly, the apical impulse is displaced downward and to the left (Kasper & Baughman, 2001). For a more extensive review of the clinical features of heart failure, see Chapter 10.

Diagnostic tests: Brain natriuretic peptide is a substance secreted from the ventricles of the heart secondary to changes in pressure. The level of brain natriuretic peptide (normal value is less than 100 pg/ml) in the blood increases when heart failure symptoms worsen, typically in the setting of volume overload, and decreases when the heart failure condition has stabilized and the patient is closer to euvolemia. A chest x-ray will be helpful to evaluate the size and shape of the cardiac silhouette, and an echocardiogram will assess the left ventricular size, mass, and function. A cardiothoracic ratio of greater than 0.5 is a good indicator of increased left ventricular volume (Givertz & Colucci, 2001).

Differential diagnoses: Signs and symptoms of CHF may be interpreted as fluid overload in the setting of multiple transfusions or hypotension in the setting of febrile neutropenia, and an underlying cardiogenic cause may not be considered. The differential diagnosis of symptoms and signs of CHF in transplant recipients is extensive and includes anything from fatigue due to the strain of the transplant process, fluid overload in the setting of transfusions, or hypotension due to sepsis or decreased oral intake in the setting of gastrointestinal upset or mucositis. Lower-extremity edema may not be a particularly helpful sign. This may occur with diminished cardiac output as well as multiple fluid challenges, low albumin, or decreased physical mobility.

Medical and nursing management: Evaluating for the cause of CHF is imperative to identifying the correct treatment algorithm, although treatment will usually start with diuresis. The initial goal in this patient population is the safe removal of excessive fluid. Once a patient's volume status is improved, slow addition of beta-blockers and angiotensin-converting enzyme inhibitors is indicated if the cause of CHF is reduced left ventricular systolic function. Currently, no definitive evidence-based guidelines exist regarding the treatment of CHF either in transplant recipients or in patients with cancer who have chemotherapy-induced heart failure. The treatment of heart failure is reviewed in Chapter 10. The management strategies discussed in this section are specific to patients who have undergone HSCT.

Fluid management is complicated in these patients for a multitude of reasons. Patients may have preexisting heart failure or may have developed heart failure and have low LVEF either from chemotherapy or from stress (SICM). The patient may also have preexisting valvular disease. During the engraftment period, patients are waiting for their blood counts to resolve, and they frequently require supportive blood products. Bruising, nosebleeds, and bleeding gums often occur in patients with thrombocytopenia. Platelet counts of less than 10,000/µl have been associated with an increase in mortality. Therefore, most centers have thresholds (platelet count of 10,000/µl) for initiating platelet transfusions in transplant recipients. Response to platelet transfusions in the post-transplant setting may not be as successful as in nontransplant patients, sometimes requiring increased platelet doses to improve counts (Gajewski, Johnson, Sandler, Sayegh, & Klumpp, 2008). Patients also may require multiple blood transfusions.

The nurse has many responsibilities in caring for this patient population. It is very important to limit the amount of fluids the patient receives while not postponing necessary treatments. A consultation with the infectious disease team can help to determine the use of broad-spectrum antibiotics and concentrating antibiotics. Unnecessary fluids should be limited; maintenance fluid may not be necessary in a patient who has sufficient oral intake. Strict intake and output records are necessary along with weight measurements, as even patients without cardiotoxicity are at risk for volume overload.

Volume management becomes even more complicated in patients who have underlying cardiac diseases such as aortic stenosis, left ventricular dysfunction, and diastolic dysfunction. Aortic stenosis is the most common acquired valvular disease. Stenosis of the aortic orifice can develop as a consequence of a congenital bicuspid anatomy or idiopathic sclerocalcific degeneration as a patient ages (Schick, 2001). This patient population may have aortic stenosis secondary to radiation. Cusps or leaflets of the valves thicken, become fibrous, and calcify. As stenosis progresses, less area is available to allow for the valve to open, eventually increasing the pressure in the left ventricle (Schick, 2001). Surgical intervention in the midst of transplant is impractical. Severity of aortic stenosis generally corresponds with a smaller valve orifice. Patients with aortic stenosis are at increased risk in the postoperative period. It remains vital to maintain appropriate intravascular filling and arterial blood pressure and to minimize the additional demands incurred on the heart. Avoidance of systemic hypotension is essential. Hypotension leads to myocardial ischemia and reduced contractility, causing further falls in blood pressure and decreased coronary perfusion (Brown & Morgan-Hughes, 2005). These patients must be monitored closely, and attempts must be made to maintain euvolemia because volume depletion can cause hemodynamic compromise. This is important to remember in febrile patients and patients with poor oral intake secondary to mucositis.

Volume management in transplant is just as difficult with left ventricular systolic or diastolic dysfunction. Diastolic dysfunction is caused by ventricular stiffness and its inability to relax. This impairs ventricular filling because the ventricle is unable to accommodate increased volume. Left ventricular end-diastolic pressure is increased, leading to pulmonary venous congestion. The mass of the left ventricle may be increased, contributing to resistance in filling (Givertz & Colucci, 2001). Patients with diastolic heart failure may present with sudden exacerbations of their symptoms and with acute pulmonary edema. Management should include control of systolic blood pressure and avoidance of fluid overload (Little, 2008). Tachycardia and arrhythmias can worsen diastolic dysfunction by decreasing filling time in the stiff ventricle. This is important for nurses to remember when taking care of post-transplant patients who are febrile and tachycardic. It is important to monitor intake and output in these patients, especially in those who are receiving fluids or frequent transfusions. Diuretics may be needed in symptomatic patients. Although these patients have a normal EF, they are at risk for heart failure.

Left ventricular systolic dysfunction is just as problematic with respect to fluid management in the transplant setting. Left ventricular systolic dysfunction is most commonly associated with prior myocardial infarction, an ischemic cardiomyopathy. However, nonischemic cardiomyopathy, weakening of the heart muscle due to other causes, is also common in this population because of prior exposure to chemotherapeutics, particularly anthracyclines, and other causes, such as long-standing hypertension or alcohol abuse. Systolic dysfunction often manifests with changes in the shape, size, and function of the heart. In systolic heart failure, reduced EF results in a decrease in stroke volume and cardiac output. Increased left ventricular end-diastolic volumes and the often-associated abnormal diastolic filling results in increased left ventricular diastolic pressure. This is significant with the patient requiring volume replacement because extreme caution must be made to keep the patient from becoming volume overloaded. If too much volume is given to the patient with left ventricular dysfunction, the patient will be unable to circulate the volume, with resulting CHF as described previously. The goals of treatment are to reduce remodeling, improve left ventricular function, and improve hemodynamic abnormalities. Medications used for this goal are predominantly beta-blockers, angiotensin-converting enzyme inhibitors, and diuretics (Chatterjee & Massie, 2007).

Mucositis is a painful complication of conditioning and radiation treatments and can occur in up to 75% patients (Cutler et al., 2005). Mucositis can be severe enough that narcotic analgesia and total parenteral nutrition are required (Cutler et al., 2005). Febrile neutropenia often experienced by patients following HSCT requires the use of broad-spectrum antibiotics prophylactically (Leger & Nevill, 2004). Neutropenic sepsis can occur, requiring multiple antibiotics and often fluid resuscitation. In all of these complications, which are not unexpected, the treatment requires IV fluid. Patients may require blood or blood products, total parenteral nutrition, antibiotics, and fluids. This adds up to a large volume intake and places patients at risk for volume overload.

Pericardial Disease

A brief summary of pericardial complications of HSCT will be discussed in this section. A detailed explanation of the management of pericarditis and pericardial effusion/tamponade was covered in Chapter 7.

Pericarditis: Pericarditis is an inflammation and irritation of the pericardium. The pericardium consists of two layers: the outer fibrinous layer, called the *parietal pericardium*, and an inner serosal membrane overlying the epicardial surface, called the *visceral pericardium*. Between these layers is a space normally containing approximately 20 ml of fluid. High-dose Cy can cause an acute form of pericarditis within 10 days of its administration (Gharib & Burnett, 2002).

Clinical features: Patients with pericarditis typically complain of sharp midsternal chest pain that worsens with lying down and is relieved by leaning forward. The pain associated with acute pericarditis may be pleuritic (changing with respiration) in nature and may radiate to the ridge of the trapezius. Physical examination may reveal the hallmark finding for pericarditis: a pericardial friction rub. Classically, this rub occurs in three phases corresponding with atrial systole, ventricular systole, and ventricular diastole and is described as a grating or scratching sound (Marinella, 1998).

Differential diagnoses: Chest pain in transplant recipients may also be associated with esophagitis or reflux, infection, pneumonia, pulmonary embolus, or myocardial injury. Hypotension and tachycardia can also be presenting symptoms of infection or sepsis, bleeding, or shock.

Pericardial effusion: Pericardial effusion is the accumulation of fluid within the pericardial space. The response of the pericardium to gradual stretching differs from its response to an acute stretch (Shabetai, 2004). If fluid accumulates rapidly, even small volumes may cause compression of the right atrium and ventricle and result in decreased left ventricular filling (Givertz & Colucci, 2001).

Clinical features: Physical findings of cardiac tamponade include tachycardia, pulsus paradoxus, and hypotension with evidence of hypoperfusion. In the nontransplant patient, careful physical examination usually can differentiate tamponade from other etiologies of hypotension and tachycardia. However, this may be more complicated in transplant recipients, in whom hypotension and tachycardia are relatively common.

Diagnostic tests: ECG is useful in diagnosing both pericarditis and pericardial effusion. Pericarditis will demonstrate diffuse ST segment elevation with PR depression (Marinella, 1998) (see Figure 9-1). ECG in a patient with a pericardial effusion may have low voltage and may also have electrical alternans due to the swinging of the heart within the fluid-filled pericardium. An ECG of a patient with tamponade usually will show tachycardia, decreased voltage, and electrical alternans (Kasper & Baughman, 2001).

Chest x-ray is useful to evaluate for an increase in the cardiac silhouette. A newly enlarged cardiac silhouette may also support the diagnosis of pericardial effusion. Echo-

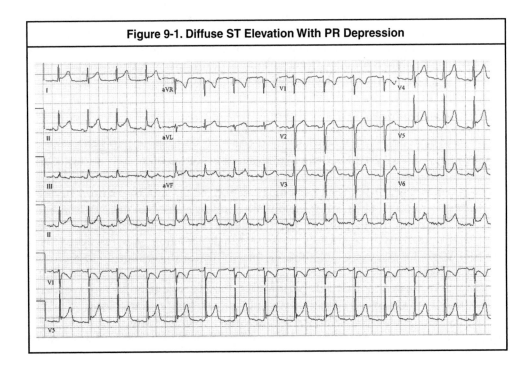

Figure 9-1. Diffuse ST Elevation With PR Depression

cardiogram will evaluate for an effusion or tamponade, confirming the diagnosis with visualization of the pericardial fluid and, in tamponade, collapse of the right ventricle in diastole (when it should be filling) and the right atrium in systole (when it should be filling) (Lopez, 2001).

Medical and nursing management: As the pain may not present in the classic form, especially because these patients may already be on pain medication, a low threshold is recommended to check the ECG, chest x-ray, computed tomography scan, or echocardiogram, depending on the clinical presentation and suspicion in each case. No data exist on the recurrence of pericarditis that is presumed to be caused by chemotherapy. Nonsteroidal anti-inflammatory drugs (NSAIDs) have been the cornerstone of treatment and continue to be widely used. Based on the results of the Colchicine for Acute Pericarditis (COPE) trial, it was determined that colchicine with NSAIDs was a safe and effective treatment for acute pericarditis, resulting in a decrease in recurrences (Imazio et al., 2005). At small doses of 1–2 mg/day, colchicine has been found to be safe even when given continuously over decades (Imazio et al., 2005). Corticosteroid therapy may have specific but rare indications, such as intolerance or contraindications to aspirin or NSAIDs, but should be considered a last resort (Imazio et al., 2005). It is important to note that conditioning renders this patient population pancytopenic for extended periods of time (Leger & Nevill, 2004). NSAIDs can cause neutropenia, agranulocytosis, aplastic anemia, and hemolytic anemia. Chronic administration of colchicine can induce bone marrow suppression including pancytopenia, thrombocytopenia, leukopenia, neutropenia, or agranulocytosis. Because of concerns regarding these side effects, transplant recipients often are not considered candidates for these treatments. In this situation, patients are treated for their pain. Steroids are used more frequently in these patients for this reason. An additional concern is that if an effusion accompanies the pericarditis, it may become hemorrhagic in the setting of severe and prolonged thrombocytopenia. Careful monitoring of the patient's status is indicated. The nurse should be aware of patients who are at risk for pericarditis and assess them for chest pain. If a patient complains of chest pain, the nurse should obtain an ECG to assist with diagnosis and further workup as indicated.

It is critical that pericardial effusions and fibrinous pericarditis are diagnosed early, as these may evolve to hemorrhagic myocarditis and cardiac tamponade. Important factors influencing the treatment of effusions are the rate at which the effusion accumulates (acute versus chronic) and whether the pericardium is scarred, adding an element of constrictive pericarditis. A chronic effusion may be followed with expectant observation (Shabetai, 2004). The nurse must recognize the signs of tamponade, as it is a medical emergency. Treatment of tamponade revolves around the removal of fluid. A pericardiocentesis can be performed by a cardiologist or surgeon, or a pericardial window, a more definitive procedure, can be performed by a surgeon (Lopez, 2001).

It is important to note that a subset of patients unexpectedly develop hemodynamic compromise within the first few hours postoperatively after pericardial fluid drainage, which can be fatal. *Paradoxical hemodynamic instability* (PHI) is defined as the development of unexpected vasopressor dependent hypotension in the immediate postoperative period requiring admission to the intensive care unit. The causes of this phenomenon remain unclear. It has been recommended that drainage of pericardial effusions be performed on a more gradual basis to reduce the chance of reexpansion pulmonary edema. It is unclear if the pathophysiology of PHI is similar to that underlying reexpansion pulmonary edema. Regardless, the nurse needs to be aware of this complication and closely monitor the patient's hemodynamic status (Wagner et al., 2011). Specific concerns with respect to transplant patients with a pericardial effusion include infection, both as an etiology for the effusion and as a risk of drainage in neutropenic patients. Effusions may become hemorrhagic in the setting of thrombocytopenia. Thrombocytopenia also complicates drainage. Transplant recipients may be hypotensive at baseline, thus complicating the diagnosis. The nurse should be alert to the diagnosis, especially in patients with chest pain.

Cardiac Dysrhythmias

Atrial Fibrillation

Pathophysiology: In A-fib, the regular impulses produced by the sinus node are overwhelmed by the rapid generated electrical discharges produced randomly by larger areas of triggering atrial tissue and/or the pulmonary veins. A-fib is usually noted 26–297 hours after the administration of melphalan with short duration of the arrhythmia (Olivieri et al., 1998). A-fib was also noted in patients who received Cy and TBI and occurred between days 0 and 79 (Murdych & Weisdorf, 2001).

Clinical features: Many of the symptoms of A-fib are subtle and nonspecific, even in the nontransplant population. Some patients can be completely asymptomatic, whereas other patients will complain of fatigue and shortness of breath or dyspnea with exertion. Palpitations are uncommonly the presenting complaint (Martin, 2001). Upon assessment, the nurse may notice an increase in the patient's heart rate when taking vital signs or an irregular rate on auscultation.

Diagnostic tests: ECG is the most useful diagnostic test and will show complete irregularity in the timing of the QRS complex in association with a baseline reflective of disorganized atrial activity or no clear atrial focus (Martin, 2001).

Differential diagnoses: Irregular rhythms noted on examination also may be secondary to supraventricular tachycardia (SVT) or ventricular tachycardia (VT).

Medical and nursing management: The treatment of A-fib in this patient population is the same as treatment in the general population and is discussed in Chapter 11. It is important to note, however, that treatment of A-fib in the HSCT setting has not been studied. Hypotension is often a complication of A-fib and patients may need fluid to treat hypotension. Efforts at controlling the patient's heart rate can be limited by the blood pressure response to the rapid rate, as well as to the agents meant to control the rate. Digoxin can be used to assist with rate control in this situation because it does not lower blood pressure; however, it takes significantly longer to work than beta-blockers and calcium channel blockers. Cardioversion, either with medications or with external defibrillation, is another treatment option. In one study, patients who developed A-fib secondary to Cy required cardioversion, indicating that medical management alone was not sufficient to control these arrhythmias (Murdych & Weisdorf, 2001). The success of maintaining normal sinus rhythm in the transplant patient often depends on the patient's underlying clinical status. The use of anticoagulation in the prevention of stroke in patients with A-fib is discussed in Chapter 12. It is important to note that there are no data specifically addressing the problems of anticoagulation in a patient following HSCT. In general, with thrombocytopenia less than 50,000 platelets, anticoagulation with warfarin, low-molecular-weight heparin, or aspirin is not considered safe. However, once the platelets have recovered, the patient's risk for stroke should be evaluated and the appropriate anticoagulation initiated.

Ventricular Dysrhythmias

Pathophysiology: Less common arrhythmias during transplant include ventricular fibrillation (V-fib), VT, and asystole. These arrhythmias all result in diminished cardiac output and are quickly lethal if untreated. Many ventricular arrhythmias occur weeks after the conditioning treatment, suggesting that although the treatments may contribute, arrhythmias in the transplant setting may just reflect seriously ill hospitalized patients who are at increased risk for cardiac arrhythmias. In a 2001 study by Murdych and Weisdorf, V-fib associated with conditioning with Cy and TBI occurred between days 0 and 8, while asystole after treatment with Cy and TBI occurred between days 0 and 22.

Clinical features: Patients with ventricular dysrhythmias may present with light-headedness, syncope, or unresponsiveness. On examination, a thready pulse or pulselessness or hypotension may be noted.

Diagnostic tests: The ECG of VT will demonstrate a wide-complex, usually monomorphic (uniform) tachycardia, though it may be polymorphic (variety of complexes) in the setting of torsades de pointes (erratic complex above and below isometric line). V-fib is similar to polymorphic VT with a constantly shifting QRS axis and amplitude secondary to multiple circulating reentrant wavelets in the ventricular myocardium, but it is significantly coarser in nature (Martin, 2001). The examples of the ECG tracings of the different ventricular dysrhythmias can be found in Chapter 13.

Differential diagnoses: The clinical picture of ventricular dysrhythmias may also be associated with asystole, cardiac tamponade, or other arrhythmias such as A-fib or SVT.

Medical and nursing management: The patient's electrolytes should be closely monitored, especially potassium and magnesium, which make the patient significantly more susceptible to problematic arrhythmias. VT, V-fib, pulseless electrical activity, and asystole all constitute medical emergencies but are not frequently encountered in the transplant setting. It is critical for the nurse to identify these life-threatening dysrhythmias, initiate appropriate interventions such as oxygenating and assessing hemodynamic stability, and alert the critical care team to initiate cardiopulmonary resuscitation (Murdych & Weisdorf, 2001) (see Table 9-4).

Table 9-4. Possible Cardiac Complications With Hematopoietic Stem Cell Transplantation				
Cardiac Diagnosis	**Physical Findings**	**Differential Diagnosis**	**Cardiac Testing**	**Intervention**
Cardiomyopathy	Dyspnea, chest pain, fatigue, or may be asymptomatic	Acute coronary syndrome, pneumonia, deconditioning	• Cardiac enzymes: elevated • Echocardiogram: abnormal wall motion • ECG: ST elevation, T-wave inversion	Medications: beta-blockers, ACE-Is, diuretics
				(Continued on next page)

(Continued on next page)

Table 9-4. Possible Cardiac Complications With Hematopoietic Stem Cell Transplantation *(Continued)*

Cardiac Diagnosis	Physical Findings	Differential Diagnosis	Cardiac Testing	Intervention
Heart failure	Dyspnea, fatigue, decreased activity, nocturnal dyspnea, lower-extremity edema, ascites, dizziness, orthostatic hypotension, coughing, wheezing, JVD, displaced atypical impulse, third heart sound	Strain of transplant, fluid overload secondary to transfusions, antibiotics, IV fluid, sepsis, deconditioning	• Brain natriuretic peptide: elevated • Chest x-ray: increased cardiothoracic ratio • Echocardiogram: increased left ventricular size, mass, decreased function	Medications (diuretics), volume restrictions if possible, strict I/O, daily weights, volume management
Pericarditis	Chest pain worse when lying down and better when sitting up, pleuritic chest pain, friction rub	Esophagitis, reflux, pneumonia, pulmonary embolus, myocardial injury	• ECG: ST segment elevation with PR depression	Medications: NSAIDs, colchicine, corticosteroids if able, pain control
Pericardial effusion	Often asymptomatic	Infection, bleeding, shock	• ECG: low-voltage electrical alternans	Monitoring for rate of accumulation
Pericardial tamponade	Tamponade, tachycardia, pulsus paradoxus, hypotension	Sepsis, bleeding, shock	• ECG: Tachycardia, low-voltage electrical alternans • Echocardiogram: evaluate size of effusion or evidence of tamponade	Pericardiocentesis, pericardial window for fluid drainage. Treat as a medical emergency.
Atrial fibrillation	Fatigue, SOB, DOE, palpitations, irregularly irregular pulse, or may be asymptomatic	SVT, VT	• ECG: irregular timing QRS complex with disorganized atrial activity	Beta-blockers, CCB, digoxin if unstable, cardioversion, IV fluid if hypotensive
V-fib, VT, and asystole	Light-headedness, syncope, unresponsiveness; on exam, a thready pulse or pulselessness may be noted with hypotension	Asystole, tamponade, atrial fibrillation, SVT	• ECG: VT wide complex, monomorphic, tachycardia • V-fib: wide QRS shifting axis and amplitude courser than VT • Asystole: flat line	Monitoring electrolytes (potassium, magnesium), CPR team. Treat as a medical emergency.

ACE-I—angiotensin-converting enzyme inhibitor; CCB—calcium channel blocker; CPR—cardiopulmonary resuscitation; DOE—dyspnea on exertion; ECG—electrocardiogram; I/O—intake/output; JVD—jugular venous distension; NSAIDs—nonsteroidal anti-inflammatory drugs; SOB—shortness of breath; SVT—supraventricular tachycardia; V-fib—ventricular fibrillation; VT—ventricular tachycardia.

Note. Based on information from Anderson et al., 2010; Huffman et al., 2010; Kasper & Baughman, 2001; Marinella, 1998; Martin, 2001; McMurray, 2010; Murdych & Weisdorf, 2001; Nussinovitch et al., 2011; Sharkey et al., 2011.

Transplant in Patients With Known Cardiac Disease

HSCT is continuing to evolve. The newer HSCT regimens, such as RIC, with improved techniques and supportive care allow more patients to receive transplantation. This includes patients with preexisting cardiac disease who used to be excluded because of concern that the underlying heart disease made the risk of transplant unmanageable.

Coronary Artery Disease

CAD often is part of the exclusion criteria for HSCT. Although these patients should be treated with caution, CAD should not prohibit patients from receiving this life-saving treatment. It is important to note that during the course of HSCT, patients are regularly taken off many of their cardiac medications including beta-blockers, statins, aspirin, and clopidogrel. A study by Stillwell et al. (2011) investigated the risk of transplants in patients with known CAD and found that patients with preexisting CAD did not have increased mortality or cardiac morbidity in the transplant setting. No statistically significant differences were seen in length of stay, cardiac events, intensive care unit admissions, or death during transplant and up to one year after. This study suggests that patients with CAD can be safely managed through transplant and should not be excluded or denied this treatment. They should, however, be monitored carefully with the assistance of a cardiology team and be restarted on cardiac medications when feasible. It is noted, though, that patients who have had a recent myocardial infarction, significantly reduced left ventricular function with severe heart failure, a large area of ischemia, uncontrolled arrhythmias, or significant angina are still not eligible for transplant because of unacceptable risk.

Cardiomyopathy

Similarly, in the past, patients with reduced LVEF were also denied eligibility for transplant. Qazilbash et al. (2009) examined the implications of allogeneic HSCT in patients whose EF was less than 45%. They concluded that patients with a low EF and good functional status can undergo transplant with acceptable risk. They did state that patients with cardiac risk factors, including CAD, myocardial infarction, smoking, hypertension, and hyperlipidemia, may be at increased risk for cardiac complications, most notably CHF and atrial fibrillation. However, no deaths related to cardiac complications occurred in this study. The final conclusion was that patients with a low EF and good functional status can be treated with transplant with an acceptable risk of cardiac complications.

It is important to note that outcomes data on patients with known cardiac disease undergoing transplant are extremely sparse. It is anticipated that as more patients with cardiac disease undergo transplant, effective peritransplant algorithms can be devised that can be instituted to safely guide these patients through this process.

Long-Term Cardiac Effects

Although getting the patients safely through transplant is the immediate goal, it is important to recognize the long-term cardiovascular effects with HSCT that can affect patients' mortality. The risk of premature death resulting from cardiac complications after HSCT was 2.3-fold higher compared with the U.S. general population (Bhatia et al., 2007). As more and more patients survive transplant, there must be continued focus on the management of the cardiac effects of transplant in the growing survivorship population.

Nonischemic Cardiomyopathy

Whether a result of chemotherapy or radiation, nonischemic cardiomyopathy may be reversible with treatment, but in some patients, it will be a long-term effect. Some patients can be considered full responders with complete recovery of their left ventricular function, whereas others may be partial responders or nonresponders. It is important that these patients know that they will be on long-term cardiac medications. The medications used are the same as for the treatment of heart failure associated with other etiologies. These medications are titrated as tolerated in an attempt to improve EF. During this titration, close follow-up is important, with blood pressure monitoring to determine if the patient is tolerating the increased medication dose and blood work to assess potassium levels and renal function. Patients should be alerted to sodium restrictions and assessment of volume status. They may need to be on diuretics temporarily or long term. It is important for these patients to know the signs of volume overload such as pedal edema, weight gain (3–5 lbs), shortness of breath, and exercise intolerance. Patients should be instructed to weigh themselves using the same scale, at the same time of day, and wearing similar clothing and to call the doctor if their weight is increasing. Patients should also be monitored with an echocardiogram to assess left ventricular response to medications. The frequency of echocardiograms is dependent upon patient symptoms and medication titration.

Development of Cardiac Risk Factors

Transplant survivors are also prone to develop cardiac risk factors. Post-transplant patients are at risk for hypothyroidism, which can contribute to diastolic hypertension, dyslipidemia, and nephrotic syndrome, which can promote dyslipidemia. GVHD is a complicated adverse effect of allogeneic transplants that can affect the liver, which has been related to severe hyperlipidemia. The medications used to treat GVHD, including immunosuppressive therapy and glucocorticoids, can contribute to elevated triglycerides and dyslipidemia. In transplant survivors, risk factors such as diabetes, dyslipidemia, and hypertension are associated with higher risk of cardiovascular events. Transplant recipients with a life expectancy of 5–10 years or more should be treated with the same recommendations as the general population to reduce morbidity and mortality from cardiovascular disease (Griffith et al., 2010).

Hypothyroidism

Hypothyroidism is one of the most common forms of endocrine dysfunction in patients following HSCT, which may be discovered years after transplant. Risk factors for the development of hypothyroidism include MA conditioning and TBI, although fractionated doses of radiation may decrease the risk. Hypothyroidism after radiation is thought to be secondary to vascular degeneration and cell death of the capillary endothelium (Felicetti et al., 2011). Subclinical hypothyroidism has been associated with increased systemic vascular resistance, arterial stiffness, altered endothelial function, increased atherosclerosis, and altered coagulability and may accelerate development of CAD. Elevated thyroid-stimulating hormone levels have been associated with an increased cardiovascular risk (Rodondi et al., 2010). These changes are caused by decreased thyroid hormone action on multiple organs including the heart, liver, and peripheral vasculature and are potentially reversible with thyroid hormone replacement. Treatment with either full dose (1.6 mcg/kg/day) or, in older adults, low-dose replacement therapy (25–50 mcg/day) with L-thyroxine has shown improvement in thyroid and cardiovascular functional measures (Klein & Danzi, 2007). Levels should be measured four to six weeks after initiation of therapy, after any change in the dose, and annually after levels become stable. Hormone requirements may increase over time if thyroid dysfunction progresses (Cooper, 2001).

Dyslipidemia

Dyslipidemia is often secondary to predisposing causes, such as obesity and familial hypercholesterolemia. In the post-transplant patient population, dyslipidemia may also be secondary to GVHD. Chronic GVHD can cause cholestatic liver disease, which causes the formation of lipoprotein X. Medications used to treat GVHD, such as immunosuppressants and glucocorticoids, can cause dyslipidemia. Glucocorticoids affect lipid metabolism and influence weight gain and hyperglycemia. Cyclosporine may interfere with bile acid synthesis, block the LDL receptor, and increase LDL by reducing the activity of lipoprotein lipase while increasing the activity of hepatic lipase (Griffith et al., 2010). No guidelines have been published for the treatment of dyslipidemia in this population, and further investigation is needed.

The role of statin therapy in the treatment of dyslipidemia is well established and is considered to be first-line treatment for elevated LDL. According to Griffith et al. (2010), statins should be considered first-line therapy for dyslipidemia in HSCT recipients. It is important to note that cyclosporins can increase some statin drug levels. For this reason, pravastatin, rosuvastatin, and fluvastatin are the preferred treatment options for patients receiving cyclosporin therapy. Liver function tests should be monitored more closely in this population, within two to four weeks after the initiation of treatment. Treatment should also be initiated for severe hypertriglyceridemia. Omega-3 fatty acids and niacin should be considered, with long-acting niacin often being better tolerated (Griffith et al., 2010). Patients should have cholesterol values and liver function tests carefully monitored with titration of medications as needed. Diabetes, an important risk factor for CAD, is also a concern in the survivorship population, as these patients may be receiving steroids for GVHD. Fasting glucose and hemoglobin A1c should be periodically evaluated.

Conclusion

HSCT is a life-saving measure for patients with a number of malignancies. Through improved transplant techniques and supportive care, this treatment option is offered to more patients, many of whom either come to transplant with underlying cardiac disease or will experience a cardiac complication with transplant. Cardiac risks are present during each phase of treatment, in addition to risks that extend into the survivorship period. Nurses are at the forefront of patient and family education, especially regarding the symptoms and signs of cardiac morbidity in the transplant setting and with the various treatment options. With a combination of expert medical and nursing care, identification and treatment of cardiac effects can be initiated to decrease morbidity and mortality in the transplant population.

References

Anderson, R., Joy, S., Carkido, A., Anthony, S., Smyntek, D., Stewart, D., … Butler, E.T. (2010). Development of a congestive heart failure protocol in a rehabilitation setting. *Rehabilitation Nursing, 35*(1), 3–7, 30. doi:10.1002/j.2048-7940.2010.tb00024.x

Bacigalupo, A., Ballen, K., Rizzo, D., Giralt, S., Lazarus, H., Ho, V., … Horowitz, M. (2009). Defining the intensity of conditioning regimens: Working definitions. *Biology of Blood and Marrow Transplantation, 15,* 1628–1633. doi:10.1016/j.bbmt.2009.07.004

Bearman, S.I., Petersen, F.B., Schor, R.A., Denney, J.D., Fisher, L.D., Appelbaum, F.R., & Buckner, C.D. (1990). Radionuclide ejection fractions in the evaluation of patients being considered for bone marrow transplantation: Risk for cardiac toxicity. *Bone Marrow Transplantation, 5,* 173–177.

Bhatia, S., Francisco, L., Carter, A., Sun, C.L., Baker, K.S., Gurney, J.G., … Weisdorf, D.J. (2007). Late mortality after allogeneic hematopoietic cell transplantation and functional status of long-term survivors: Report from the Bone Marrow Transplant Survivor Study. *Blood, 110,* 3784–3792.

Braverman, A.C., Antin, J.H., Plappert, M.T., Cook, E.F., & Lee, R.T. (1991). Cyclophosphamide cardiotoxicity in bone marrow transplantation: A prospective evaluation of new dosing regimens. *Journal of Clinical Oncology, 9,* 1215–1223.

Brown, J., & Morgan-Hughes, N.J. (2005). Aortic stenosis and non-cardiac surgery. *Continuing Education in Anaesthesia, Critical Care and Pain, 5*(1), 1–4. doi:10.1093/bjaceaccp/mki001

Broxmeyer, H.E. (2011). Insights into the biology of cord blood stem/progenitor cells. *Cell Proliferation, 44*(Suppl. 1), 55–59. doi:10.1111/j.1365-2184.2010.00728.x

Buccheri, G., Ferrigno, D., & Tamburini, M. (1996). Karnofsky and ECOG performance status scoring in lung cancer: A prospective, longitudinal study of 536 patients from a single institution. *European Journal of Cancer, 32A,* 1135–1141. doi:10.1016/0959-8049(95)00664-8

Buckner, C.D. (1999). Autologous bone marrow transplants to hematopoietic stem cell support with peripheral blood stem cells: A historical perspective. *Journal of Hematotherapy, 8,* 233–236. doi:10.1089/106161299320244

Carella, A.M., Beltrami, G., Scalzulli, P.R., Carella A.M., Jr., & Corsetti, M.T. (2004). Alemtuzumab can successfully treat steroid-refractory acute graft-versus-host disease (aGVHD). *Bone Marrow Transplantation, 33,* 131–132. doi:10.1038/sj.bmt.1704322

Chatterjee, K., & Massie, B. (2007). Systolic and diastolic heart failure: Differences and similarities. *Journal of Cardiac Failure, 13,* 569–576. doi:10.1016/j.cardfail.2007.04.006

Chow, E.J., Mueller, B.A., Baker, K.S., Cushing-Haugen, K.L., Flowers, M.E., Martin, P.J., … Lee, S.J. (2011). Cardiovascular hospitalizations and mortality among recipients of hematopoietic stem cell transplantation. *Annals of Internal Medicine, 155,* 21–32. doi:10.1059/0003-4819-155-1-201107050-00004

Cooper, D.S. (2001). Clinical practice. Subclinical hypothyroidism. *New England Journal of Medicine, 345,* 260–265. doi:10.1056/NEJM200107263450406

Corradini, P., Zallio, F., Mariotti, J., Farina, L., Bregni, M., Valagussa, P., … Olivieri, A. (2005). Effect of age and previous autologous transplantation on nonrelapse mortality and survival in patients treated with reduced-intensity conditioning and allografting for advanced hematologic malignancies. *Journal of Clinical Oncology, 23,* 6690–6698. doi:10.1200/JCO.2005.07.070

Cutler, C., Li, S., Kim, H.T., Laglenne, P., Szeto, K.C., Hoffmeister, L., … Antin, J.H. (2005). Mucositis after allogeneic hematopoietic stem cell transplantation: A cohort study of methotrexate- and non-methotrexate-containing graft-versus-host disease prophylaxis regimens. *Biology of Blood and Marrow Transplantation, 11,* 383–388. doi:10.1016/j.bbmt.2005.02.006

Felicetti, F., Manicone, R., Corrias, A., Manieri, C., Biasin, E., Bini, I., … Brignardello, E. (2011). Endocrine late effects after total body irradiation in patients who received hematopoietic cell transplantation during childhood: A retrospective study from a single institution. *Journal of Cancer Research and Clinical Oncology, 137,* 1343–1348. doi:10.1007/s00432-011-1004-2

Gajewski, J.L., Johnson, V.V., Sandler, S.G., Sayegh, A., & Klumpp, T.R. (2008). A review of transfusion practice before, during, and after hematopoietic progenitor cell transplantation. *Blood, 112,* 3036–3047. doi:10.1182/blood-2007-10-118372

Gharib, M.I., & Burnett, A.K. (2002). Chemotherapy-induced cardiotoxicity: Current practice and prospects of prophylaxis. *European Journal of Heart Failure, 4,* 235–242. doi:10.1016/S1388-9842(01)00201-X

Giralt, S., Logan, B., Rizzo, D., Zhang, M.J., Ballen, K., Emmanouilides, C., ... Weisdorf, D. (2007). Reduced-intensity conditioning for unrelated donor progenitor cell transplantation: Long-term follow-up of the first 285 reported to the National Marrow Donor Program. *Biology of Blood and Marrow Transplantation, 13,* 844–852. doi:10.1016/j.bbmt.2007.03.011

Givertz, M.M., & Colucci, W.S. (2001). Heart failure. In J. Noble (Ed.), *Textbook of primary care medicine* (3rd ed., pp. 578–596). St. Louis, MO: Mosby.

Gottdiener, J.S., Appelbaum, F.R., Ferrans, V.J., Deisseroth, A., & Ziegler, J. (1981). Cardiotoxicity associated with high-dose cyclophosphamide therapy. *Archives of Internal Medicine, 141,* 758–763.

Griffith, M.L., Savani, B.N., & Boord, J.B. (2010). Dyslipidemia after allogeneic hematopoietic stem cell transplantation: Evaluation and management. *Blood, 116,* 1197–1204. doi:10.1182/blood-2010-03-276576

Hamadani, M., Craig, M., Awan, F.T., & Devine, S.M. (2010). How we approach patient evaluation for hematopoietic stem cell transplantation. *Bone Marrow Transplantation, 45,* 1259–1268. doi:10.1038/bmt.2010.94

Hertenstein, B., Stefanic, M., Schmeiser, T., Scholz, M., Goller, V., Clausen, M., ... Kochs, M. (1994). Cardiac toxicity of bone marrow transplantation: Predictive value of cardiologic evaluation before transplant. *Journal of Clinical Oncology, 12,* 998–1004.

Huffman, C., Wagman, G., Fudim, M., Zolty, R., & Vittorio, T. (2010). Reversible cardiomyopathies—A review. *Transplantation Proceedings, 42,* 3673–3678. doi:10.1016/j.transproceed.2010.08.034

Imazio, M., Bobbio, M, Cecchi, E., Demarie, D., Demichelis, D., Pomari, F., ... Trinchero, R. (2005). Colchicine in addition to conventional therapy for acute pericarditis: Results of the Colchicine for Acute pericarditis (COPE) trial. *Circulation, 112,* 2012–2016. doi:10.1161/CIRCULATIONAHA.105.542738

Kasper, E.K., & Baughman, K.L. (2001). Myocardial and pericardial disease. In J. Noble (Ed.), *Textbook of primary care medicine* (3rd ed., pp. 615–623). St. Louis, MO: Mosby.

Klein, I., & Danzi, S. (2007). Thyroid disease and the heart. *Circulation, 116,* 1725–1735. doi:10.1161/CIRCULATIONAHA.106.678326

Leger, C.S., & Nevill, T.J. (2004). Hematopoietic stem cell transplantation: A primer for the primary care physician. *Canadian Medical Association Journal, 170,* 1569–1577. doi:10.1503/cmaj.1011625

Lenihan, D.J., Alencar, A.J., Yang, D., Kurzrock, R., Keating M.J., & Duvic, M. (2004). Cardiac toxicity of alemtuzumab in patients with mycosis fungoides/Sézary syndrome. *Blood, 104,* 655–658. doi:10.1182/blood-2003-07-2345

Lilly, L.S. (2001). Ischemic heart disease. In J. Noble (Ed.), *Textbook of primary care medicine* (3rd ed., pp. 545–570). St. Louis, MO: Mosby.

Little, W.C. (2008). Heart failure with a normal left ventricular ejection fraction: Diastolic heart failure. *Transactions of the American Clinical and Climatological Association, 119,* 93–99.

Lopez, A.M. (2001). Management of oncologic emergencies. In J. Noble (Ed.), *Textbook of primary care medicine* (3rd ed., pp. 1084–1092). St. Louis, MO: Mosby.

Marinella, M.A. (1998). Electrocardiographic manifestations and differential diagnosis of acute pericarditis. *American Family Physician, 57,* 699–704.

Martin, D.T. (2001). Arrhythmias. In J. Noble (Ed.), *Textbook of primary care medicine* (3rd ed., pp. 525–537). St. Louis, MO: Mosby.

McMurray, J.J. (2010). Clinical practice. Systolic heart failure. *New England Journal of Medicine, 362,* 228–238. doi:10.1056/NEJMcp0909392

Morandi, P., Ruffini, P.A., Benvenuto, G.M., Raimondi, R., & Fosser, V. (2005). Cardiac toxicity of high-dose chemotherapy. *Bone Marrow Transplantation, 35,* 323–334. doi:10.1038/sj.bmt.1704763

Murdych, T., & Weisdorf, D.J. (2001). Serious cardiac complications during bone marrow transplantation at the University of Minnesota, 1977–1997. *Bone Marrow Transplantation, 28,* 283–287. doi:10.1038/sj.bmt.1703133

National Cancer Institute. (2011a, September). Adult acute myeloid leukemia treatment (PDQ®). Retrieved from http://www.cancer.gov/cancertopics/pdq/treatment/adultAML/Patient

National Cancer Institute. (2011b, July). Plasma cell neoplasms (including multiple myeloma) treatment (PDQ®). Retrieved from http://www.cancer.gov/cancertopics/pdq/treatment/ myeloma/Patient

National Institutes of Health. (2009). Stem cell information. Retrieved from http://stemcells.nih.gov/info/basics/defaultpage

National Marrow Donor Program. (2011, July). Evaluating adult patients prior to hematopoietic cell transplant. Retrieved from http://www.marrow.org/PHYSICIAN/Tx_Indications_Timing_Referral/Evaluating_Adult_Patients_Prio/index.html

Ng, M.K.C., & Celermajer, D.S. (2004). Glucocorticoid treatment and cardiovascular disease. *Heart, 90,* 829–830. doi:10.1136/hrt.2003.031492

Niehof, M., & Borlak, J. (2011). HNF4alpha dysfunction as a molecular rational for cyclosporine induced hypertension. *PLoS One, 6,* e16319. doi:10.1371/journal.pone.0016319

Nussinovitch, U., Goitein, O., Nussinovitch, N., & Altman, A. (2011). Distinguishing a heart attack from the "broken heart syndrome" (Takotsubo cardiomyopathy). *Journal of Cardiovascular Nursing, 26,* 524–529. doi:10.1097/JCN.0b013e31820e2a90

Oshima, K., Sakata-Yanagimoto, M., Asano-Mori, Y., Izutsu, K., Watanabe, T., Shoda, E., … Kanda, Y. (2005). Cardiac complications after haploidentical HLA-mismatched hematopoietic stem cell transplantation using in vivo alemtuzumab. *Bone Marrow Transplantation, 36,* 821–824. doi:10.1038/sj.bmt.1705145

Olivieri, A., Corvatta, L., Montanari, M., Brunori, M., Offidani, M., Ferretti, G.F., … Leoni, P. (1998). Paroxysmal atrial fibrillation after high-dose melphalan in five patients autotransplanted with blood progenitor cells. *Bone Marrow Transplantation, 21,* 1049–1053. doi:10.1038/sj.bmt.1701217

Pilgrim, T.M., & Wyss, T.R. (2008). Takotsubo cardiomyopathy or transient left ventricular apical ballooning syndrome: A systematic review. *International Journal of Cardiology, 124,* 283–292. doi:10.1016/j.ijcard.2007.07.002

Qazilbash, M.H., Amjad, A.I., Qureshi, S., Qureshi, S.R., Saliba, R.M., Khan, Z.U., … Champlin, R.E. (2009). Outcome of allogeneic hematopoietic stem cell transplantation in patients with low left ventricular ejection fraction. *Biology of Blood and Marrow Transplantation, 15,* 1265–1270. doi:10.1016/j.bbmt.2009.06.001

Reece, D.E., Bredeson, C., Perez, W.S., Jagannath, S., Zhang, M.J., Ballen, K.K., … Vesole, D.H. (2003). Autologous stem cell transplantation in multiple myeloma patients < 60 vs ≥ 60 years of age. *Bone Marrow Transplantation, 32,* 1135–1143. doi:10.1038/sj.bmt.1704288

Ritchie, D.S., Seymour, J.F., Roberts, A.W., Szer, J., & Grigg, A.P. (2001). Acute left ventricular failure following melphalan and fludarabine conditioning. *Bone Marrow Transplantation, 28,* 101–103. doi:10.1038/sj.bmt.1703098

Rodondi, N., den Elzen, W.P., Bauer, D.C., Cappola, A.R., Razvi, S., Walsh, J.P., … Gussekloo, J. (2010). Subclinical hypothyroidism and the risk of coronary heart disease and mortality. *JAMA, 304,* 1365–1374. doi:10.1001/jama.2010.1361

Sakata-Yanagimoto, M., Kanda, Y., Nakagawa, M., Asano-Mori, Y., Kandabashi, K., Izutsu, K., … Hirai, H. (2004). Predictors for severe cardiac complications after hematopoietic stem cell transplantation. *Bone Marrow Transplantation, 33,* 1043–1047. doi:10.1038/sj.bmt.1704487

Schag, C.C., Heinrich, R.L., & Ganz, P.A. (1984). Karnofsky performance status revisited: Reliability, validity and guidelines. *Journal of Clinical Oncology, 2,* 187–193.

Schick, E.C. (2001). Valvular heart disease. In J. Noble (Ed.), *Textbook of primary care medicine* (3rd ed., pp. 596–608). St. Louis, MO: Mosby.

Shabetai, R. (2004). Pericardial effusion: Haemodynamic spectrum. *Heart, 90,* 255–256. doi:10.1136/hrt.2003.024810

Sharkey, S.W., Lesser, J.R., & Maron, B.J. (2011). Takotsubo (stress) cardiomyopathy. *Circulation, 124,* e460–e462. doi:10.1161/CIRCULATIONAHA.111.052662

Slavin, S., Nagler, A., Naparstek, E., Kapelushnik, Y., Aker, M., Cividalli, G., … Or, R. (1998). Nonmyeloablative stem cell transplantation and cell therapy as an alternative to conventional bone marrow transplantation with lethal cytoreduction for the treatment of malignant and nonmalignant hematologic diseases. *Blood, 91,* 756–763.

Souverein, P.C., Berard, A., Van Staa, T.P., Cooper, C., Egberts, A.C.G., Leufkens, H.G.M., & Walker, B.R. (2004). Use of oral glucocorticoids and risk of cardiovascular and cerebrovascular disease in a population based case-control study. *Heart, 90,* 859–865. doi:10.1136/hrt.2003.020180

St. Jude Children's Research Hospital. (2011). Stem cell/bone marrow transplant—Historical perspective (1970s–present). Retrieved from http://www.stjude.org/stjude/v/index.jsp?vgnextoid=8370fa2454e70110VgnVCM1000001e0215acRCRD&vgnextchannel=761bbfe82e118010VgnVCM1000000e2015acRCRD

Stillwell, E.E., Wessler, J.D., Rebolledo, B.J., Steingart, R.M., Petrlik, E.L., Jakubowski, A.A., & Schaffer, W.L. (2011). Retrospective outcome data for hematopoietic stem cell transplantation in patients with concurrent coronary artery disease. *Biology of Blood and Marrow Transplantation, 17,* 1182–1186. doi:10.1016/j.bbmt.2010.12.698

Wagner, P.L., McAleer, E., Stillwell, E., Bott, M., Rusch, V.W., Schaffer, W., & Huang, J. (2011). Pericardial effusions in the cancer population: Prognostic factors after pericardial window and the impact of paradoxical hemodynamic instability. *Journal of Thoracic and Cardiovascular Surgery, 141,* 34–38. doi:10.1016/j.jtcvs.2010.09.015

Yeh, E.T., Tong, A.T., Lenihan, D.J., Yusuf, S.W., Swafford, J., Champion, C., ... Ewer, M.S. (2004). Cardiovascular complications of cancer therapy: Diagnosis, pathogenesis, and management. *Circulation, 109*, 3122–3131. doi:10.1161/01.cir.0000133187.74800.b9

Zangari, M., Henzlova, M.J., Ahmad, S., Scigliano, E., Isola, L., Platnik, J., ... Fruchtman, S.M. (1999). Predictive value of left ventricular ejection fraction in stem cell transplantation. *Bone Marrow Transplantation, 23*, 917–920. doi:10.1038/sj.bmt.1701734

CHAPTER 10

Heart Failure in Patients With Cancer

Anecita P. Fadol, PhD, RN, FNP-BC, FAANP

Introduction

Heart failure (HF) is a dreaded complication for patients with cancer and survivors that can result from the cardiotoxic effects of many antineoplastic agents, especially anthracyclines (Ewer, Swain, Cardinale, Fadol, & Suter, 2011), high-dose cyclophosphamide (Carver et al., 2007), and trastuzumab (Ewer & Ewer, 2008). Because of the advances in cancer detection and cancer treatment, the number of individuals living years after their cancer diagnosis has increased steadily, and hence the likelihood of developing HF secondary to cardiotoxicity has increased. The concurrence of HF and cancer in the same patient presents a complex array of physiologic, psychological, social, and healthcare delivery issues, making management a challenge.

The prevalence of HF in patients with cancer is not clearly established, but data from the oncology literature indicate that more than half of all patients exposed to anthracyclines will show some degree of cardiac dysfunction 10–20 years after treatment and that 5% of those patients will develop overt HF (Steinherz, Steinherz, Tan, Heller, & Murphy, 1991). Cancer survivors who develop late anthracycline-induced cardiotoxicity with New York Heart Association (NYHA) class III or IV HF have a poor prognosis, with a one-year mortality of 40% and a two-year mortality of 60% (Felker et al., 2000). However, the clinical magnitude of this diagnosis is unknown. The overall incidence may be underestimated because even when patients with cancer are admitted to the hospital for HF exacerbation, cancer—not HF—is the primary coding diagnosis listed. Thus, when an insurance claims database is queried to track statistical data for hospital admissions, an HF diagnosis may not be documented.

Understanding the epidemiology and pathophysiology of HF, recognizing the possible etiologies, identifying the early signs and symptoms, and using the available diagnostic modalities are essential for devising effective prevention strategies and implementing therapeutic approaches to effectively manage HF and improve a patient's quality of life. This chapter addresses these issues to assist the clinician in managing the complex issues of HF in patients with cancer.

What Is Heart Failure?

HF is a complex clinical syndrome that can result from any structural or cardiac disorder that impairs the ability of the ventricle to fill or eject blood (Hunt et al., 2005). The clinical syndrome of HF is the final pathway for a myriad of diseases that affect the heart. HF syndrome is characterized by manifestations of intravascular and interstitial volume overload and inadequate tissue perfusion: fatigue, shortness of breath, and lower-extremity edema, which are the cardinal signs of HF.

Terms such as *cardiac arrest, myocardial infarction, cardiomyopathy*, and *cardiotoxicity* do not represent HF, but they may be easily confused. Myocardial infarction, also known as a heart attack, is the death of the heart muscle from the sudden blockage of a coronary artery usually caused by a blood clot. Cardiac arrest, or *asystole*, refers to situations in which there is no cardiac output. These conditions are not HF per se but can result in HF or sudden cardiac death. Cardiomyopathy, on the other hand, refers to disorders of the heart muscle, which can be ischemic (decreased blood supply to the cardiac muscle) or nonischemic (secondary to the effects of cancer therapies, including chemotherapeutic agents, radiation, and targeted therapy) (see Chapters 2, 3, and 4). Cardiotoxicity, which is defined by the National Cancer Institute (n.d.) as "toxicity that affects the heart," can result from cancer treatments such as chemotherapy, radiation therapy, or biologic therapy. Chemotherapy can cause reversible or irreversible damage to cardiomyocytes, resulting in cardiotoxicity that may manifest as subclinical heart disease, mild left ventricular (LV) dysfunction, or overt HF. The term *congestive heart failure* is sometimes used when the body tissues become congested because of the heart's inability to meet the metabolic demands of the body. In this scenario, cardiac output is low and the body becomes congested with fluid, manifesting symptoms of shortness of breath, fatigue, abdominal bloating, or lower-extremity edema. Because not all patients with HF experience pulmonary and systemic congestion, this term is not frequently used today.

Causes of Heart Failure in Patients With Cancer

The most common cause of HF in the general population is coronary artery disease resulting in ischemic cardiomyopathy (Hunt et al., 2005). In patients with cancer, the risk for developing HF is increased as a result of conventional risk factors (see Figure 10-1) as well as nonischemic cardiomyopathy associated with antineoplastic agents (see Table 10-1). In addition, several comorbid conditions (see Figure 10-2) in a patient with cancer can result in HF. Thus, almost any form of cardiovascular disease and any of these comorbid conditions may eventually lead to impairment of LV function, resulting in HF.

Pathophysiology of Heart Failure

The pathophysiology of HF resulting from the adverse effects of cancer therapy is heterogeneous. Identification of single potential mechanisms is difficult because the majority of patients with cancer are not only treated with a multitude of cancer drugs but also may have been exposed to potentially cardiotoxic radiation therapy. The patho-

---

Figure 10-1. Risk Factors for the Development of Heart Failure in Patients With Cancer

- Hypertension
- Ischemic heart disease
- Cardiotoxic agents (e.g., anthracycline, trastuzumab)
- Diabetes mellitus/metabolic syndrome
- Obesity

- Familial history/genetic markers
- Low ejection fraction
- Impaired diastolic function
- Left ventricular hypertrophy
- Radiation treatment to left side of chest

Note. Based on information from Carver et al., 2007; Swain et al., 2003.

Table 10-1. Antineoplastic Agents That Can Cause Heart Failure

Agent	Incidence (%)
Anthracyclines	
Doxorubicin	3–26
Epirubicin	0.9–3.3
Idarubicin	5–18
Alkylating agents	
Cyclophosphamide	7–28
Ifosfamide	17
Anthraquinone	
Mitoxantrone	2.6–13
Antitumor antibiotic	
Mitomycin	15.3*
Antimetabolite	
Clofarabine	27
Antimicrotubule agent	
Docetaxel	2.3–8
Proteasome inhibitor	
Bortezomib	2.5
Monoclonal antibody tyrosine kinase inhibitors	
Bevacizumab	1–3.8
Trastuzumab	2–28
Small-molecule tyrosine kinase inhibitor	
Dasatinib	2–4
Imatinib	0.5–1.7
Lapatinib	0.2–2.2
Sunitinib	4–11
Sorafenib	< 1

*When used in combination with doxorubicin

Note. Based on information from Clinical Pharmacology, 2010; Guarneri et al., 2006; Khakoo et al., 2008; Pai & Nahata, 2000; Swain et al., 2003; Thompson Reuters Micromedex, 2011; Yeh & Bickford, 2009.

From "Cardiovascular Adverse Events Associated With Cancer Therapy," by A. Fadol and T. Lech, 2011, *Journal of the Advanced Practitioner in Oncology, 2,* p. 235. Copyright 2011 by Harborside Press. Reprinted with permission.

Figure 10-2. Comorbid Conditions That Can Cause Heart Failure

- Amyloidosis
- Cardiotoxic chemotherapy
- Coronary artery disease
- Endocarditis, myocarditis
- Hemochromatosis
- Hypertension

- Mantle radiation to the chest
- Persistent tachycardia
- Pericardial disease
- Stress induced (takotsubo cardiomyopathy)
- Sepsis
- Thyroid disorders

Note. Based on information from Boufidou et al., 2010; Ewer & Lippman, 2005; Giampaolo et al., 2011; Hunt et al., 2005; Martinelli et al., 2011; Murphy & Oudit, 2010; Prasad et al., 2008.

From "Cardiovascular Adverse Events Associated With Cancer Therapy," by A. Fadol and T. Lech, 2011, *Journal of the Advanced Practitioner in Oncology, 2,* p. 237. Copyright 2011 by Harborside Press. Reprinted with permission.

---

physiologic mechanisms leading to chemotherapy-induced cardiomyopathy ultimately resulting in HF are mainly associated with myocardial cell loss, due to either apoptosis or necrosis. Anthracyclines are among the best-characterized chemotherapeutic agents leading to myocardial cell loss (Lipshultz et al., 1995; Singal & Iliskovic, 1998). Some of the new biologic anticancer drugs associated with cardiomyopathy and HF include targeted therapies such as trastuzumab, imatinib, and bevacizumab (Drímal, Zúrová-Nedelcevová, Knezl, Sotníková, & Navarová, 2006; Kerkelä et al., 2006; Slamon et al., 2001). The incidence of HF is increased when trastuzumab is combined with other anticancer agents such as anthracyclines or paclitaxel. Paclitaxel induces myofibrillar structural damage secondary to basal phosphorylation of the Erk1/2 kinase and increased oxidative stress (Pentassuglia et al., 2007). The resulting ventricular dysfunction can occur in patients with decreased or normal ejection fraction (EF) and is classified as either systolic or diastolic dysfunction. Please refer to Chapters 2 and 3 for further discussion of the pathophysiologic mechanisms of cardiomyopathy that can potentially result in HF.

Stages of Heart Failure

In 2001, the American College of Cardiology (ACC) and the American Heart Association (AHA) developed a new approach to the classification of HF and identified four stages in HF development (see Table 10-2) that emphasized both the evolution and the progression of the disease (Hunt et al., 2005). This classification is intended to guide clinicians in the early identification of established risk factors and structural prerequisites for the development of HF and in the suggested therapeutic interventions even before the appearance of LV dysfunction or HF symptoms. Stage A includes patients who have risk factors (e.g., hypertension, coronary artery disease, diabetes mellitus) that can predispose for the development of HF but who do not yet demonstrate LV dysfunction or hypertrophy. Patients with cancer who have previously received antineoplastic agents with potential cardiotoxic adverse effects or radiation to the left side of the chest are included in stage A. Stage B includes those patients who have demonstrated LV hypertrophy, impaired LV function, or both but are asymptomatic. Stage C includes patients with current or past symptoms of HF associated with underlying structural disease, whereas stage D consists of patients with refractory HF who might be eligible for advanced HF treatment (e.g., mechanical circulatory support, cardiac transplantation) or for end-of-life care or hospice care. Similar to the staging system for cancer, in the HF staging approach, patients would be expected to advance from one stage to the next unless progression of the

Stage	Description	Patient Characteristics	Therapy
A	High risk for developing HF but without structural heart disease or symptoms of HF	HTN, coronary artery disease, diabetes mellitus, metabolic syndrome, family history of cardiomyopathy, cardiotoxic chemotherapy	Treat HTN and lipids, TLC, smoking cessation, dose modification or discontinuation of chemotherapy
B	Structural heart disease but asymptomatic	Previous myocardial infarction, LVH, low LVEF, asymptomatic valvular disease	All measures in stage A; ACE-I or ARB, and beta-blockers in appropriate patients
C	Structural heart disease with prior or current symptoms	Known structural heart disease, shortness of breath, fatigue, reduced exercise tolerance	All measures in stages A and B; diuretics, aldosterone antagonist, hydralazine, CRT, AICD in selected patients
D	Refractory end-stage HF	Marked symptoms at rest despite maximum medical therapy	All measures in stages A, B, and C; decision on appropriate level of care (compassionate end-of-life, hospice, chromic inotropes, permanent mechanical support)

Table 10-2. Stages of Heart Failure

ACE-I—angiotensin-converting enzyme inhibitor; AICD—automatic implantable cardioverter defibrillator; ARB—angiotensin receptor blocker; CRT—cardiac resynchronization therapy; HF—heart failure; HTN—hypertension; LVEF—left ventricular ejection fraction; LVH—left ventricular hypertrophy; TLC—therapeutic lifestyle changes

Note. Based on information from Hunt et al., 2009.

disease was slowed or stopped by treatment. The ACC/AHA classification system was intended to complement but not replace the NYHA functional classification, which is based primarily on the severity of symptoms (Hunt et al., 2005).

Classification of Heart Failure

Several classification methods for HF exist. Possible classification categories include type of onset, side of the heart involved, strength of ventricular contraction, and degree of functional impairment.

Type of Onset

Acute heart failure: The term *acute heart failure* is often used to describe de novo HF or decompensation of chronic HF. This type of onset is commonly referred to as *acute decompensated heart failure* (ADHF) to describe exacerbated HF characterized by increases in symptoms such as dyspnea, fatigue, and fluid retention. ADHF is not a single phenomenon but a group of syndromes that can include hypertensive crisis, pulmonary edema, cardiogenic shock, worsening chronic HF, and advanced or end-stage HF (Fleisher et al., 2007). Precipitating factors for ADHF include uncontrolled hypertension, acute coronary syndrome, arrhythmias, infectious process, pericardial disease, cardiotoxic agents, fluid overload, and nonadherence to prescribed medications or dietary restrictions (Fadol, 2006). Patients with cancer presenting to the emergency department with ADHF are often hemodynamically unstable and have severe symptoms of dyspnea and fluid overload (Fadol, 2006).

Chronic heart failure: Chronic HF is the end result of a long sequence of events of clinical syndromes caused by cardiac dysfunction. In cancer survivors, most cases of chronic HF occur as an end result of late-onset chronic progressive cardiomyopathy secondary to anthracycline-based chemotherapy. This condition can manifest with symptoms after one year to decades after initiation of therapy (Bristow et al., 1978; Pai & Nahata, 2000; Silber, 2004).

Side of the Heart Involved

Left-sided heart failure: Left-sided HF, or LV failure, involves failure on the left side of the heart, which pumps blood to the systemic circulation, thus resulting in congestion of the pulmonary vasculature. The congestion manifests in predominantly respiratory symptoms, including shortness of breath on exertion and, in severe cases, dyspnea at rest. Other symptoms include orthopnea (increased breathlessness when lying flat), which is measured by the number of pillows required to lie comfortably, and paroxysmal nocturnal dyspnea (nighttime attack of severe breathlessness, usually occurring several hours after lying in bed). The patient may resort to sleeping while sitting up in a recliner. Easy fatigability and exercise intolerance are common symptoms related to respiratory compromise. Common signs indicating LV failure include a laterally displaced apical pulse as a result of an enlarged heart, a gallop rhythm due to increased blood flow, and increased intracardiac pressure. Heart murmurs may indicate the presence of valvular heart disease, as either a cause (e.g., aortic stenosis) or a result (e.g., mitral regurgitation) of HF. Rales or crackles are heard initially in the lung bases and, in severe cases, throughout the lung fields when pulmonary edema is present. Tachypnea (increased rate and work of breathing) is a common sign as fluid starts to flood the alveoli. Cyanosis, which suggests hypoxemia, is a late sign of extremely severe pulmonary edema.

Right-sided heart failure: Right-sided HF may manifest with similar symptoms as left-sided HF, but on physical examination patients may present with pitting peripheral edema, ascites, hepatomegaly, and elevated jugular venous pressure, which is a marker of fluid overload.

Strength of Ventricular Contraction

Systolic heart failure: Systolic HF, or systolic dysfunction, is characterized by the inability of the ventricles to eject an adequate volume of blood during systole as a result of reduced pumping power of the heart. The myocardial damage can lead to weakening of the heart muscle and dilation of the left ventricle, resulting in enlargement of the heart (cardiomegaly) (see Figure 10-3). Enlargement results in a decreased amount of blood being ejected from the ventricle during a contraction, resulting in an EF less than 50%. The EF is the amount of blood being ejected from the ventricle during a contraction; the normal value is 50%–70% (Pfisterer, Battler, & Zaret, 1985). As the EF diminishes, the pressure increases, resulting in pulmonary congestion. In general, systolic HF is caused by dysfunction or destruction of the cardiac myocytes or their molecular components being damaged by inflammation (myocarditis), infiltration (amyloidosis) (Boufidou et al., 2010), pharmacologic agents (e.g., ethanol and cocaine) (George & Figueredo, 2011), or toxins causing intracellular damage and oxidative stress (e.g., an-

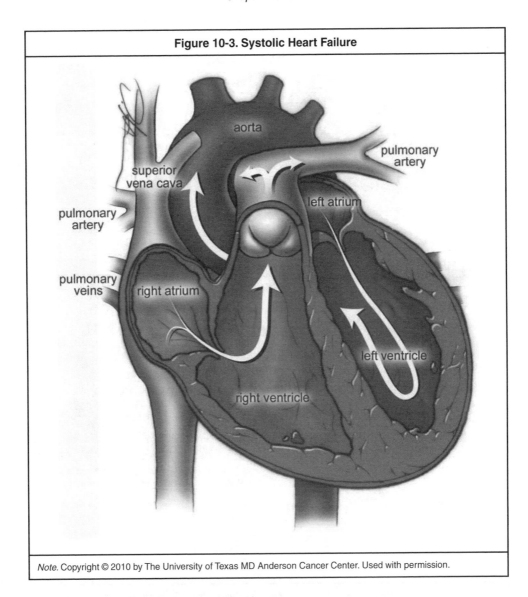

Figure 10-3. Systolic Heart Failure

thracyclines and other antineoplastic agents) (Bristow et al., 1978). In some patients, LV dysfunction may occur as a combination of both systolic and diastolic dysfunction.

Diastolic heart failure: Diastolic HF is also known as HF with preserved LV function with normal EF (greater than 50%). This type of dysfunction occurs when the left ventricle is unable to fill sufficiently during diastole because of the inability of the heart to relax, thereby inhibiting the ventricles from filling adequately (see Figure 10-4). Patients may be completely asymptomatic at rest, but they are very sensitive to increases in heart rate, fever, volume overload or dehydration, or tachyarrhythmia (e.g., atrial fibrillation with rapid ventricular response that can result in flash pulmonary edema). Because of the stiff ventricles, the pressure needed to fill the chamber is increased, resulting in pulmonary congestion and decreased cardiac output, which in turn results in diastolic HF (Swedberg et al., 2005). Following chemotherapy, 50% of asymptomatic patients with normal LVEF have diastolic dysfunc-

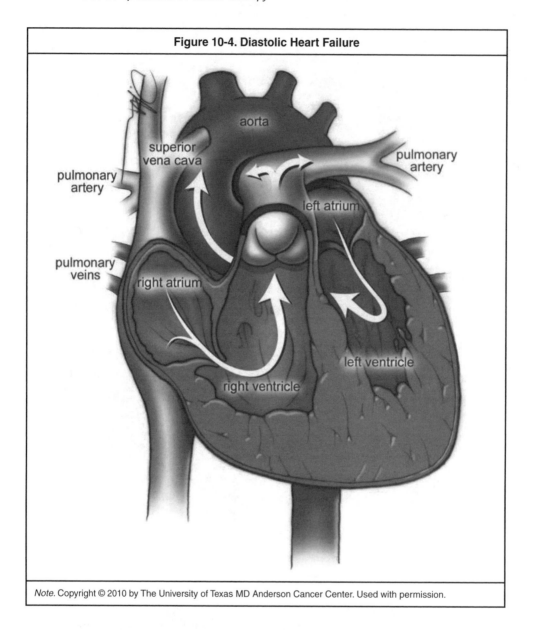

Figure 10-4. Diastolic Heart Failure

tion on echocardiogram (Tjeerdsma et al., 1999). The left ventricle in HF with pre-served LVEF may be characterized by LV hypertrophy, concentric remodeling and in-creased extracellular matrix, abnormal calcium handling, abnormal relaxation and filling, or decreased diastolic distensibility (Gwathmey et al., 1987; Pearlman, Weber, Janicki, Pietra, & Fishman, 1982; Zile & Brutsaert, 2002). In prospective studies, ap-proximately half of the patients with HF have normal or near-normal resting LVEF (Philbin, Rocco, Lindenmuth, Ulrich, & Jenkins, 2000; Smith, Masoudi, Vaccarino, Radford, & Krumholz, 2003; Vasan et al., 1999). HF with preserved LVEF is particu-larly prevalent among older adults, women, and patients with a history of long-stand-ing hypertension (Chen, Lainchbury, Senni, Bailey, & Redfield, 2002; Senni & Red-field, 2001; Smith et al., 2003).

Degree of Functional Impairment

The NYHA functional classification of patients with cardiac diseases was developed in 1928 on the basis of clinical severity and prognosis (Criteria Committee of the New York Heart Association, 1994). Once a diagnosis of HF is established, the symptoms may be used to classify the severity of the HF and to monitor the effects of therapy. This system assigns patients to one of four functional classes depending on the degree of the symptoms: an NYHA class I patient will experience symptoms only at certain levels of exertion (mild symptoms), class II on ordinary exertion (mild), class III on less than ordinary exertion (moderate), and class IV with HF symptoms even at rest (severe) (see Table 10-3). This classification is based on subjective symptoms, and grading is based on the clinician's judgment. However, the relationship between symptoms and the severity of cardiac dysfunction appears to be poor (Cleland et al., 2003; Fadol et al., 2008; Marantz et al., 1988), especially among patients with cancer (Fadol et al., 2008). The symptoms may be related to prognosis, particularly if they are persistent even after therapy (Adams & Zannad, 1998). Although the functional class of the patient tends to deteriorate over time, the severity of symptoms can fluctuate with dietary indiscretion and noncompliance with medications, especially diuretics.

Initial Evaluation for Possible Heart Failure Diagnosis in Patients With Cancer

Most cancer survivors who develop HF seek medical attention with complaints of reduced exercise tolerance due to shortness of breath or fatigue, sometimes with associated lower-extremity edema. Most of the time, shortness of breath and fatigue occur at rest or during exercise and may be attributed inappropriately by the patient or the healthcare provider to aging, history of cancer, or treatments received, including chemotherapy and radiation. In the inpatient setting, the majority of patients with cancer are evaluated for possible HF after they become symptomatic.

Table 10-3. New York Heart Association (NYHA) Functional Classification	
NYHA Class	**Patient Symptoms**
I (mild)	No limitation of physical activity No undue fatigue, palpitation, or dyspnea
II (mild)	Slight limitation of physical activity Comfortable at rest Less than ordinary activity results in fatigue, palpitation, or dyspnea
III (moderate)	Marked limitation of physical activity Comfortable at rest Less than ordinary activity results in palpitation, fatigue, or dyspnea
IV (severe)	Unable to carry out physical activity without discomfort Symptoms of cardiac insufficiency at rest Physical activity causes increased discomfort
Note. Based on information from Criteria Committee of the New York Heart Association, 1994.	

The initial evaluation of a patient with cancer with suspected LV dysfunction should aim to identify the etiology of HF, assess the nature and severity of symptoms, determine the functional impairment, and, in collaboration with the oncologist, establish a prognosis to guide the cancer therapy and support the patient in decision making regarding treatments and life plan. The evaluation should include a detailed history, physical examination, and diagnostic workup (see Figure 10-5).

The healthcare provider should inquire about a history of hypertension, diabetes mellitus, dyslipidemia, tobacco use, rheumatic fever, heart murmur or congenital heart disease, and coronary, valvular, or peripheral vascular disease; personal or family history of myopathy; sleep-disturbed breathing; and all cancer treatments received, including mediastinal radiation treatments and doses and types of chemotherapy (especially anthracyclines, trastuzumab, and high-dose cyclophosphamide). HF may occur years after exposure to anthracyclines (Bird & Swain, 2008) or mediastinal irradiation (Cutter, Darby, & Yusuf, 2011). The cardiac workup should include determination of cardiac function, etiology of HF (ischemic versus nonischemic), risk of life-threatening dysrhythmias, exacerbating factors, and barriers to adherence and compliance with medical management. The history and physical evaluation should also include specific considerations of noncardiac diseases, such as collagen vascular disease, bacterial or parasitic infection, obesity, thyroid disorders, amyloidosis, hemochromatosis, and pheochromocytoma.

The physical examination should evaluate the fluid or volume status of a patient with HF during the initial visit and at every follow-up examination. At each visit, documentation should include the patient's body weight; sitting and standing blood pressure levels; degree of jugular venous distension (JVD); presence of elevated jugular venous pressure; and presence and severity of organ congestion (pulmonary rales and hepatomegaly), lower-extremity edema, and ascites. The most reliable sign of volume overload is JVD (Cesario, Clark, & Maisel, 1998; Leier & Binkley, 1998; Marius-Nunez et al., 1996). JVD can be accentuated by abdominal compression eliciting the hepatojugular reflux (see Figure 10-6), which is elevated in many patients with chronically elevated left-sided filling pressures (Drazner et al., 1999). The presence of JVD and a third heart sound has been shown to have prognostic significance (Drazner, Rame, Stevenson, & Dries, 2001). Patients with peripheral edema should be considered to have volume overload, although the possibility of noncardiac issues such as hypoalbuminemia,

---

Figure 10-5. Initial Evaluation of Patients With Cancer With Left Ventricular Dysfunction

- History: coronary artery disease, myocardial infarction, hypertension, diabetes mellitus, dyslipidemia, valvular disease, chemotherapy, radiation therapy, sleep-disordered breathing, thyroid problems, family history
- Physical examination: shortness of breath, fatigue, edema, symptoms of embolic events, symptoms of possible cerebral hypoperfusion (syncope, light-headedness, dizziness)
- Diagnostic tests: electrocardiogram, echocardiogram, chest x-ray
- Laboratory examinations: complete blood count, electrolytes, brain natriuretic peptide, blood urea nitrogen, creatinine, thyroid-stimulating hormone, thyroxine
- Determination of clinical severity: New York Heart Association classification, Eastern Cooperative Oncology Group criteria
- Determination of the etiology of heart failure: ischemic versus nonischemic
- Evaluation for life-threatening dysrhythmia
- Identification of exacerbating factors for heart failure
- Identification of barriers to adherence and compliance

which is present in many patients with cancer, should be ruled out. In contrast, most patients with chronic HF and those with end-stage disease who have markedly elevated left-sided filling pressures do not have peripheral edema and rales. The cardiac filling pressures can be measured with right heart catheterization or a central venous catheter. The presence of rales generally reflects the rapid onset of HF rather than the degree of volume overload.

The signs and symptoms of HF (see Figure 10-7) are difficult to use in ascertaining the exact etiology, whether they are from the cancer, a side effect of cancer treatment,

---

Figure 10-6. Hepatojugular Reflux

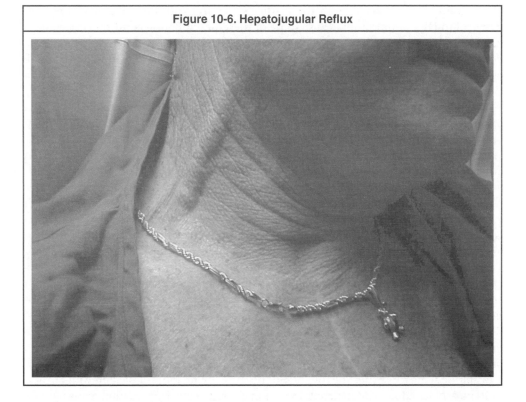

Figure 10-7. Signs and Symptoms of Heart Failure

Signs
- Edema (lower-extremity swelling, abdominal ascites)
- Jugular venous distention
- Hepatomegaly (enlarged liver)
- Abnormal heart sound (S_3 gallop, murmurs)
- Tachycardia
- Changes in blood pressure (hypotension)
- Decreased oxygen saturation
- Tachycardia (rapid heart rate)
- Tachypnea (rapid respiratory rate)
- Abnormal lung sounds (crackles)
- Changes in skin appearance (color, moisture)

Symptoms
- Fatigue, weakness, exercise intolerance
- Dyspnea (shortness of breath)
- Orthopnea (increased dyspnea when lying flat)
- Paroxysmal nocturnal dyspnea (waking up at night because of shortness of breath)
- Increased abdominal girth, bloating
- Frequent coughing (especially when lying flat)
- Sudden weight gain
- Lack of appetite

or due to HF or other comorbid conditions. Any patient receiving cardiotoxic chemo-therapy or complaining of paroxysmal nocturnal dyspnea, orthopnea, recent onset of exertional dyspnea, or increasing fatigue should undergo evaluation for HF.

Diagnostic Tests for Chronic Heart Failure in Patients With Cancer

In addition to a comprehensive history and physical examination, the identification of the conditions responsible for the cardiac structural and functional abnormalities that lead to HF is important because some of these precipitating conditions are potentially treatable or reversible. Appropriate intervention, such as coronary revascularization, may improve cardiac function in patients with cardiomyopathy of ischemic etiology. To confirm a suspected diagnosis of HF, the initial patient evaluation should include a complete diagnostic workup (see Figure 10-8).

Diagnosis is the first essential step in the provision of good management of HF in a patient with cancer because of the heterogeneous presentation, causes, pathophysiology, prognosis, and treatment of HF. The purposes of the diagnostic evaluation of patients with HF are to evaluate the etiologic processes, differentiate the cardiac abnormalities from other system malfunctions, establish the symptom severity, provide prognostic information to the oncologists, and lay the groundwork for medical and pharmacologic therapy.

Establishing a diagnosis of HF in a patient with cancer is a complex process because it is a cluster of syndromes and each syndrome is of varied etiology. The diagnosis of HF relies on clinical judgment based on patient history, physical examination, and appropriate investigations. A clinician recognizes HF not by a single measurement but rather by a cluster of features that includes subjective and objective components. Those components include the signs and symptoms of HF and objective evidence of a cardiac abnormality from an echocardiogram, ventriculogram, or other form of cardiac diagnostic testing. In an at-risk group such as patients who have received cancer therapy with potential cardiotoxic side effects, symptoms alert the clinician to a possible diagnosis of HF, which must be confirmed by further investigation. Integration of the diagnostic evaluation with the clinical presentation (see Table 10-4) is necessary for a correct diagnosis. Once the diagnosis of HF is established, the cause must be sought out. Because the majority of patients with HF and cancer are older adults, concomitant diseases may complicate diagnosis and management.

The diagnostic tests used to evaluate LV dysfunction include endomyocardial biopsy (EMB), echocardiography, radionuclide ventriculography, and cardiac biomarkers.

Figure 10-8. Assessment Process to Establish a Heart Failure Diagnosis in a Patient With Cancer

- Perform a comprehensive history and physical examination.
- Obtain history of treatments received for cancer therapy.
- Determine the etiology of heart failure (e.g., ischemic versus nonischemic).
- Classify the presenting syndrome (e.g., acute versus chronic, systolic versus diastolic).
- Identify concomitant disease relevant to heart failure (e.g., amyloidosis, hemochromatosis).
- Evaluate for presence of coronary artery disease and valvular problems.
- Assess severity of symptoms.
- Perform diagnostic and interventional procedures as needed (e.g., cardiac catheterization).

Table 10-4. Diagnostic Tests for Heart Failure	
Diagnostic Test	**Purpose**
Electrocardiogram	To detect arrhythmias (premature ventricular contractions) or atrial fibrillation, which may cause or exacerbate heart failure
Chest x-ray	To evaluate for pulmonary edema, pleural effusion, and cardiomegaly
Echocardiogram	To detect decrease in left ventricular ejection fraction, valvular problems, and wall motion abnormalities; longitudinal strain used for early detection of cardiotoxicity
Nuclear imaging	To detect the location and severity of coronary artery disease
Coronary arteriography	To evaluate the blockages in the coronary arteries
Endomyocardial biopsy	To diagnose anthracycline-induced CMP; endomyocardial biopsies demonstrate sarcoplasmic reticulum dilation, vacuole formation, myofibrillar dropout, and necrosis
Cardiovascular magnetic resonance imaging	To detect coronary artery calcification
Cardiac biomarkers (troponin I and N-terminal pro-BNP)	Elevated troponin level signals myocardial damage after chemotherapy; increased troponin level associated with increased incidence of cardiac events
Thyroid function	To evaluate for hypothyroidism/hyperthyroidism as the heart failure etiology
Viral titers	To evaluate causes of myocarditis, endocarditis, and pericarditis (cytomegalovirus, echovirus, parvovirus, and adenovirus)
Blood cultures	To define organisms in sepsis-related heart failure
Iron studies	To evaluate for hemochromatosis resulting in heart failure

BNP—brain natriuretic peptide; CMP—cardiomyopathy

Note. Based on information from Cardinale et al., 2004; Sawaya et al., 2011; Steinherz & Yahalom, 2001; Urbanova et al., 2006.

From "Cardiovascular Adverse Events Associated With Cancer Therapy," by A. Fadol and T. Lech, 2011, *Journal of the Advanced Practitioner in Oncology, 2,* p. 238. Copyright 2011 by Harborside Press. Reprinted with permission.

Endomyocardial Biopsy

EMB is an invasive diagnostic technique used for patients who present with abnormal systolic or diastolic function. It is considered the most sensitive and specific tool for diagnosing and monitoring anthracycline-induced cardiotoxicity (Mason, Bristow, Billingham, & Daniels, 1978), but it is difficult to perform this invasive test in all patients undergoing chemotherapy (Yeh, 2006). EMB is not indicated in the routine evaluation of cardiomyopathy (Hunt et al., 2009). The procedure involves insertion of a bioptome into the right internal jugular vein with fluoroscopic guidance to obtain a sample from more than one region of the right ventricular septum. At least four or five samples are obtained and submitted for transmission electron microscopy, particularly if anthracycline-induced cardiotoxicity is suspected. EMB also can provide diagnostic information about certain conditions associated with unexplained HF (Cooper et al., 2007).

Multigated Acquisition Scan

Before echocardiography technology improved in the past decade, multigated acquisition (MUGA) scans were the most commonly used modality for monitoring LVEF in patients with cancer. A MUGA scan has low interobserver variability and generates an exact value of the EF as opposed to a range, which is often reported in echocardiography. However, MUGA scans yield data for only LVEF and left ventricle size. In patients with cancer who develop cardiotoxicity, many other factors can have profound effects on LVEF, including states of adrenergic stimulation, volume status (preload and afterload), systemic vascular resistance, valvular problems, and adrenal insufficiency. Patients undergoing chemotherapy are particularly at risk for hypovolemia secondary to chemotherapy-associated adverse effects (e.g., nausea, vomiting, diarrhea), anemia, and sympathetic stimulation from anxiety or fear.

Echocardiography

With improvements in imaging quality in the past two decades, echocardiography has become the choice of many clinicians in monitoring for LV function. The advantages of using this technique are that it does not use ionizing radiation, it is a noninvasive way to monitor LV function similar to a MUGA scan, and it provides a more comprehensive cardiac assessment beyond LVEF measurement, including assessment of chamber size, valvular function, pericardial abnormalities, and diastolic dysfunction (Witteles, Fowler, & Telli, 2011). A recent study showed that measurement of longitudinal strain on echocardiograms can predict the development of cardiotoxicity in patients treated with anthracycline and trastuzumab (Sawaya et al., 2011).

Cardiac Magnetic Resonance Imaging

Cardiac magnetic resonance imaging (MRI) is another diagnostic test that can be used to monitor LV dysfunction resulting from cancer therapy. MRI is a noninvasive test that uses radio waves, magnets, and a computer to create detailed pictures of the heart. MRI does not expose the patient to ionizing radiation, and it offers the most reproducible assessment of LVEF. In addition, if gadolinium contrast is administered, the presence of regions of delayed enhancement may reveal the earliest sign of myocardial injury and thus allow for early intervention before reductions in LVEF are apparent (Wassmuth et al., 2001). However, MRI cannot be performed with patients who have metal devices, and gadolinium contrast cannot be safely administered in patients with significant renal dysfunction. In addition, cardiac MRI requires expensive equipment and technical expertise and is not readily available in most institutions.

Cardiac Biomarkers

The cardiac biomarkers that have been studied for monitoring HF in patients with cancer are brain natriuretic peptide (BNP) and troponin I. BNP is a neurohormone that is elevated in response to volume overload. The usefulness of BNP in the diagnosis of chronic HF with patients who do not have cancer is well established (Maisel et al., 2001). For patients with cancer, high levels of BNP have been shown to correlate with LV function during chemotherapy (Cardinale et al., 2000; Meinardi et al., 2001; Nousiainen et al., 1999) and hematopoietic stem cell transplantation (Snowden et al., 2000). Routine BNP measurement could be useful in monitoring LV function during chemotherapy, but further investigation is needed. BNP levels are usually higher for hospitalized patients with signs of volume overload and tend to decrease during aggressive therapy for decompensation. However, it cannot be assumed that BNP levels can be used effectively as the only target when therapy is adjusted for HF decompensation in patients with cancer.

Troponin I may be useful in the early detection of cardiotoxicity, before a reduction in LV function occurs (Lipshultz et al., 1997). In a study of 204 patients who were undergoing high-dose chemotherapy for aggressive malignancies, the elevation of troponin I during chemotherapy accurately predicted the development of future LVEF depression (Cardinale et al., 2000). Conversely, patients whose troponin I remained low during chemotherapy and in the months following treatment had excellent prognoses in terms of cardiac function. A similar finding was noted in a recent study of 43 women diagnosed with breast cancer who received anthracycline and trastuzumab and were monitored with echocardiography and cardiac biomarkers (high-sensitivity cardiac troponin I and N-terminal pro-BNP) at three time points (baseline and three and six months during chemotherapy) (Sawaya et al., 2011). The results of the study showed that elevated troponin I at three months ($p < 0.02$) and decreased longitudinal strain between baseline and three months ($p < 0.02$) were predictive of patients who developed cardiotoxicity at six months (Sawaya et al., 2011). However, further studies are needed before routine screening with the troponin I biomarker is used in clinical practice.

Management of Heart Failure in Patients With Cancer

The discussion regarding the management of HF is divided into the acute and chronic phases. These phases are considered separately because the treatment and pharmacologic management are different for each.

Acute Decompensated Heart Failure

The goal of ADHF management is hemodynamic stabilization and improvement of the clinical signs and symptoms. Patients with ADHF who present in the emergency department usually are hemodynamically unstable and belong to one of the three clinical profiles: (a) patients with volume overload, as manifested by pulmonary congestion, systemic congestion, or both, (b) patients with hypotension, renal insufficiency, or shock syndrome (or a combination) resulting from severely low EF, and (c) patients with signs and symptoms of both fluid overload and shock (Hunt et al., 2009).

ADHF is a common and potentially fatal cause of acute respiratory distress. HF may be new or an exacerbation of chronic disease. ADHF can be precipitated by several factors (Fadol, 2006; Tsuyuki et al., 2001) (see Figure 10-9). The clinical syndrome is characterized by the development of acute dyspnea with elevated cardiac filling pressures (pulmonary capillary wedge pressure, central venous pressure) or by cardiogenic pulmonary edema (Ware & Matthay, 2005). ADHF is usually due to LV systolic or diastolic dysfunction. Patients with ADHF most commonly present with cough, dyspnea, and fatigue that escalate rapidly and become severe and may or may not be associated with chest discomfort.

Figure 10-9. Precipitants of Acute Decompensated Heart Failure

- Patient-related factors
  - Nonadherence to medications
  - Excessive salt intake
  - Physical and environmental stressors
- Cardiac-related factors
  - Cardiac arrhythmias (atrial fibrillation, ventricular arrhythmias, bradyrhythmias)
  - Uncontrolled hypertension
  - Acute myocardial infarction
  - Valvular disease, worsening mitral regurgitation
- Adverse effects of medications
  - Steroids
  - Chemotherapy (doxorubicin, cyclophosphamide)
  - Nonsteroidal anti-inflammatory drugs
  - Thiazolidinediones

Note. Based on information from Fadol, 2006; Tsuyuki et al., 2001.

Initial assessment should include a brief, focused history and a physical examination to evaluate the signs and symptoms of HF, as well as contributing factors, comorbidities, and differential diagnoses (see Figure 10-10), so that appropriate interventions can be administered expeditiously to improve the clinical status; otherwise, the patient's condition can worsen. In the oncology population, accurately differentiating patients with ADHF is a diagnostic challenge because the presenting symptoms of dyspnea, fatigue, and volume overload are nonspecific and can be caused by the cancer, cancer therapy, or both (Fadol, 2006). The differential diagnosis is complicated further by many other conditions that can mimic HF (see Figure 10-11). ADHF can be precipitated by medication noncompliance, cardiac dysrhythmias, dietary indiscretion, or antineoplastic agents. However, data from the Acute Decompensated Heart Failure National Registry (ADHERE) indicate that 30% of patients hospitalized with HF have a history of renal insufficiency and 20% of the patients have serum creatinine levels greater than 2 mg/dl (Adams et al., 2005). Acute renal failure or renal insufficiency should be considered in these patients because of the nephrotoxic effects of many antineoplastic agents.

Although patient history and physical examination findings may provide important clues regarding the underlying etiology, invasive and noninvasive testing are necessary to provide a definitive diagnosis of HF (see Figure 10-12). Routine use of invasive hemodynamic monitoring in patients with ADHF is not recommended; however, it may be helpful to determine intracardiac filling pressures in patients who are in respiratory distress or have clinical evidence of hypoperfusion. Urgent coronary angiography may be indicated for patients with ADHF and acute coronary syndrome. Management of acute coronary syndrome is discussed in Chapter 5.

No clinical practice guidelines have been developed for the management of ADHF for patients with concurrent cancer diagnoses; hence, the management is largely based on empirical evidence, expert consensus, retrospective in-hospital data, and observational level of evidence. The most commonly used pharmacologic agents for ADHF are listed in Table 10-5. After hemodynamic stabilization is achieved in the emergency department, the patient may be admitted to the hospital for continuous monitoring and management until clinically stable. In some cases, patients may be discharged home after adequate response to diuretics and resolution of symptoms. A critical component

Figure 10-10. Assessment for Acute Decompensated Heart Failure

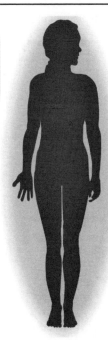

Overall Appearance
Skin color, temperature, turgor, shortness of breath, acute respiratory distress using accessory muscles to breathe

Vital Signs
Hypotension, tachycardia, tachypnea, decreased oxygen saturation

Physical Exam
Confusion, decreased alertness, JVD, S_3 or S_4, new or changed murmurs, check for irregular heartbeats, hepatomegaly, ascites, weight gain, lower-extremity pitting edema

Identify Precipitating Factors
Dietary indiscretion, nonadherence to medications, iatrogenic volume overload, chemotherapy adverse effect, cardiac arrhythmias, renal failure

Diagnostic Tests
ECG, chest x-ray, echocardiogram, labs (BMP, CBC, BNP, cardiac panel, thyroid panel, ABGs), Swan-Ganz catheter, cardiac catheterization

Differential Diagnosis
Pulmonary embolism, AMI, pleural/pericardial effusion, pneumonia, COPD exacerbation, pneumothorax

ABGs—arterial blood gases; AMI—acute myocardial infarction; BMP—basic metabolic panel; BNP—brain natriuretic peptide; CBC—complete blood count; COPD—chronic obstructive pulmonary disease; ECG—electrocardiogram; JVD—jugular venous distension

Figure 10-11. Differential Diagnosis for Acute Decompensated Heart Failure

- Acute myocardial infarction
- Acute pericardial effusion
- Acute pleural effusion
- Acute adverse reaction from chemotherapy administration
- Chronic obstructive pulmonary disease exacerbation
- Lung cancer

- Pneumonia
- Pulmonary embolism
- Severe hypoalbuminemia
- Tension pneumothorax
- Thyroid disease
- Renal failure

Note. Based on information from Tsuyuki et al., 2001.

Figure 10-12. Recommended Diagnostic Tests for Acute Decompensated Heart Failure

- Arterial blood gases
- Basic metabolic profile
- Brain natriuretic peptide
- Complete blood count
- Liver function test

- Thyroid profile
- Electrocardiogram
- Chest x-ray
- Echocardiogram

Table 10-5. Pharmacologic Therapy for Acute Decompensated Heart Failure

Drug	Method of Administration Bolus Rate	Infusion Rate	Indications
Diuretics			
Furosemide	20–80 mg IV	2–10 mg/hr	To correct volume overload, decrease pulmonary congestion, and achieve euvolemia
Torsemide			
Catecholamines			
Dobutamine	–	2–20 mcg/kg/min	Peripheral hypoperfusion refractory to volume replacement and diuretics
Dopamine	–	5–10 mcg/kg/min	Hypotension, renal perfusion
Vasodilators			
Nitroglycerine	–	5–10 mcg/min	Venodilator that can potentiate the effect of diuretics
Nesiritide	2 mcg/kg	0.01–0.03 mcg/kg/min	Adjunctive therapy for ADHF To promote diuresis and natriuresis
Phosphodiesterase inhibitor			
Milrinone	25–75 mcg/kg over 10–20 min	0.375–0.75 mcg/kg/min	Peripheral hypoperfusion refractory to diuretics and vasodilators. Preferred to dobutamine in patients on beta-blocker therapy.
Calcium sensitizer			
Levosimendan	6–24 mcg/kg over 10 min	0.05–0.2 mcg/kg/min	Symptomatic, low cardiac output, HF secondary to systolic HF without severe hypotension

Note. Based on information from DiDomenico et al., 2004; Fadol, 2006.

of care coordination at discharge and transition to home care is providing the patient and caregiver with written discharge instructions and educational materials that address the discharge medications, activity level, follow-up appointments, weight monitoring, and steps to take if symptoms worsen (Bonow et al., 2005). The Centers for Medicare and Medicaid Services recommend that prior to discharge, the four core performance measures (LVEF, angiotensin-converting enzyme [ACE] inhibitor use, tobacco cessation, and discharge instructions; see Table 10-6) be discussed with the patient and documented in the patient's medical record. The performance measures are standards of care that are designed to assess and subsequently improve the quality of medical care. ACC recommends the use of beta-blockers and anticoagulation agents as performance measures as well.

Chronic Heart Failure

Patients with chronic HF usually are managed in the outpatient setting in specialty clinics or by primary care providers. Once the diagnosis of HF has been made, health-

Table 10-6. Heart Failure Core Measures

Set Measure ID #	Performance Measure	Measure Description
HF-1	Discharge instruction	Prior to discharge, patients should have written instructions or educational materials given addressing all the following: activity level, diet, discharge medications, follow-up appointment, weight monitoring, what to do when symptoms worsen, and contact information for the outpatient clinic.
HF-2	Evaluation of left ventricular systolic (LVS) function	Documentation that LVS function was assessed during hospitalization
HF-3	Angiotensin-converting enzyme (ACE) inhibitor or angiotensin receptor blocker (ARB) for LVS dysfunction	Documentation that ACE inhibitor/ARB (if without contraindications) was prescribed at hospital discharge
HF-4	Adult smoking cessation advice/counseling	Patients with heart failure and history of smoking were given advice or counseling during hospital stay.

Note. Based on information from Joint Commission, 2011.

care providers should focus on the clinical assessment of the patient during the initial presentation and during subsequent visits. The frequency of the clinic visits may range from weekly to every six months depending on the functional status, signs, and symptoms and on whether the patient is undergoing chemotherapy treatment with potential cardiotoxic adverse effects. Ongoing review of the patient's clinical status is critical to the appropriate selection and monitoring of treatment. The review should include assessment of functional capacity and volume status, laboratory evaluation, assessment of prognosis, and other significant parameters. An outpatient clinic visit checklist for patients with chronic HF is outlined in Table 10-7. The major goals for chronic HF management are to (a) prevent the development of ADHF, (b) prevent progression and initiate reversal of cardiac remodeling, and (c) manage symptoms to improve patients' quality of life. To achieve these goals, it is of utmost importance that patients with cancer who have HF receive standard HF medications as recommended by clinical practice guidelines and as tolerated by physiologic and clinical parameters. In addition to optimum pharmacologic therapy, nonpharmacologic treatment strategies have proved to be effective in many HF management programs.

Pharmacologic Therapy

The goals of pharmacologic therapy for patients with cancer who also have HF are to improve survival, slow the progression of disease, alleviate symptoms, and minimize risk factors. There is a paucity of clinical guidelines specific for patients with cancer who have HF because most cardiac-based investigations exclude this patient population. However, the principles for treating HF apply to all patients, and several studies have shown the cardioprotective benefit of HF medications for the oncolo-

Table 10-7. Outpatient Visit Checklist for Patients With Heart Failure	
Activity	**Measurement**
Left ventricular systolic (LVS) function assessment	Documentation that LVS had been assessed (echocardiogram, multigated acquisition scan, or cardiac catheterization)
Evaluation of heart failure etiology (ischemic versus non-ischemic)	Documentation that patient had undergone diagnostic workup to evaluate for ischemic etiology
Cancer treatment received	Documentation of type and total dosage of chemotherapy, radiation, and other cardiotoxic treatment received
Assessment of clinical signs and symptoms of volume overload	Completion of a physical examination pertaining to volume overload status assessment at each outpatient visit, and documentation of weight to assess change in volume status
Assessment of activity level	Evaluation of impact of heart failure on activity level at each outpatient visit
Laboratory assessment	Documentation of laboratory results (electrolytes, blood urea nitrogen, creatinine, brain natriuretic peptide, magnesium, lipid panel, thyroid panel)
Electrocardiogram assessment	Evaluation of dysrhythmia and QT prolongation, and assessment for cardiac resynchronization therapy placement
Recommended heart failure medications	Documentation of angiotensin-converting enzyme inhibitor, angiotensin receptor blocker, or beta-blockers for patients with LVS dysfunction or patients with atrial fibrillation. For patients with atrial fibrillation, warfarin, aspirin, or dabigatran (Pradaxa®) based on $CHADS_2$ score is recommended for anticoagulation.
Patient education	Reinforcement of patient education on daily weight monitoring, symptoms, and compliance with medical regimen, smoking cessation, and therapeutic lifestyle changes

gy population (Cardinale et al., 2006; Kalay et al., 2006). The ACC, AHA, and Heart Failure Society of America (HFSA) clinical practice guidelines recommend that all patients with HF should be on ACE inhibitors and beta-blockers unless contraindicated, as these medications have been shown in numerous randomized clinical trials to improve survival, increase quality of life, and reduce mortality (MERIT-HF Study Group, 1999; SOLVD Investigators, 1991). Table 10-8 outlines the ACC/AHA/HFSA clinical guideline (Hunt et al., 2005) recommendations for pharmacologic therapy for chronic HF.

Angiotensin-Converting Enzyme Inhibitors

ACE inhibitors are recommended for all patients with current or prior symptoms of HF and reduced LVEF, unless contraindicated (Hunt et al., 2009). ACE inhibitors decrease the conversion of angiotensin I to angiotensin II (a potent vasoconstrictor), thereby minimizing the physiologic effects of angiotensin II and decreasing the degradation of bradykinin. Bradykinin promotes vasodilation in the vascular endothelium and causes natriuresis in the kidney.

The beneficial effects of ACE inhibitors for HF include improvements in survival, less severe symptoms, reverse of remodeling, and a lower rate of hospitalization (Khalil, Basher, Brown, & Alhaddad, 2001; Munzel & Keaney, 2001). An ongoing clinical trial has been designed to evaluate whether the combined treatment of enalapril (an ACE inhibitor) and carvedilol (a beta-blocker) can prevent LV dysfunction in patients recently diagnosed with acute leukemia and in patients with other malignant hemopathies who underwent autologous peripheral blood stem cell transplantation (Bosch et al., 2011).

The most common adverse effects of ACE inhibitors are hypotension and dizziness, particularly among patients with cancer who may have borderline low systolic blood

Table 10-8. Recommended Medications for the Treatment of Heart Failure			
Drug	**Starting Dose**	**Target Dose**	**Maximum Dose**
Angiotensin-converting enzyme inhibitors			
Captopril (Capoten®)	6.25–12.5 mg 3x/day	50 mg 3x/day	100 mg 3x/day
Enalapril (Vasotec®)	2.5 mg 2x/day	20 mg 2x/day	40 mg/day
Fosinopril (Monopril®)	2.5–5 mg/day	20 mg/day	40 mg/day
Lisinopril (Zestril®, Prinivil®)	2.5–5 mg/day	20 mg/day	40 mg/day
Quinapril (Accupril®)	5 mg 2x/day	20 mg 2x/day	20 mg 2x/day
Ramipril (Altace®)	1.25–2.5 mg/day	10 mg/day	10 mg/day
Trandolapril (Mavik®)	1 mg/day	4 mg/day	8 mg/day
Angiotensin receptor blockers			
Candesartan (Atacand®)	4 mg/day	32 mg/day	32 mg/day
Valsartan (Diovan®)	40 mg 2x/day	160 mg 2x/day	320 mg/day
Beta-blockers			
Carvedilol (Coreg®)	3.125 mg 2x/day	25 mg 2x/day	50 mg/day (weight > 85 kg)
Carvedilol phosphate (Coreg CR®)	10 mg/day	80 mg/day	80 mg/day
Metoprolol succinate (Toprol XL®)	25 mg 2x/day	100 mg/day	100 mg/day
Bisoprolol (Zebeta®)	1.25 mg/day	10 mg/day	10 mg/day
Aldosterone antagonists			
Eplerenone (Inspra®)	25 mg/day	50 mg/day	50 mg/day
Spironolactone (Aldactone®)	25 mg/day	50 mg/day	50 mg/day
Cardiac glycoside			
Digitalis (Lanoxin®)	0.125 mg/day	0.25 mg/day	0.25 mg /day
Direct-acting vasodilator			
Hydralazine + isosorbide dinitrate (BiDil®)	37.5 mg and 20 mg (1 tablet) 3x/day	37.5 mg and 20 mg (2 tablets) 3x/day	37.5 mg and 20 mg (2 tablets) 3x/day

Note. Based on information from Hunt et al., 2005.

From "Cardiovascular Adverse Events Associated With Cancer Therapy," by A. Fadol and T. Lech, 2011, *Journal of the Advanced Practitioner in Oncology, 2,* p. 237. Copyright 2011 by Harborside Press. Reprinted with permission.

pressure related to multiple factors, such as hypovolemia (a result of decreased fluid intake, nausea, and vomiting due to adverse effects of cancer therapy). These adverse effects may limit the dose of ACE inhibitors. Regardless, ACE inhibitors should be started at a low dose because most randomized trials have shown no difference in mortality between patients receiving high-dose or low-dose ACE inhibitors (Packer et al., 1999; Tang et al., 2002).

Other potential adverse effects of ACE inhibitors are worsening renal function, hyperkalemia, cough, and angioedema. A significant increase in serum creatinine with the use of ACE inhibitors has been observed for 15%–30% of patients with severe HF (Giles et al., 1989). ACE inhibitors should not be started simultaneously with nephrotoxic chemotherapeutic agents.

Coughing secondary to ACE inhibitors is nonproductive and is accompanied by a persistent and annoying "tickle" in the back of the throat. The coughing usually occurs within the first months of therapy and disappears within one or two weeks of discontinuation. The frequency of cough is approximately 5%–10% among White patients of European descent and nearly 50% among Chinese patients (Woo & Nicholls, 1995).

Angioedema is a life-threatening situation characterized by a self-limited, localized subcutaneous (or submucosal) swelling that results from extravasation of fluid into interstitial tissues. Angioedema may occur in isolation, be accompanied by urticaria, or be a component of anaphylaxis. Angioedema occurs in less than 1% of patients taking an ACE inhibitor and more frequently among African Americans (Hunt et al., 2009). ACE inhibitors should not be initiated for a patient with a history of angioedema.

Nursing Considerations for Patients Receiving Angiotensin-Converting Enzyme Inhibitors

- Patients should be educated about the possible adverse effects of ACE inhibitors, especially angioedema.
- Patients receiving ACE inhibitors should be monitored closely for signs of hypotension (such as dizziness or near-syncope) and for deteriorating renal function.
- Renal function should be checked within one or two weeks after initiation of therapy, especially in the presence of preexisting hypotension or hyponatremia and for patients who are taking potassium supplementation or potassium-sparing diuretics.
- Close monitoring of serum potassium is required. Potassium levels and renal function should be checked at three days and seven days after initiation of therapy and at least monthly for the first three months.

Angiotensin Receptor Blockers

Angiotensin receptor blockers are recommended as an alternative for patients with current or prior symptoms of HF and reduced LVEF who cannot tolerate ACE inhibitors (Hunt et al., 2009) because of cough or angioedema. The use of the angiotensin receptor blocker candesartan was shown to improve outcomes among patients with preserved LVEF who were ACE-inhibitor intolerant (Granger et al., 2003). Many of the considerations for angiotensin receptor blockers are similar to those for ACE inhibitors.

Beta-Adrenergic Receptor Blockers

The primary action of beta-blockers is to counteract the harmful effects of the sympathetic nervous system that are activated during the pathophysiologic process of HF.

Beta-blockers should be used with all patients in stable condition who are clinically eu-volemic and have no recent HF exacerbations. The beta-blockers carvedilol, metopro-lol succinate, and bisoprolol have been shown to be effective in reducing the risk of death in patients with chronic HF (CIBIS-II Investigators and Committees, 1999; Dar-gie, 2001; Packer et al., 2001).

The beneficial effects of beta-blockers include improvements in survival, morbid-ity, EF, remodeling, and quality of life as well as reductions in rate of hospitalization, incidence of sudden cardiac death (Bristow, 2000; Foody, Farrell, & Krumholz, 2002; Poole-Wilson et al., 2003), and anthracycline-induced cardiotoxicity (Cardinale, Co-lombo, & Cipolla, 2008; Kalay et al., 2006; MERIT-HF Study Group, 1999). Because of the favorable effects of beta-blockers on survival and disease progression, treatment with these agents should be initiated as soon as LV dysfunction is diagnosed. Patients with a current or recent history of fluid retention require diuretics to maintain sodi-um and fluid balance and to prevent the exacerbation of fluid retention that can ac-company the initiation of beta-blocker therapy (Epstein & Braunwald, 1966; Gaffney & Braunwald, 1963).

Beta-blockers should not be used (or should be used with extreme caution) in pa-tients who have reactive airway disease, diabetes with frequent episodes of hypogly-cemia, or bradyrhythmia or heart block unless a pacemaker is used as well (Jessup & Brozena, 2003).

Nursing Considerations for Patients Receiving Beta-Blockers

- To increase compliance with therapy, patients should be educated about the poten-tial side effects of beta-blockers, such as generalized fatigue and weakness at the ini-tiation or uptitration of treatment.
- Because initiation of beta-blocker therapy can cause fluid retention (Epstein & Braunwald, 1966; Gaffney & Braunwald, 2000), which is usually asymptomatic, pa-tients should be monitored closely for weight increases and worsening of signs and symptoms of HF.
- Beta-blockers should be initiated at very low doses and gradually titrated as tolerated as indicated by blood pressure, heart rate, and symptoms.
- Patients should be monitored closely for symptoms of hypotension, bradycardia, heart block, weight gain, and fluid retention.
- To decrease the incidence of hypotensive episodes, beta-blockers should be taken with food and at a separate time from ACE inhibitors.
- Patients should be advised that clinical responses to the drug are generally de-layed and may require two to three months to become apparent (Massie, Kramer, & Haughom, 1981).
- Abrupt withdrawal of treatment with beta-blockers can lead to clinical deterioration and should be avoided (Waagstein, Caidahl, Wallentin, Bergh, & Hjalmarson, 1989) unless the patient is severely hypotensive or in cardiogenic shock.

Diuretics

Patients with LV dysfunction may need diuretics to prevent volume overload and ex-acerbation of HF. Treatment should be individualized based on response to therapy and degree of fluid overload. A patient discharged from the hospital with diuretics should be followed up in the clinic at least one week after discharge to check for volume sta-tus and electrolyte abnormalities. Bumetanide and furosemide are the most common-ly used loop diuretics. The bioavailability of bumetanide is approximately twice that of furosemide and is 40–50 times more potent on a milligram-per-milligram basis; bumetanide can also be administered intravenously (Jain, Massie, Gattis, Klein, & Gheorghiade, 2003).

Excessive use of diuretics may result in electrolyte abnormalities and worsening renal function, although such effects occur because of changes in renal hemodynamics rather than nephrotoxicity. Diuretic agents may increase the incidence of digitalis toxicity both by decreasing the glomerular filtration rate secondary to volume depletion and by inducing hypokalemia and hypomagnesemia, and these electrolyte disturbances may lower the threshold for proarrhythmic events (Jain et al., 2003). If a patient exhibits resistance to diuretics, an oral thiazide diuretic or spironolactone may be combined with a loop diuretic for a synergistic effect. If all diuretic strategies are unsuccessful, an ultrafiltration strategy may be reasonable. Ultrafiltration moves water and solutes across a semipermeable membrane to reduce volume overload. Because the electrolyte concentration is similar to that of plasma, relatively more sodium can be removed by ultrafiltration than by diuretics (Costanzo, Saltzberg, O'Sullivan, & Sobotka, 2005).

Nursing Considerations for Patients Receiving Diuretics
- The patient's weight should be monitored daily to evaluate for volume overload and diuretic dose adjustment.
- Patients on daily diuretics should be monitored for hypotension, electrolyte levels (especially potassium and magnesium), and renal function.

Digitalis

The digitalis glycoside (digoxin) inhibits the sodium-potassium adenosine triphosphatase (ATPase) in cardiac cells, resulting in increased cardiac contractility (Akera, Baskin, Tobin, & Brody, 1973). Several placebo-controlled trials have shown that digoxin can improve symptoms, quality of life, and exercise tolerance in patients with mild to moderate HF (Cohn et al., 1988; Uretsky et al., 1993). These benefits resulted regardless of the underlying rhythm (normal sinus rhythm or atrial fibrillation), cause of HF (ischemic or nonischemic), or concomitant therapy (with or without ACE inhibitors).

Digoxin should be considered for patients with persistent symptoms of HF despite therapy with diuretics, ACE inhibitors or angiotensin receptor blockers, and beta-blockers (Gheorghiade & Ferguson, 1991; Rahimtoola, 2004). Digoxin is not indicated as primary therapy for the stabilization of patients with acute exacerbation of HF symptoms, including fluid retention or hypotension. Low doses (0.125 mg daily or every other day) should be used initially if the patient is older than 70, has impaired renal function, or has a lean body mass (Jelliffe & Brooker, 1974). In a retrospective analysis of the Digitalis Investigation Group trial, risk-adjusted mortality increased as the plasma digoxin concentration exceeded 1 ng/ml (Rathore, Curtis, Wang, Bristow, & Krumholz, 2003). The major side effects included cardiac arrhythmias (e.g., ectopic and reentrant cardiac rhythms and heart block), gastrointestinal symptoms (e.g., anorexia, nausea, vomiting), and neurologic complaints (e.g., visual disturbances, disorientation, confusion). Overt digoxin toxicity is commonly associated with serum digoxin levels greater than 2 ng/ml. The concomitant use of clarithromycin, erythromycin, amiodarone, itraconazole, cyclosporine, verapamil, or quinidine can increase the serum concentration and may increase the likelihood of digoxin toxicity (Bizjak & Mauro, 1997; Hager et al., 1979; Juurlink, Mamdani, Kopp, Laupacis, & Redelmeier, 2003).

Nursing Considerations for Patients Receiving Digitalis
- Patients should not be given digoxin if they have significant sinus or atrioventricular block, unless the block has been addressed in a permanent pacemaker.
- Digoxin should be used cautiously in patients taking other drugs that can depress sinus or atrioventricular nodal function or affect digoxin levels (e.g., amiodarone or a beta-blocker).
- Patients should be monitored for signs and symptoms of digoxin toxicity when it is administered concomitantly with certain medications (listed previously).

Aldosterone Receptor Antagonists

Addition of an aldosterone antagonist is recommended for selected patients with moderate or severe symptoms of HF and reduced LVEF who can be carefully monitored for preserved renal function and normal potassium concentration. Spironolactone is the most widely used aldosterone antagonist. In a large-scale clinical trial, low doses of spironolactone (12.5 mg daily) added to ACE inhibitors for patients with NYHA class IV HF symptoms reduced the risk of death from 46% to 35% over two years, with a 35% reduction in HF hospitalization and improvement in functional class (Pitt et al., 1999). Eplerenone is a newer aldosterone antagonist that has been shown to decrease mortality from 13.6% to 11.8% at one year. Gynecomastia and other antiandrogen effects are generally not seen with eplerenone compared with spironolactone (Pitt et al., 2001). In circumstances in which monitoring for hyperkalemia and renal dysfunction will not be feasible, these risks may outweigh the benefits of using aldosterone antagonists.

Nursing Considerations for Patients Receiving Aldosterone Receptor Antagonists
- The major risk in using aldosterone antagonists is hyperkalemia due to inhibition of potassium excretion.
- Renal function must be monitored. Aldosterone antagonists should not be given when creatinine clearance is less than 30 ml/min.
- Patients must be monitored for possible increased diuresis after the addition of an aldosterone antagonist to other diuretic therapy, even though it has a relatively weak diuretic effect.

Drugs to Avoid in Patients With Heart Failure

Antiarrhythmic Agents

Some antiarrhythmic agents have cardiodepressant and proarrhythmic effects and therefore should be avoided by patients with HF. Of the available antiarrhythmic agents, only amiodarone and dofetilide have been shown to not adversely affect survival (Torp-Pedersen et al., 1999).

Calcium Channel Blockers

Calcium channel blockers can lead to worsening HF and have been associated with an increased risk of cardiovascular events (Packer, Kessler, & Lee, 1987). Of the available calcium channel blockers, only the vasoselective ones (e.g., amlodipine) have been shown to not adversely affect survival (Elkayam, 1998; McKelvie et al., 1995; Packer et al., 1987, 1996; Reed et al., 2004; Torp-Pedersen et al., 1999).

Nonsteroidal Anti-Inflammatory Agents

Nonsteroidal anti-inflammatory agents (NSAIDs) can cause sodium retention and peripheral vasoconstriction and can attenuate the efficacy and enhance the toxicity of diuretics and ACE inhibitors (Herchuelz et al., 1989). NSAIDs have been associated with an increase in the incidence of new HF and hospitalization for HF (Page & Henry, 2000).

Nonpharmacologic Treatment Strategies

Patient Education

Patient and family education is a critical intervention that should be reinforced with every clinic visit. Education and counseling should be provided regarding compliance with medications, dietary management, daily weight monitoring, alcohol restriction, physical activity, symptom monitoring, avoidance of NSAIDs, and early detection of symptoms of HF exacerbation. In addition to pharmacologic agents, behavioral modification (specifically with regard to dietary guidelines and exercise training) should be encouraged. Compliance with medications and dietary restrictions is most likely if the patient understands the pathophysiology and treatment and receives encouragement and positive reinforcement from healthcare providers. In a recent study, patients who received an education intervention had a lower risk of rehospitalization, lower risk of death, and lower cost of care (Hunt et al., 2009).

Dietary Modifications

Excessive salt and fluid intake are important factors in causing ADHF, which may precipitate hospitalizations. Dietary modification is a major challenge because patients with cancer have decreased appetite, eat less, and may experience nausea and vomiting as side effects of cancer therapy. Cachexia is one of the most frequent effects of malignancy, and weight loss in excess of 5% of premorbid weight has been noted for more than half of patients with cancer (Tisdale, 2002). Patients should be instructed on the relationship between sodium and fluid retention, and the importance of sodium restriction must be stressed. It is recommended that sodium intake be restricted to 2,000 mg/day to prevent volume overload (Thomas & Harrah, 2000). Using salt while cooking instead of adding it at the table and avoiding salty foods are usually sufficient to achieve this goal.

Activity

Physical activity should be encouraged except during periods of acute exacerbation, when physical rest is recommended. Patients should be advised on how to carry out daily physical activity and leisure activities that do not induce symptoms. Exercise improves skeletal function and overall functional capacity. The most recent data have shown that exercise training by patients with HF and preserved EF improved physical functioning, diastolic function, and overall quality of life (Edelmann et al., 2011).

Weight Monitoring

Patients should be advised to monitor their daily weight and, in case of a sudden unexpected weight gain (more than 2 lbs/day for two consecutive days or more than

5 lbs/week), to alert their healthcare provider for possible adjustment of the diuretic dose.

Alcohol Intake

Moderate alcohol intake (one beer or one or two glasses of wine per day) is permitted except in cases of alcoholic cardiomyopathy, in which case alcohol consumption is prohibited.

Smoking Cessation

Smoking should always be discouraged. Referral should be made to a smoking cessation program with a comprehensive approach to help the patient to stop smoking.

Symptom Management in Patients With Cancer and Heart Failure

HF and cancer are progressive diseases with debilitating symptoms resulting from both the disease and the cancer treatments. The presence of HF in a patient with cancer or vice versa is likely to have a substantial impact on symptoms and quality of life. Management of symptoms presents a challenge to patients, families, and healthcare providers throughout the entire trajectory of the disease process (Fadol et al., 2008). Despite optimal medical therapy, some patients do not improve with treatment and continue to experience recurrent symptoms that not only diminish quality of life but also lead to frequent visits to the emergency department and more frequent hospital admissions. Early identification of symptoms and timely intervention are critical components of cost-effective disease management to improve quality of life. For many patients with HF, improvement in symptoms rather than longer survival is a preferred therapeutic outcome (Stanek, Oates, McGhan, Denofrio, & Loh, 2000).

The goals of symptom management are the same irrespective of the diagnosis. A full assessment of the patient, intervention to reverse any reversible factors, and palliation of irreversible situations (e.g., end-stage HF and cancer) are applicable to oncology and cardiology alike. It is important that the medical management of HF is optimized because optimization has a major effect on both symptom control and survival. Using a symptom assessment instrument such as the MD Anderson Symptom Inventory–Heart Failure (MDASI-HF) (Fadol et al., 2008) (see Figure 10-13) will facilitate the early identification of symptoms and prompt timely intervention to prevent HF exacerbation. All practitioners involved in the management of these patients need to develop skills that include a full holistic assessment of symptoms, teamwork, and collaboration with patients, families, caregivers, and other healthcare professionals to adequately manage symptoms and improve patients' quality of life.

Conclusion

As a complication of cancer therapy or as a comorbid condition in cancer, HF can significantly affect both survival and quality of life. Multiple chemotherapeutic regimens

Figure 10-13. MD Anderson Symptom Inventory–Heart Failure Instrument

Date: _____   Institution:_____

Participant Initials: _____   Hospital Chart #:_____

Participant Number: _____

Part I. How **severe** are your symptoms?

People with cancer frequently have symptoms that are caused by their disease or by their treatment. Patients with heart failure may have similar symptoms. We ask you to rate how severe the following symptoms have been *in the last 24 hours.* Please fill in the circle below from 0 (symptom has not been present) to 10 (the symptom was as bad as you can imagine it could be) for each item.

	NOT PRESENT										AS BAD AS YOU CAN IMAGINE
	0	1	2	3	4	5	6	7	8	9	10
1. Your **pain** at its WORST?	○	○	○	○	○	○	○	○	○	○	○
2. Your **fatigue (tiredness)** at its WORST?	○	○	○	○	○	○	○	○	○	○	○
3. Your **nausea** at its WORST?	○	○	○	○	○	○	○	○	○	○	○
4. Your **disturbed sleep** at its WORST?	○	○	○	○	○	○	○	○	○	○	○
5. Your feeling of being **distressed (upset)** at its WORST?	○	○	○	○	○	○	○	○	○	○	○
6. Your **shortness of breath** at its WORST?	○	○	○	○	○	○	○	○	○	○	○
7. Your problem with **remembering things** at its WORST?	○	○	○	○	○	○	○	○	○	○	○
8. Your problem with **lack of appetite** at its WORST?	○	○	○	○	○	○	○	○	○	○	○
9. Your feeling **drowsy (sleepy)** at its WORST?	○	○	○	○	○	○	○	○	○	○	○
10. Your having a **dry mouth** at its WORST?	○	○	○	○	○	○	○	○	○	○	○
11. Your feeling **sad** at its WORST?	○	○	○	○	○	○	○	○	○	○	○
12. Your **vomiting** at its WORST?	○	○	○	○	○	○	○	○	○	○	○
13. Your **numbness or tingling** at its WORST?	○	○	○	○	○	○	○	○	○	○	○

Page 1 of 2

MDASI-HF - August, 2008

(Continued on next page)

Figure 10-13. MD Anderson Symptom Inventory–Heart Failure Instrument *(Continued)*

Date: _____   Institution: _____

Participant Initials: _____   Hospital Chart #: _____

Participant Number: _____

Heart Failure (HF)	NOT PRESENT 0	1	2	3	4	5	6	7	8	AS BAD AS YOU CAN IMAGINE 9	10
14. Your problem with **abdominal bloating** at its WORST?	O	O	O	O	O	O	O	O	O	O	O
15. Your problem with **ankle swelling** at its WORST?	O	O	O	O	O	O	O	O	O	O	O
16. Your difficulty **sleeping without adding more pillows under your head** at its WORST?	O	O	O	O	O	O	O	O	O	O	O
17. Your problem with **lack of energy** at its WORST?	O	O	O	O	O	O	O	O	O	O	O
18. Your problem with **racing heartbeat (palpitation)** at its WORST?	O	O	O	O	O	O	O	O	O	O	O
19. Your problem with **nighttime cough** at its WORST?	O	O	O	O	O	O	O	O	O	O	O
20. Your problem with **waking up at night with difficulty breathing** at its WORST?	O	O	O	O	O	O	O	O	O	O	O
21. Your problem with **sudden weight gain** at its WORST?	O	O	O	O	O	O	O	O	O	O	O

Part II. How have your symptoms **interfered** with your life?

Symptoms frequently interfere with how we feel and function. How much have your symptoms interfered with the following items **in the last 24 hours**:

	Did not Interfere 0	1	2	3	4	5	6	7	8	Interfered Completely 9	10
22. General **activity**?	O	O	O	O	O	O	O	O	O	O	O
23. **Mood**?	O	O	O	O	O	O	O	O	O	O	O
24. **Work** (including work around the house)**?**	O	O	O	O	O	O	O	O	O	O	O
25. **Relations** with other people?	O	O	O	O	O	O	O	O	O	O	O
26. **Walking**?	O	O	O	O	O	O	O	O	O	O	O
27. **Enjoyment** of life?	O	O	O	O	O	O	O	O	O	O	O

Page 2 of 2

MDASI-HF - August, 2008

have been implicated as the cause of damage to the myocardial cells, thereby resulting in HF. In some cases this damage may take months or years to become apparent. Prevention of HF is critical, and timely intervention is paramount for patients who have already developed HF to prevent exacerbation and improve quality of life. To achieve better care for patients, open communication among cardiology, oncology, patients, and caregivers should be fostered with mutual understanding and learning.

References

Adams, K.F., Jr., Fonarow, G.C., Emerman, C.L., LeJemtel, T.H., Costanzo, M.R., Abraham, W.T., ... Horton, D.P. (2005). Characteristics and outcomes of patients hospitalized for heart failure in the United States: Rationale, design, and preliminary observations from the first 100,000 cases in the Acute Decompensated Heart Failure National Registry (ADHERE). *American Heart Journal, 149,* 209–216. doi:10.1016/j.ahj.2004.08.005

Adams, K.F., Jr., & Zannad, F. (1998). Clinical definition and epidemiology of advanced heart failure. *American Heart Journal, 135,* S204–S215. doi:10.1016/S0002-8703(98)70251-0

Akera, T., Baskin, S.I., Tobin, T., & Brody, T.M. (1973). Ouabain: Temporal relationship between the inotropic effect and the in vitro binding to, and dissociation from, (Na + + K +)-activated ATPase. *Naunyn-Schmiedeberg's Archives of Pharmacology, 277,* 151–162. doi:10.1007/BF00501156

Bird, B.R., & Swain, S.M. (2008). Cardiac toxicity in breast cancer survivors: Review of potential cardiac problems. *Clinical Cancer Research, 14,* 14–24. doi:10.1158/1078-0432.CCR-07-1033

Bizjak, E.D., & Mauro, V.F. (1997). Digoxin-macrolide drug interaction. *Annals of Pharmacotherapy, 31,* 1077–1079.

Bonow, R.O., Bennett, S., Casey, D.E., Jr., Ganiats, T.G., Hlatky, M.A., Konstam, M.A., ... Spertus, J.A. (2005). ACC/AHA clinical performance measures for adults with chronic heart failure: A report of the American College of Cardiology/American Heart Association Task Force on Performance Measures (Writing Committee to Develop Heart Failure Clinical Performance Measures) endorsed by the Heart Failure Society of America. *Journal of the American College of Cardiology, 46,* 1144–1178. doi:10.1016/j.jacc.2005.07.012

Bosch, X., Esteve, J., Sitges, M., de Caralt, T.M., Domènech, A., Ortiz, J.T., ... Rovira, M. (2011). Prevention of chemotherapy-induced left ventricular dysfunction with enalapril and carvedilol: Rationale and design of the OVERCOME trial. *Journal of Cardiac Failure, 17,* 643–648. doi:10.1016/j.cardfail.2011.03.008

Boufidou, A., Mantziari, L., Paraskevaidis, S., Karvounis, H., Nenopoulou, E., Manthou, M.E., ... Parcharidis, G. (2010). An interesting case of cardiac amyloidosis initially diagnosed as hypertrophic cardiomyopathy. *Hellenic Journal of Cardiology, 51,* 552–557.

Bristow, M.R. (2000). Beta-adrenergic receptor blockade in chronic heart failure. *Circulation, 101,* 558–569. doi:10.1161/01.CIR.101.5.558

Bristow, M.R., Thompson, P.D., Martin, R.P., Mason, J.W., Billingham, M.E., & Harrison, D.C. (1978). Early anthracycline cardiotoxicity. *American Journal of Medicine, 65,* 823–832. doi:10.1016/0002-9343(78)90802-1

Cardinale, D., Colombo, A., & Cipolla, C.M. (2008). Prevention and treatment of cardiomyopathy and heart failure in patients receiving cancer chemotherapy. *Current Treatment Options in Cardiovascular Medicine, 10,* 486–495. doi:10.1007/s11936-008-0041-x

Cardinale, D., Colombo, A., Sandri, M.T., Lamantia, G., Colombo, N., Civelli, M., ... Cipolla, C.M. (2006). Prevention of high-dose chemotherapy-induced cardiotoxicity in high-risk patients by angiotensin-converting enzyme inhibition. *Circulation, 114,* 2474–2481. doi:10.1161/CIRCULATIONAHA.106.635144

Cardinale, D., Sandri, M.T., Colombo, A., Colombo, N., Boeri, M., Lamantia, G., ... Cipolla, C.M. (2004). Prognostic value of troponin I in cardiac risk stratification of cancer patients undergoing high-dose chemotherapy. *Circulation, 109,* 2749–2754. doi:10.1161/01.CIR.0000130926.51766.CC

Cardinale, D., Sandri, M.T., Martinoni, A., Tricca, A., Civelli, M., Lamantia, G., ... Fiorentini, C. (2000). Left ventricular dysfunction predicted by early troponin I release after high-dose chemotherapy. *Journal of the American College of Cardiology, 36,* 517–522. doi:10.1016/S0735-1097(00)00748-8

Carver, J.R., Shapiro, C.L., Ng, A., Jacobs, L., Schwartz, C., Virgo, K.S., ... Vaughn, D.J. (2007). American Society of Clinical Oncology clinical evidence review on the ongoing care of adult cancer survivors: Cardiac and pulmonary late effects. *Journal of Clinical Oncology, 25,* 3991–4008. doi:10.1200/JCO.2007.10.9777

Cesario, D., Clark, J., & Maisel, A. (1998). Beneficial effects of intermittent home administration of the inotrope/vasodilator milrinone in patients with end-stage congestive heart failure: A preliminary study. *American Heart Journal, 135,* 121–129. doi:10.1016/S0002-8703(98)70352-7

Chen, H.H., Lainchbury, J.G., Senni, M., Bailey, K.R., & Redfield, M.M. (2002). Diastolic heart failure in the community: Clinical profile, natural history, therapy, and impact of proposed diagnostic criteria. *Journal of Cardiac Failure, 8,* 279–287. doi:10.1054/jcaf.2002.128871

CIBIS-II Investigators and Committees. (1999). The Cardiac Insufficiency Bisoprolol Study II (CIBIS-II): A randomised trial. *Lancet, 353,* 9–13. doi:10.1016/S0140-6736(98)11181-9

Cleland, J.G., Swedberg, K., Follath, F., Komajda, M., Cohen-Solal, A., Aguilar, J.C., ... Mason, J. (2003). The EuroHeart Failure survey programme—A survey on the quality of care among patients with heart failure in Europe. Part 1: Patient characteristics and diagnosis. *European Heart Journal, 24,* 442–463. doi:10.1016/S0195-668X(02)00823-0

Clinical Pharmacology. (2010). Online database. Retrieved from http://www.clinicalpharmacology.com

Cohn, J., Hawkins, M., Levine, H., Naughton, J., Rapaport, E., Goldstein, S., ... Petey, K. (1988). Comparative effects of therapy with captopril and digoxin in patients with mild to moderate heart failure. The Captopril-Digoxin Multicenter Research Group. *JAMA, 259,* 539–544. doi:10.1001/jama.1988.03720040031022

Cooper, L.T., Baughman, K.L., Feldman, A.M., Frustaci, A., Jessup, M., Kuhl, U., ... Virmani, R. (2007). The role of endomyocardial biopsy in the management of cardiovascular disease: A scientific statement from the American Heart Association, the American College of Cardiology, and the European Society of Cardiology. *Circulation, 116,* 2216–2233. doi:10.1161/CIRCULATIONAHA.107.186093

Costanzo, M.R., Saltzberg, M., O'Sullivan, J., & Sobotka, P. (2005). Early ultrafiltration in patients with decompensated heart failure and diuretic resistance. *Journal of the American College of Cardiology, 46,* 2047–2051. doi:10.1016/j.jacc.2005.05.099

Criteria Committee of the New York Heart Association. (1994). *Nomenclature and criteria for diagnosis of diseases of the heart and great vessels* (9th ed.). Boston, MA: Little, Brown.

Cutter, D.J., Darby, S.C., & Yusuf, S.W. (2011). Risks of heart disease after radiotherapy. *Texas Heart Institute Journal, 38,* 257–258.

Dargie, H.J. (2001). Effect of carvedilol on outcome after myocardial infarction in patients with left-ventricular dysfunction: The CAPRICORN randomised trial. *Lancet, 357,* 1385–1390. doi:10.1016/S0140-6736(00)04560-8

DiDomenico, R.J., Park, H.Y., Southworth, M.R., Eyrich, H.M., Lewis, R.K., Finley, J.M., & Schumock, G.T. (2004). Guidelines for acute decompensated heart failure treatment. *Annals of Pharmacotherapy, 38,* 649–660. doi:101345/aph.1D481

Drazner, M.H., Hamilton, M.A., Fonarow, G., Creaser, J., Flavell, C., & Stevenson, L.W. (1999). Relationship between right and left-sided filling pressures in 1000 patients with advanced heart failure. *Journal of Heart and Lung Transplantation, 18,* 1126–1132. doi:10.1056/NEJMoa010641

Drazner, M.H., Rame, J.E., Stevenson, L.W., & Dries, D.L. (2001). Prognostic importance of elevated jugular venous pressure and a third heart sound in patients with heart failure. *New England Journal of Medicine, 345,* 574–581.

Drímal, J., Zúrová-Nedelcevová, J., Knezl, V., Sotníková, R., & Navarová, J. (2006). Cardiovascular toxicity of the first line cancer chemotherapeutic agents: Doxorubicin, cyclophosphamide, streptozotocin and bevacizumab. *Neuro Endocrinology Letters, 27*(Suppl. 2), 176–179.

Edelmann, F., Gelbrich, G., Dungen, H.D., Fröhling, S., Wachter, R., Stahrenberg, R., ... Pieske, B. (2011). Exercise training improves exercise capacity and diastolic function in patients with heart failure with preserved ejection fraction results of the Ex-DHF (Exercise training in Diastolic Heart Failure) pilot study. *Journal of the American College of Cardiology, 58,* 1780–1791. doi:10.1016/j.jacc.2011.06.054

Elkayam, U. (1998). Calcium channel blockers in heart failure. *Cardiology, 89*(Suppl. 1), 38–46. doi:10.1159/000047278

Epstein, S.E., & Braunwald, E. (1966). The effect of beta adrenergic blockade on patterns of urinary sodium excretion: Studies in normal subjects and in patients with heart disease. *Annals of Internal Medicine, 65,* 20–27.

Ewer, M.S., Swain, S.M., Cardinale, D., Fadol, A., & Suter, T.M. (2011). Cardiac dysfunction after cancer treatment. *Texas Heart Institute Journal, 38,* 248–252.

Ewer, M.S., & Lippman, S.M. (2005). Type II chemotherapy-related cardiac dysfunction: Time to recognize a new entity. *Journal of Clinical Oncology, 23,* 2900–2902. doi:10.1200/JCO.2005.05.827

Ewer, S.M., & Ewer, M.S. (2008). Cardiotoxicity profile of trastuzumab. *Drug Safety, 31,* 459–467. doi:10.2165/00002018-200831060-00002

Fadol, A. (2006). Management of acute decompensated heart failure in patients with cancer. *Clinical Journal of Oncology Nursing, 10,* 731–736. doi:10.1188/06.CJON.731-736

Fadol, A., Mendoza, T., Gning, I., Kernicki, J., Symes, L., Cleeland, C.S., & Lenihan, D. (2008). Psychometric testing of the MDASI-HF: A symptom assessment instrument for patients with cancer and concurrent heart failure. *Journal of Cardiac Failure, 14,* 497–507. doi:10.1016/j.cardfail.2008.01.012

Felker, G.M., Thompson, R.E., Hare, J.M., Hruban, R.H., Clemetson, D.E., Howard, D.L., … Kasper, E.K. (2000). Underlying causes and long-term survival in patients with initially unexplained cardiomyopathy. *New England Journal of Medicine, 342,* 1077–1084. doi:10.1056/NEJM200004133421502

Fleisher, L.A., Beckman, J.A., Brown, K.A., Calkins, H., Chaikof, E.L., Fleischmann, K.E., … Robb, J.F. (2007). ACC/AHA 2006 guideline update on perioperative cardiovascular evaluation for noncardiac surgery: Focused update on perioperative beta-blocker therapy—A report of the American College of Cardiology/American Heart Association Task Force on Practice Guidelines (Writing Committee to Update the 2002 Guidelines on Perioperative Cardiovascular Evaluation for Noncardiac Surgery). *Anesthesia and Analgesia, 104,* 15–26. doi:10.1213/01.ane.0000243335.31748.22

Foody, J.M., Farrell, M.H., & Krumholz, H.M. (2002). Beta-blocker therapy in heart failure: Scientific review. *JAMA, 287,* 883–889. doi:10.1001/jama.287.7.883

Gaffney, T.E., & Braunwald, E. (1963). Importance of the adrenergic nervous system in the support of circulatory function in patients with congestive heart failure. *American Journal of Medicine, 34,* 320–324. doi:10.1016/0002-9343(63)90118-9

George, A., & Figueredo, V.M. (2011). Alcoholic cardiomyopathy: A review. *Journal of Cardiac Failure, 17,* 844–849. doi:10.1016/j.cardfail.2011.05.008

Gheorghiade, M., & Ferguson, D. (1991). Digoxin. A neurohormonal modulator in heart failure? *Circulation, 84,* 2181–2186. doi:10.1161/01.CIR.84.5.2181

Giampolo, M., Seldin, D.C., & Gertz, M.A. (2011). Amyloidosis: Pathogenesis and new therapeutic options. *Journal of Clinical Oncology, 29,* 1924–1933.

Giles, T.D., Katz, R., Sullivan, J.M., Wolfson, P., Haugland, M., Kirlin, P., … Chiaramida, A. (1989). Short- and long-acting angiotensin-converting enzyme inhibitors: A randomized trial of lisinopril versus captopril in the treatment of congestive heart failure. The Multicenter Lisinopril-Captopril Congestive Heart Failure Study Group. *Journal of the American College of Cardiology, 13,* 1240–1247. doi:10.1016/0735-1097(89)90294-5

Granger, C.B., McMurray, J.J., Yusuf, S., Held, P., Michelson, E.L., Olofsson, B., … Swedberg, K. (2003). Effects of candesartan in patients with chronic heart failure and reduced left-ventricular systolic function intolerant to angiotensin-converting-enzyme inhibitors: The CHARM-Alternative trial. *Lancet, 362,* 772–776. doi:10.1016/S0140-6736(03)14284-5

Guarneri, V., Lenihan, D.J., Valero, V., Durand, J.B., Broglio, K., Hess, K.R., & Esteva, F.J. (2006). Long-term cardiac tolerability of trastuzumab in metastatic breast cancer: The MDACC experience. *Journal of Clinical Oncology, 24,* 4107–4115. doi:10.1200/JCO.2005.04.9551

Gwathmey, J.K., Copelas, L., MacKinnon, R., Schoen, F.J., Feldman, M.D., Grossman, W., & Morgan, J.P. (1987). Abnormal intracellular calcium handling in myocardium from patients with end-stage heart failure. *Circulation Research, 61,* 70–76. doi:10.1161/01.RES.61.1.70

Hager, W.D., Fenster, P., Mayersohn, M., Perrier, D., Graves, P., Marcus, F.I., & Goldman, S. (1979). Digoxin-quinidine interaction—Pharmacokinetic evaluation. *New England Journal of Medicine, 300,* 1238–1241. doi:10.1056/NEJM197905313002202

Herchuelz, A., Derenne, F., Deger, F., Juvent, M., Van Ganse, E., Staroukine, M., … Douchamps, J. (1989). Interaction between nonsteroidal anti-inflammatory drugs and loop diuretics: Modulation by sodium balance. *Journal of Pharmacology and Experimental Therapeutics, 248,* 1175–1181.

Hunt, S.A., Abraham, W.T., Chin, M.H., Feldman, A.M., Francis, G.S., Ganiats, T.G., … Riegel, B. (2005). ACC/AHA 2005 guideline update for the diagnosis and management of chronic heart failure in the adult: A report of the American College of Cardiology/American Heart Association Task Force on Practice Guidelines (Writing Committee to Update the 2001 Guidelines for the Evaluation and Management of Heart Failure): Developed in collaboration with the American College of Chest Physicians and the International Society for Heart and Lung Transplantation: Endorsed by the Heart Rhythm Society. *Circulation, 112,* e154–e235. doi:10.1161/CIRCULATIONAHA.105.167586

Hunt, S.A., Abraham, W.T., Chin, M.H., Feldman, A.M., Francis, G.S., Ganiats, T.G., … Yancy, C.W. (2009). 2009 focused update incorporated into the ACC/AHA 2005 Guidelines for the Diagnosis and Management of Heart Failure in Adults: A report of the American College of Cardiology Foundation/American Heart Association Task Force on Practice Guidelines: Developed in collaboration with the

International Society for Heart and Lung Transplantation. *Circulation, 119*, e391–e479. doi:10.1161/CIRCULATIONAHA.109.192065

Jain, P., Massie, B.M., Gattis, W.A., Klein, L., & Gheorghiade, M. (2003). Current medical treatment for the exacerbation of chronic heart failure resulting in hospitalization. *American Heart Journal, 145*(Suppl. 2), S3–S17. doi:10.1067/mhj.2003.149

Jelliffe, R.W., & Brooker, G. (1974). A nomogram for digoxin therapy. *American Journal of Medicine, 57*, 63–68. doi:10.1016/0002-9343(74)90769-4

Jessup, M., & Brozena, S. (2003). Heart failure. *New England Journal of Medicine, 348*, 2007–2018. doi:10.1056/NEJMra021498

Joint Commission. (2011). Heart failure core measure set. Retrieved from http://www.jointcommission.org/assets/1/6/Heart%20Failure.pdf

Juurlink, D.N., Mamdani, M., Kopp, A., Laupacis, A., & Redelmeier, D.A. (2003). Drug-drug interactions among elderly patients hospitalized for drug toxicity. *JAMA, 289*, 1652–1658. doi:10.1001/jama.289.13.1652

Kalay, N., Basar, E., Ozdogru, I., Er, O., Cetinkaya, Y., Dogan, A., … Ergin, A. (2006). Protective effects of carvedilol against anthracycline-induced cardiomyopathy. *Journal of the American College of Cardiology, 48*, 2258–2262. doi:10.1016/j.jacc.2006.07.052

Kerkelä, R., Grazette, L., Yacobi, R., Iliescu, C., Patten, R., Beahm, C., … Force, T. (2006). Cardiotoxicity of the cancer therapeutic agent imatinib mesylate. *Nature Medicine, 12*, 908–916. doi:10.1038/nm1446

Khakoo, A.Y., Kassiotis, C.M., Tannir, N., Plana, J.C., Halushka, M., Bickford, C., … Lenihan, D.J. (2008). Heart failure associated with sunitinib malate: A multitargeted receptor tyrosine kinase inhibitor. *Cancer, 112*, 2500–2508. doi:10.1002/cncr.23460

Khalil, M.E., Basher, A.W., Brown, E.J., Jr., & Alhaddad, I.A. (2001). A remarkable medical story: Benefits of angiotensin-converting enzyme inhibitors in cardiac patients. *Journal of the American College of Cardiology, 37*, 1757–1764. doi:10.1016/S0735-1097(01)01229-3

Leier, C.V., & Binkley, P.E. (1998). Parenteral inotropic support for advanced congestive heart failure. *Progress in Cardiovascular Diseases, 41*, 207–224. doi:10.1016/S0033-0620(98)80056-X

Lipshultz, S.E., Lipsitz, S.R., Mone, S.M., Goorin, A.M., Sallan, S.E., Sanders, S.P., … Colan, S.D. (1995). Female sex and drug dose as risk factors for late cardiotoxic effects of doxorubicin therapy for childhood cancer. *New England Journal of Medicine, 332*, 1738–1743. doi:10.1056/NEJM199506293322602

Lipshultz, S.E., Rifai, N., Sallan, S.E., Lipsitz, S.R., Dalton, V., Sacks, D.B., & Ottlinger, M.E. (1997). Predictive value of cardiac troponin T in pediatric patients at risk for myocardial injury. *Circulation, 96*, 2641–2648. doi:10.1161/01.CIR.96.8.2641

Maisel, A.S., Koon, J., Krishnaswamy, P., Kazenegra, R., Clopton, P., Gardetto, N., … De Maria, A. (2001). Utility of B-natriuretic peptide as a rapid, point-of-care test for screening patients undergoing echocardiography to determine left ventricular dysfunction. *American Heart Journal, 141*, 367–374. doi:10.1067/mhj.2001.113215

Marantz, P.R., Tobin, J.N., Wassertheil-Smoller, S., Steingart, R.M., Wexler, J.P., Budner, N., … Wachspress, J. (1988). The relationship between left ventricular systolic function and congestive heart failure diagnosed by clinical criteria. *Circulation, 77*, 607–612. doi:10.1161/01.CIR.77.3.607

Marius-Nunez, A.L., Heaney, L., Fernandez, R.N., Clark, W.A., Ranganini, A., Silber, E., & Denes, P. (1996). Intermittent inotropic therapy in an outpatient setting: A cost-effective therapeutic modality in patients with refractory heart failure. *American Heart Journal, 132*, 805–808. doi:10.1016/S0002-8703(96)90315-4

Martinelli, N., Carleo, P., Girelli, D., & Olivieri, O. (2011). An unusual heart failure: Cardiac amyloidosis due to light-chain myeloma. *Circulation, 123*, e583–e584. doi:10.1161/CIRCULATIONAHA.110.011601

Mason, J.W., Bristow, M.R., Billingham, M.E., & Daniels, J.R. (1978). Invasive and noninvasive methods of assessing Adriamycin cardiotoxic effects in man: Superiority of histopathologic assessment using endomyocardial biopsy. *Cancer Treatment Reports, 62*, 857–864.

Massie, B., Kramer, B., & Haughom, F. (1981). Postural hypotension and tachycardia during hydralazine–isosorbide dinitrate therapy for chronic heart failure. *Circulation, 63*, 658–664. doi:10.1161/01.CIR.63.3.658

McKelvie, R.S., Teo, K.K., McCartney, N., Humen, D., Montague, T., & Yusuf, S. (1995). Effects of exercise training in patients with congestive heart failure: A critical review. *Journal of the American College of Cardiology, 25*, 789–796. doi:10.1016/0735-1097(94)00428-S

Meinardi, M.T., van Veldhuisen, D.J., Gietema, J.A., Dolsma, W.V., Boomsma, F., van den Berg, M.P., … van der Graaf, W.T. (2001). Prospective evaluation of early cardiac damage induced by epirubicin-containing adjuvant chemotherapy and locoregional radiotherapy in breast cancer patients. *Journal of Clinical Oncology, 19*, 2746–2753.

MERIT-HF Study Group. (1999). Effect of metoprolol CR/XL in chronic heart failure: Metoprolol CR/ XL Randomised Intervention Trial in Congestive Heart Failure (MERIT-HF). *Lancet, 353,* 2001–2007. doi:10.1016/S0140-6736(99)04440-2

Munzel, T., & Keaney, J.F., Jr. (2001). Are ACE inhibitors a "magic bullet" against oxidative stress? *Circulation, 104,* 1571–1574. doi:10.1161/hc3801.095585

Murphy, C.J., & Oudit, G.Y. (2010). Iron-overload cardiomyopathy: Pathophysiology, diagnosis, and treatment. *Journal of Cardiac Failure, 16,* 888–900. doi:10.1016/j.cardfail.2010.05.009

National Cancer Institute. (n.d.). Cardiotoxicity. In *Dictionary of cancer terms.* Retrieved from http:// www.cancer.gov/dictionary?CdrID=44004

Nousiainen, T., Jantunen, E., Vanninen, E., Remes, J., Vuolteenaho, O., & Hartikainen, J. (1999). Natriuretic peptides as markers of cardiotoxicity during doxorubicin treatment for non-Hodgkin's lymphoma. *European Journal of Haematology, 62,* 135–141. doi:10.1111/j.1600-0609.1999.tb01734.x

Packer, M., Coats, A.J., Fowler, M.B., Katus, H.A., Krum, H., Mohacsi, P., ... DeMets, D.L. (2001). Effect of carvedilol on survival in severe chronic heart failure. *New England Journal of Medicine, 344,* 1651–1658. doi:10.1056/NEJM200105313442201

Packer, M., Kessler, P.D., & Lee, W.H. (1987). Calcium-channel blockade in the management of severe chronic congestive heart failure: A bridge too far. *Circulation, 75*(6, Pt. 2), V56–V64.

Packer, M., O'Connor, C.M., Ghali, J.K., Pressler, M.L., Carson, P.E., Belkin, R.N., ... DeMets, D.L. (1996). Effect of amlodipine on morbidity and mortality in severe chronic heart failure. Prospective Randomized Amlodipine Survival Evaluation Study Group. *New England Journal of Medicine, 335,* 1107–1114. doi:10.1056/NEJM199610103351504

Packer, M., Poole-Wilson, P.A., Armstrong, P.W., Cleland, J.G., Horowitz, J.D., Massie, B.M., ... Uretsky, B.F. (1999). Comparative effects of low and high doses of the angiotensin-converting enzyme inhibitor, lisinopril, on morbidity and mortality in chronic heart failure. ATLAS Study Group. *Circulation, 100,* 2312–2318. doi:10.1161/01.CIR.100.23.2312

Page, J., & Henry, D. (2000). Consumption of NSAIDs and the development of congestive heart failure in elderly patients: An underrecognized public health problem. *Archives of Internal Medicine, 160,* 777–784. doi:10.1001/archinte.160.6.777

Pai, V.B., & Nahata, M.C. (2000). Cardiotoxicity of chemotherapeutic agents: Incidence, treatment and prevention. *Drug Safety, 22,* 263–302. doi:10.2165/00002018-200022040-00002

Pearlman, E.S., Weber, K.T., Janicki, J.S., Pietra, G.G., & Fishman, A.P. (1982). Muscle fiber orientation and connective tissue content in the hypertrophied human heart. *Laboratory Investigation, 46,* 158–164.

Pentassuglia, L., Timolati, F., Seifriz, F., Abudukadier, K., Suter, T.M., & Zuppinger, C. (2007). Inhibition of ErbB2/neuregulin signaling augments paclitaxel-induced cardiotoxicity in adult ventricular myocytes. *Experimental Cell Research, 313,* 1588–1601. doi:10.1016/j.yexcr.2007.02.007

Pfisterer, M.E., Battler, A., & Zaret, B.L. (1985). Range of normal values for left and right ventricular ejection fraction at rest and during exercise assessed by radionuclide angiocardiography. *European Heart Journal, 6,* 647–655.

Philbin, E.F., Rocco, T.A., Jr., Lindenmuth, N.W., Ulrich, K., & Jenkins, P.L. (2000). Systolic versus diastolic heart failure in community practice: Clinical features, outcomes, and the use of angiotensin-converting enzyme inhibitors. *American Journal of Medicine, 109,* 605–613. doi:10.1016/ S0002-9343(00)00601-X

Pitt, B., Williams, G., Remme, W., Martinez, F., Lopez-Sendon, J., Zannad, F., ... Kleiman, J. (2001). The EPHESUS trial: Eplerenone in patients with heart failure due to systolic dysfunction complicating acute myocardial infarction. Eplerenone Post-AMI Heart Failure Efficacy and Survival Study. *Cardiovascular Drugs and Therapy, 15,* 79–87. doi:10.1056/NEJM199909023411001

Pitt, B., Zannad, F., Remme, W.J., Cody, R., Castaigne, A., Perez, A., ... Wittes, J. (1999). The effect of spironolactone on morbidity and mortality in patients with severe heart failure. Randomized Aldactone Evaluation Study Investigators. *New England Journal of Medicine, 341,* 709–717. doi:10.1056/ NEJM199909023411001

Poole-Wilson, P.A., Swedberg, K., Cleland, J.G., Di Lenarda, A., Hanrath, P., Komajda, M., ... Skene, A. (2003). Comparison of carvedilol and metoprolol on clinical outcomes in patients with chronic heart failure in the Carvedilol or Metoprolol European Trial (COMET): Randomised controlled trial. *Lancet, 362,* 7–13. doi:10.1016/S0140-6736(03)13800-7

Prasad, A., Lerman, A., & Rihal, C.S. (2008). Apical ballooning syndrome (Tako-Tsubo or stress cardiomyopathy): A mimic of acute myocardial infarction. *American Heart Journal, 155,* 408–417. doi:10.1016/j.ahj.2007.11.008

Rahimtoola, S.H. (2004). Digitalis therapy for patients in clinical heart failure. *Circulation, 109,* 2942–2946. doi:10.1161/01.CIR.0000132477.32438.03

Rathore, S.S., Curtis, J.P., Wang, Y., Bristow, M.R., & Krumholz, H.M. (2003). Association of serum digoxin concentration and outcomes in patients with heart failure. *JAMA, 289,* 871–878. doi:10.1001/jama.289.7.871

Reed, S.D., Friedman, J.Y., Velazquez, E.J., Gnanasakthy, A., Califf, R.M., & Schulman, K.A. (2004). Multinational economic evaluation of valsartan in patients with chronic heart failure: Results from the Valsartan Heart Failure Trial (Val-HeFT). *American Heart Journal, 148,* 122–128. doi:10.1016/j.ahj.2003.12.040

Sawaya, H., Sebag, I.A., Plana, J.C., Januzzi, J.L., Ky, B., Cohen, V., & Scherrer-Crosbie, M. (2011). Early detection and prediction of cardiotoxicity in chemotherapy-treated patients. *American Journal of Cardiology, 107,* 1375–1380. doi:10.1016/j.amjcard.2011.01.006

Senni, M., & Redfield, M.M. (2001). Heart failure with preserved systolic function. A different natural history? *Journal of the American College of Cardiology, 38,* 1277–1282. doi:10.1016/S0735-1097(01)01567-4

Silber, J.H. (2004). Can dexrazoxane reduce myocardial injury in anthracycline-treated children with acute lymphoblastic leukemia? *Nature Clinical Practice Oncology, 1,* 16–17. doi:10.1038/ncponc0023

Singal, P.K., & Iliskovic, N. (1998). Doxorubicin-induced cardiomyopathy. *New England Journal of Medicine, 339,* 900–905. doi:10.1056/NEJM199809243391307

Slamon, D.J., Leyland-Jones, B., Shak, S., Fuchs, H., Paton, V., Bajamonde, A., ... Norton, L. (2001). Use of chemotherapy plus a monoclonal antibody against HER2 for metastatic breast cancer that overexpresses HER2. *New England Journal of Medicine, 344,* 783–792. doi:10.1056/NEJM200103153441101

Smith, G.L., Masoudi, F.A., Vaccarino, V., Radford, M.J., & Krumholz, H.M. (2003). Outcomes in heart failure patients with preserved ejection fraction: Mortality, readmission, and functional decline. *Journal of the American College of Cardiology, 41,* 1510–1518. doi:10.1016/S0735-1097(03)00185-2

Snowden, J.A., Hill, G.R., Hunt, P., Carnoutsos, S., Spearing, R.L., Espiner, E., & Hart, D.N.J. (2000). Assessment of cardiotoxicity during haemopoietic stem cell transplantation with plasma brain natriuretic peptide. *Bone Marrow Transplantation, 26,* 309–313. doi:10.1038/sj.bmt.1702507

SOLVD Investigators. (1991). Effect of enalapril on survival in patients with reduced left ventricular ejection fractions and congestive heart failure. *New England Journal of Medicine, 325,* 293–302. doi:10.1056/NEJM199108013250501

Stanek, E.J., Oates, M.B., McGhan, W.F., Denofrio, D., & Loh, E. (2000). Preferences for treatment outcomes in patients with heart failure: Symptoms versus survival. *Journal of Cardiac Failure, 6,* 225–232. doi:10.1054/jcaf.2000.9503

Steinherz, L.J., Steinherz, P.G., Tan, C.T., Heller, G., & Murphy, M.L. (1991). Cardiac toxicity 4 to 20 years after completing anthracycline therapy. *JAMA, 266,* 1672–1677. doi:10.1001/jama.1991.03470120074036

Steinherz, L.J., & Yahalom, J. (2001). Cardiac toxicity. In S. Hellman, V.T. DeVita Jr., & S.A. Rosenberg (Eds.), *Cancer: Principles and practice of oncology* (6th ed., pp. 2904–2921). Philadelphia, PA: Lippincott Williams & Wilkins.

Swain, S.M., Whaley, F.S., & Ewer, M.S. (2003). Congestive heart failure in patients treated with doxorubicin: A retrospective analysis of three trials. *Cancer, 97,* 2869–2879.

Swedberg, K., Cleland, J., Dargie, H., Drexler, H., Follath, F., Komajda, M., ... Remme, W.J. (2005). Guidelines for the diagnosis and treatment of chronic heart failure: Executive summary (update 2005): The Task Force for the Diagnosis and Treatment of Chronic Heart Failure of the European Society of Cardiology. *European Heart Journal, 26,* 1115–1140. doi:10.1093/eurheartj/ehi204

Tang, W.H., Vagelos, R.H., Yee, Y.G., Benedict, C.R., Willson, K., Liss, C.L., & Fowler, M.B. (2002). Neurohormonal and clinical responses to high- versus low-dose enalapril therapy in chronic heart failure. *Journal of the American College of Cardiology, 39,* 70–78. doi:10.1016/S0735-1097(01)01714-4

Thomas, D.J., & Harrah, B.F. (2000). A new look at heart failure. *Home Healthcare Nurse, 18,* 164–170. doi:10.1097/00004045-200003000-00006

Thomson Reuters Micromedex. (2011). Retrieved from http://www.micromedex.com

Tisdale, M.J. (2002). Cachexia in cancer patients. *Nature Reviews Cancer, 2,* 862–871. doi:10.1038/nrc927

Tjeerdsma, G., Meinardi, M.T., van Der Graaf, W.T., van Den Berg, M.P., Mulder, N.H., Crijns, H.J., ... van Veldhuisen, D.J. (1999). Early detection of anthracycline induced cardiotoxicity in asymptomatic patients with normal left ventricular systolic function: Autonomic versus echocardiographic variables. *Heart, 81,* 419–423.

Torp-Pedersen, C., Møller, M., Bloch-Thomsen, P.E., Køber, L., Sandøe, E., Egstrup, K., ... Camm, A.J. (1999). Dofetilide in patients with congestive heart failure and left ventricular dysfunction. Danish Investigations of Arrhythmia and Mortality on Dofetilide Study Group. *New England Journal of Medicine, 341,* 857–865. doi:10.1056/NEJM199909163411201

Tsuyuki, R.T., McKelvie, R.S., Arnold, J.M., Avezum, A., Jr., Barretto, A.C., Carvalho, A.C., … Yusuf, S. (2001). Acute precipitants of congestive heart failure exacerbations. *Archives of Internal Medicine, 161,* 2337–2342. doi:10.1001/archinte.161.19.2337

Urbanova, D., Urban, L., Carter, A., Maasova, D., & Mladosievicova, B. (2006). Cardiac troponins—Biochemical markers of cardiac toxicity after cytostatic therapy. *Neoplasma, 53,* 183–190.

Uretsky, B.F., Young, J.B., Shahidi, F.E., Yellen, L.G., Harrison, M.C., & Jolly, M.K. (1993). Randomized study assessing the effect of digoxin withdrawal in patients with mild to moderate chronic congestive heart failure: Results of the PROVED trial. PROVED Investigative Group. *Journal of the American College of Cardiology, 22,* 955–962. doi:10.1016/0735-1097(93)90403-N

Vasan, R.S., Larson, M.G., Benjamin, E.J., Evans, J.C., Reiss, C.K., & Levy, D. (1999). Congestive heart failure in subjects with normal versus reduced left ventricular ejection fraction: Prevalence and mortality in a population-based cohort. *Journal of the American College of Cardiology, 33,* 1948–1955. doi:10.1016/S0735-1097(99)00118-7

Waagstein, F., Caidahl, K., Wallentin, I., Bergh, C.H., & Hjalmarson, A. (1989). Long-term beta-blockade in dilated cardiomyopathy. Effects of short- and long-term metoprolol treatment followed by withdrawal and readministration of metoprolol. *Circulation, 80,* 551–563. doi:10.1161/01.CIR.80.3.551

Ware, L.B., & Matthay, M.A. (2005). Clinical practice. Acute pulmonary edema. *New England Journal of Medicine, 353,* 2788–2796. doi:10.1056/NEJMcp052699

Wassmuth, R., Lentzsch, S., Erdbruegger, U., Schulz-Menger, J., Doerken, B., Dietz, R., & Friedrich, M.G. (2001). Subclinical cardiotoxic effects of anthracyclines as assessed by magnetic resonance imaging—A pilot study. *American Heart Journal, 141,* 1007–1013. doi:10.1067/mhj.2001.115436

Witteles, R.M., Fowler, M.B., & Telli, M.L. (2011). Chemotherapy-associated cardiotoxicity: How often does it really occur and how can it be prevented? *Heart Failure Clinics, 7,* 333–344. doi:10.1016/j.hfc.2011.03.005

Woo, K.S., & Nicholls, M.G. (1995). High prevalence of persistent cough with angiotensin converting enzyme inhibitors in Chinese. *British Journal of Clinical Pharmacology, 40,* 141–144.

Yeh, E.T.H. (2006). Cardiotoxicity induced by chemotherapy and antibody therapy. *Annual Review of Medicine, 57,* 485–498. doi:10.1146/annurev.med.57.121304.131240

Yeh, E.T., & Bickford, C.L. (2009). Cardiovascular complications of cancer therapy: Incidence, pathogenesis, and management. *Circulation, 109,* 3122–3131. doi:10.1161/01.CIR.0000133187.74800.B9

Zile, M.R., & Brutsaert, D.L. (2002). New concepts in diastolic dysfunction and diastolic heart failure: Part II: Causal mechanisms and treatment. *Circulation, 105,* 1503–1508. doi:10.1161/hc1202.105290

CHAPTER 11

Atrial Dysrhythmias and Atrioventricular Blocks

Sheryl W. Murphy, RN, BSN, MSN, FNP, and Edgar C. Salire, MSN, NP-C

Introduction

Atrial dysrhythmias are a common condition of aging and a major cause of hospital admission and morbidity (Chugh, Blackshear, Shen, Hammill, & Gersh, 2001). These dysrhythmias may manifest as atrial fibrillation, atrial flutter, supraventricular tachycardia, sick sinus syndrome, or atrioventricular blocks (first-, second-, or third-degree). Atrial fibrillation, which is often benign in the general population, can carry a higher postoperative mortality and readmission rate for patients undergoing noncardiac surgeries (van Diepen, Bakal, McAlister, & Ezekowitz, 2011). Various cancer treatments such as chemotherapy, surgery, and radiation may precipitate the occurrence of atrial dysrhythmias. It is essential for oncology nurses to have a basic understanding of the underlying mechanisms and management strategies for atrial dysrhythmias and atrioventricular blocks. Providing appropriate care can minimize morbidity and mortality as patients undergo cancer treatment. This chapter will review basic electrocardiogram (ECG) interpretation to foster interpretation skills to detect atrial dysrhythmias. A review of the pathophysiology, risk factors, and medical management including pharmacologic therapy and nursing considerations for atrial dysrhythmias and atrioventricular blocks (AVBs) will follow.

Basic Electrocardiogram Interpretation

The ECG represents a recording of cardiac electrical activity. The P-wave deflection reflects depolarization of the atria. The QRS complex represents ventricular depolarization, and the T wave/U wave represents ventricular repolarization (see Figure 11-1). Basic ECG analysis should proceed in a systematic and thorough pattern each time an ECG is interpreted (see Figure 11-2). Calculations are made to determine the rate and intervals, allowing rhythm identification. The paper used for ECG tracing is divid-

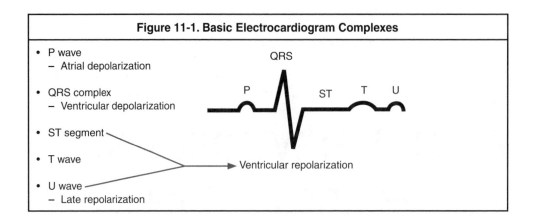

Figure 11-1. Basic Electrocardiogram Complexes

- P wave
  - Atrial depolarization

- QRS complex
  - Ventricular depolarization

- ST segment

- T wave

→ Ventricular repolarization

- U wave
  - Late repolarization

QRS

P   ST   T   U

Figure 11-2. Analysis for Electrocardiogram Interpretation

- Heart rate
- P-wave morphology and amplitude
- Relationship between the P wave and the QRS complex
- PR interval
- QRS width/voltage

- R wave progression in the precordial leads
- Abnormal Q waves
- ST segment
- T wave
- U wave
- Pacemaker spikes

---

ed by thick and thin lines into large (5 × 5 mm) and small (1 × 1 mm) squares. Heart rate, intervals, and the relationship between P waves and QRS complexes are basic determinations used in interpreting ECGs.

At a paper speed of 25 mm/second, which is the most commonly used speed and the one that will be used in this chapter, the width of one of the large squares corresponds to 0.20 seconds and that of a small square to 0.04 seconds. Amplitude is determined by counting the number of vertical small squares from peak to baseline. Five small squares equal 0.5 mV. The PR interval, QRS complex width, and QT interval can be calculated using these measurement standards. To calculate the PR interval, measure the number of small squares from the beginning of the P wave to the beginning of the QRS complex and multiply by 0.04 seconds. A normal PR interval is less than 0.12–0.20 seconds. The QT interval is measured by counting the number of small squares from the beginning of the QRS complex to the end of the T wave and multiplying by 0.04 seconds. The ECG machine will calculate a corrected QT interval based on a formula to take into account the effect of heart rate on the lengthening or shortening of the QT interval. The normal QT interval at 70 beats per minute (bpm) is 0.42 seconds. The QRS complex is measured by counting the number of small squares from the beginning of the Q wave to the end of the S wave and multiplying by 0.04 seconds. A normal QRS complex is 0.06–0.10 seconds. The rate can be determined using the "rule of 300." The heart rate equals 300 divided by the number of heavy vertical lines between R waves. The distance from one R wave falling in a heavy vertical line to the next R wave is measured in numbers of heavy vertical lines. An interval of one line correlates to a rate of 300/1 = 300 bpm, two lines to 300/2 = 150 bpm, three lines to 300/3 = 100 bpm, and four lines to 300/4 = 75 bpm. Once the rate and intervals have been calculated, a rhythm can be determined. Normal sinus rhythm (NSR) will show a P wave prior to each QRS complex, a PR interval less than 0.20 seconds, and a QRS complex less than 0.12 seconds (*ECG Interpretation Made Incredibly Easy!*, 2011) (see Figure 11-3).

Atrial Fibrillation

Atrial fibrillation (A-fib) is the most common of the atrial dysrhythmias (Go et al., 2001). The ECG finding for A-fib is an absence of discrete P waves and an "irregularly irregular" ventricular rate (see Figure 11-4).

Pathophysiology and Classification

In NSR, an impulse forms in the sinoatrial node (SAN), progresses through the atrioventricular (AV) junctional node, and travels through the His-Purkinje fibers and bundle branches, stimulating the ventricles to contract. A-fib is an example of an abnormal impulse formation arrhythmia in which the ectopic beats (any beat originating outside of the SAN) progress through the AV node faster than the sinus beats, leaving an irregularly irregular rhythm and variable rate. A-fib is believed to initiate from chaotic impulse formation in atrial tissues, most likely near the pulmonary veins. Heart rate then depends on how many of these extra impulse formations are conducted through the AV node. Patients may have tachycardia (heart rate faster than 100 bpm) or bradycardia (less than 60 bpm) (Beheiry, Al-Ahmad, & Natale, 2011).

A-fib is classified into three categories: paroxysmal, persistent, and permanent, as defined by consensus statements from the American College of Cardiology/American Heart Association/European Society of Cardiology committee of experts on the treatment of patients with A-fib (Fuster et al., 2001; Onaitis, D'Amico, Zhao, O'Brien, & Harpole, 2010). *Paroxysmal A-fib* is an episode of A-fib that self-terminates without medications or cardioversion and can last from seconds to days. *Persistent A-fib* is an episode of

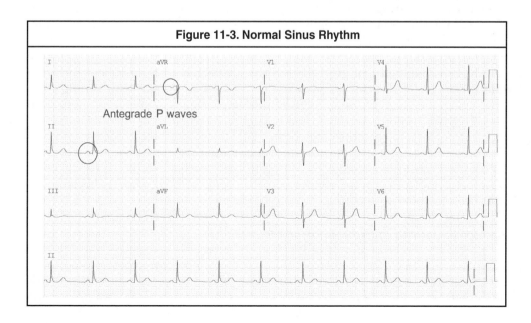

Figure 11-3. Normal Sinus Rhythm

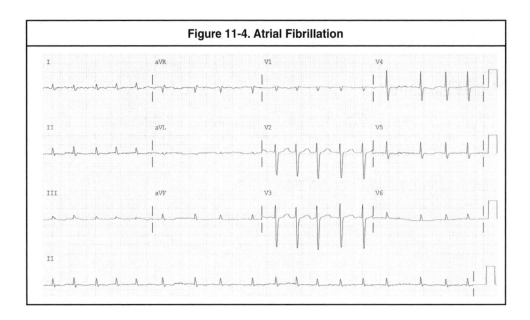

A-fib that requires medication or cardioversion to convert back to NSR. *Permanent A-fib* is A-fib that is refractory to conversion to NSR despite medication or cardioversion (electrical or chemical).

General Atrial Fibrillation Risk Factors

Risk factors in the general population for developing A-fib include older age, pre-existing cardiovascular heart disease, high blood pressure, thyroid disorders, sleep apnea, electrolyte or metabolic imbalances, pericardial disease, pulmonary embolism, emotional stress, and binge drinking. A-fib is a general disease of aging and carries a significant morbidity and mortality risk. The annual risk rates for ischemic stroke associated with A-fib from the Framingham study were 1.5% for people age 50–59 and 23.5% for those age 80–89 (Fuster et al., 2001). Total mortality is about doubled in patients with A-fib compared with NSR. An estimated 2.2 million Americans will have A-fib at some point in their lives (Fuster et al., 2001). Thromboembolic events are a side effect of A-fib that can be catastrophic or lengthen hospital stay. During an A-fib episode, the atria quiver and do not fully empty their blood contents with each systole, or contraction. The left atrium has a pouch (left atrial appendage) that is at high risk for forming thrombus when the atria do not fully empty their blood content with each systole. Clots forming in this left atrial appendage are at risk for dislodging and causing a thromboembolic event, whether that is a stroke, heart attack, pulmonary embolism, or any arterial embolic event (Beheiry et al., 2011; Fuster et al., 2001; Onaitis et al., 2010).

Cancer and Atrial Fibrillation Risk Factors

A-fib is responsible for significant morbidity in postoperative patients with cancer. These arrhythmias cause tachycardia that is sometimes difficult to treat, leading to longer hospital stays and higher costs (Ciriaco, Mazzone, Canneto, & Zannini, 2000; Hollings et al., 2010; Murthy et al., 2003; Onaitis et al., 2010; Roselli et al., 2005). Treating the underlying cause of the A-fib and concurrently managing it usually will terminate the arrhythmia.

Patients who have had a lung cancer resection have a 13%–20% chance of developing postoperative A-fib (Ciriaco et al., 2000; Onaitis et al., 2010). The peak onset of A-fib in these patients is postoperative day 2 (Ciriaco et al., 2000; Roselli et al., 2005). Risk factors for surgical patients to develop A-fib are both patient related and procedure related. Older age, male sex, and preexisting cardiovascular disease are patient-related risk factors for the development of postoperative A-fib in patients with lung cancer (Ciriaco et al., 2000; Hollings et al., 2010; Onaitis et al., 2010; Roselli et al., 2005). Procedure-related risk factors include pneumonectomy or lobectomy (Ciriaco et al., 2000; Roselli et al., 2005), whereas minor resections are less of a risk factor.

Surgical patients with esophageal cancer have a 20%–25% chance of developing postoperative A-fib (Murthy et al., 2003). Risk factors for these patients are also both patient and procedure related. Older age and male sex are commonly reported predictors of postoperative A-fib (Ma et al., 2006; Murthy et al., 2003). Pulmonary issues are a predisposing risk factor for postoperative A-fib in patients following esophagectomy. Conditions such as chronic obstructive pulmonary disease and postoperative hypoxia can increase the risk of developing postoperative A-fib (Ma et al., 2006; Murthy et al., 2003). Anastomotic leakage and surgical sepsis are further factors contributing to postoperative A-fib in these patients (Murthy et al., 2003).

Limited data exist on the incidence of postoperative A-fib in patients with colorectal cancer undergoing elective colectomy. One study found that 4.4% of patients developed postoperative A-fib (Siu et al., 2005). Patients undergoing an open colectomy are more likely to develop postoperative A-fib than those undergoing a laparoscopic colectomy. Elevated neutrophil count on postoperative day 1 was also an independent predictor of postoperative A-fib (Siu et al., 2005).

Patients undergoing hematopoietic stem cell transplantation have a 12% risk of developing post-transplant A-fib (Hidalgo et al., 2004). Non-Hodgkin lymphoma is the most common diagnosis, with A-fib occurring at a median of six days after transplant and lasting about three days. Older age and preexisting cardiovascular conditions are additional risk factors for this patient population (Hidalgo et al., 2004).

Chemotherapeutic agents are not commonly reported as precipitators for A-fib. A few case reports have described A-fib developing during or shortly after gemcitabine administration (Tavil, Arslan, Okyay, Sen, & Boyaci, 2007). Case reports linking infusion of the chemotherapy agents doxorubicin (Montella et al., 2005), docetaxel (Palma et al., 2002), cisplatin (Menard, Martinet, & Lamy, 1991), and melphalan (Olivieri et al., 1998) to induction of A-fib have appeared in the literature, but such cases have not been extensively studied and appear to be rare.

Medical Management and Nursing Considerations

The treatment of A-fib follows one of two strategies. Attempts to maintain NSR (*rhythm control strategy*) are one option. The second strategy is to allow A-fib to continue and control the ventricular rate (*rate control strategy*). The Atrial Fibrillation Follow-Up Investigation of Rhythm Management (AFFIRM) trial, a landmark study published in 2002 of nearly 10,000 patients without cancer who had paroxysmal A-fib, found that morbidity and mortality outcomes were the same whether a rate control or a rhythm control strategy was employed (Olshansky et al., 2004). The rate control strategy had a potential advantage of fewer toxic drug side effects.

Rate Control Strategy

Rate control is based on suppression of the AV node to control the rate of the ventricles in response to the A-fib. A resting heart rate of less than 110 bpm in a patient with a stable left ventricular ejection fraction of greater than 40% is the goal (Wann et al., 2011a). Medications commonly used for rate control include beta-blockers, calcium channel blockers (nondihydropyridine), and digoxin. Table 11-1 describes IV medications frequently prescribed in the acute care setting for rate control of A-fib and atrial flutter (AFL).

Table 11-2 describes medications commonly used in the outpatient setting for rate control in A-fib. Bradycardia and heart blocks occur more frequently in older adult patients as an unwanted side effect of these medications.

Rhythm Control Strategy

Prior to attempting rhythm control, treatment of precipitating factors or reversible causes of A-fib is recommended. Antiarrhythmic therapy is not indicated in patients with advanced sinus node or AV node disease unless they have a functioning implanted pacemaker. Consideration must also be made as to how long the patient has been in A-fib when rhythm control is being considered. Current practice is that in A-fib of less than 48 hours' duration, rhythm control is safe to attempt without increasing the risk for a thromboembolic event. If the patient has been in A-fib greater than 48 hours, an evaluation for thrombus in the heart, especially the left atrial appendage, should be completed prior to attempting cardioversion. A transesophageal echocardiogram (TEE) is performed to evaluate for cardiac thrombus prior to attempting conversion to NSR. The patient must have nothing by mouth for at least six hours prior to the TEE. If no thrombus is seen in the left atrial appendage, a rhythm control strategy can be safely pursued. If thrombus is observed, the clinicians should abort the cardioversion attempt and use a rate control strategy. The patient undergoes therapeutic levels of full-dose anticoagulation for at least three weeks prior to another cardioversion attempt. A TEE is then repeated, and if there is no cardiac thrombus, cardioversion is attempted. Medications can be used to maintain NSR once conversion to NSR has occurred. Table 11-3 summarizes commonly prescribed antiarrhythmics used to maintain NSR (Fuster et al., 2011).

Patients with congestive heart failure are more susceptible to proarrhythmic effects of antiarrhythmic drugs. Amiodarone and dofetilide have demonstrated safety for this subset of patients with A-fib. Patients with left ventricular hypertrophy should be given a trial of amiodarone or sotalol for antiarrhythmic effect. If these medications fail to convert A-fib or AFL to NSR, cardioversion may be attempted. Cardioversion can be mechanical with direct current cardioversion (DCCV) or chemical with ibutilide (Fuster et al., 2011).

DCCV requires cardiac monitoring, external defibrillator pads, and a synchronized shock at 50–100 joules. Sedation is usually given, as the shock can be quite painful and distressing to a patient. Some facilities use a mild anesthetic to make the patient lightly unconscious. Other facilities use conscious-sedation drugs, which render the patient quite drowsy but not fully unconscious (Fuster et al., 2011).

Table 11-1. Rate Control IV Medications for Atrial Fibrillation and Atrial Flutter

Medication	Onset	Loading Dose	Maintenance Dose	Side Effects	Nursing Considerations
Metoprolol (beta-blocker)	5 min	2.5–5 mg every 5 minutes up to 3 doses	NA	Hypotension, bradycardia, heart block, wheezing	Continuous cardiac monitoring. BP every 5 minutes after each dose × 2–3 readings; hold for SBP < 90 mm Hg or HR < 60 bpm.
Diltiazem (calcium channel blocker)	2–7 min	0.25 mg/kg over 2 min	5–15 mg/hr drip	Hypotension, heart block	Continuous cardiac monitoring. BP every 5 minutes after bolus then hourly; contraindicated for patients with CHF; hold for SBP < 90 mm Hg or HR < 60 bpm.
Esmolol (beta-blocker)	5 min	0.5 mg/kg over 1 min	0.05–0.2 mg/kg/min	Hypotension, bradycardia, heart block, wheezing	Continuous cardiac monitoring. BP every 5 minutes after initial bolus then hourly; hold for SBP < 90 mm Hg or HR < 60 bpm.
Verapamil (calcium channel blocker)	3–5 min	0.075–0.15 mg/kg over 2 min	NA	Hypotension, heart block	Continuous cardiac monitoring. BP every 5 minutes × 1 hour then hourly; contraindicated for patients with CHF; hold for SBP < 90 mm Hg or HR < 60 bpm.
Propranolol (beta-blocker)	5 min	0.15 mg/kg	NA	Hypotension, bradycardia, heart block, wheezing	Continuous cardiac monitoring. BP every 5 minutes × 2–3 readings then routine; hold for SBP < 90 mm Hg or HR < 60 bpm.
Digoxin (AV nodal blocking agent)	2 hrs	0.5 mg over 5 min. Half dose for elderly or renal impairment: 0.25 mg over 5 min	0.25 mg IV every 6 hrs × 2 doses. Half dose: 0.125 mg every 6 hrs × 2 doses	Digitalis toxicity, heart block, bradycardia	Continuous cardiac monitoring. Hold for HR < 60 bpm.

AV—atrioventricular; BP—blood pressure; bpm—beats per minute; CHF—congestive heart failure; HR—heart rate; NA—not applicable; SBP—systolic blood pressure

Note. Based on information from Wann et al., 2011b.

Table 11-2. Rate Control Oral Medications for Atrial Fibrillation and Atrial Flutter

Medication	Onset	Loading Dose	Maintenance Dose	Side Effects	Nursing Considerations
Metoprolol tartrate (beta-blocker)	4–6 hrs	NA	25–100 mg every 12 hrs	Hypotension, bradycardia, heart block, wheezing	Teach patient to hold for SBP < 90 mm Hg or HR < 60 bpm.
Propranolol (beta-blocker)	60–90 min	NA	80–240 mg daily in divided doses	Hypotension, bradycardia, heart block, wheezing	Teach patient to hold for SBP < 90 mm Hg or HR < 60 bpm.
Digoxin (AV nodal blocking agent)	2 hrs	0.25 mg every 2 hrs up to 1.5 mg; half dose for elderly or renal impairment	0.125–0.25 mg daily	Digitalis toxicity, heart block, bradycardia	Teach patient to hold for HR < 60 bpm, about digoxin toxicity symptoms (i.e., nausea and vomiting, bright yellow halo around lights).
Diltiazem (calcium channel blocker)	2–4 hrs	NA	120–360 mg daily in divided doses	Hypotension, heart block	Contraindicated for patients with CHF or systolic dysfunction. Teach patient to hold for SBP < 90 mm Hg or HR < 60 bpm.
Verapamil (calcium channel blocker)	1–2 hrs	NA	120–360 mg daily in divided doses, slow release not as effective	Hypotension, heart block	Contraindicated for patients with CHF or systolic dysfunction. Teach patient to hold for SBP < 90 mm Hg or HR < 60 bpm.
Amiodarone (antiarrhythmic with some beta-blocker properties)	1–3 weeks	400 mg BID × 1 week, then 400 mg am and 200 mg pm × 1 week, then 200 mg BID × 4–6 weeks	200 mg daily	Pulmonary toxicity, heart block, hypo- or hyperthyroidism, skin discoloration, corneal deposits, abnormal liver enzymes, drug interactions	Teach patient to hold for HR < 60 bpm, wear sunscreen or clothing to shield skin from sun, and obtain baseline and yearly pulmonary function testing/TSH/free T4/AST/ALT and ophthalmology examination.

ALT—alanine aminotransferase; AST—aspartate transaminase; AV—atrioventricular; BID—twice a day; BP—blood pressure; bpm—beats per minute; CHF—congestive heart failure; HR—heart rate; NA—not applicable; SBP—systolic blood pressure; TSH—thyroid-stimulating hormone

Note. Based on information from Wann et al., 2011b.

Table 11-3. Commonly Prescribed Antiarrhythmics to Maintain Normal Sinus Rhythm in Patients With Atrial Fibrillation and Atrial Flutter

Medication	Loading Dose	Usual Maintenance Dose	Side Effects	Nursing Considerations
Amiodarone	400 mg BID × 1 week, then 400 mg am and 200 mg pm × 1 week, then 200 mg BID × 4–6 weeks	200 mg daily	Pulmonary toxicity, heart block, hypo- or hyperthyroidism, skin discoloration, corneal deposits, abnormal liver enzymes, drug interactions	Teach patient to hold for HR < 60 bpm, wear sunscreen or clothing to shield skin from sun, and obtain yearly pulmonary function testing/TSH/free T4/AST/ALT.
Dofetilide	Requires 72-hour hospital stay for cardiac monitoring for loading dose. ECG within 2 hours after each dose to measure QT interval for prolongation. Dose is adjusted for renal impairment and QT interval response during in-hospital initiation phase.	500–1,000 mcg every 12 hrs	Torsades des pointes	Keep electrolytes in therapeutic range. Must be taken 12 hours apart to keep therapeutic blood levels and avoid toxicity.
Flecainide	Requires 72-hour hospital stay for cardiac monitoring for loading dose. ECG within 2 hours after each dose to measure QT interval for prolongation.	200–300 mg daily in divided doses 12 hours apart	Ventricular tachycardia, CHF, enhanced AV nodal conduction causing a faster rate response	Keep electrolytes in therapeutic range. Must be taken 12 hours apart to keep therapeutic blood levels and avoid toxicity.
Propafenone	NA	450–900 mg daily in divided doses 12 hours apart	Ventricular tachycardia, CHF, enhanced AV nodal conduction causing a faster rate response	Keep electrolytes in therapeutic range. Must be taken 12 hours apart to keep therapeutic blood levels and avoid toxicity.
Sotalol	Requires 72-hour hospital stay for cardiac monitoring for loading dose. ECG within 2 hours after each dose to measure QT interval for prolongation. Dose is adjusted for renal impairment and QT interval response during in-hospital initiation phase.	240–360 mg daily in divided doses every 12 hours	Torsades des pointes, CHF, bradycardia	Teach patient to hold for HR < 60 bpm. Must be taken 12 hours apart to keep therapeutic blood levels and avoid toxicity.

ALT—alanine aminotransferase; AST—aspartate transaminase; AV—atrioventricular; BID—twice a day; bpm—beats per minute; CHF—congestive heart failure; HR—heart rate; NA—not applicable; TSH—thyroid-stimulating hormone

Note. Based on information from Wann et al., 2011b.

Ibutilide is a potassium channel blocker that is given as 1 mg in 50 ml of normal saline infusion over 10 minutes. Utmost attention is paid to electrolyte replacement prior to administering this medication because of the potential side effect of torsades des pointes being heightened in the setting of hypokalemia or hypomagnesemia. Full advanced cardiac life support equipment and trained individuals should be available in the suite when this medication is infused. Serum potassium should be greater than 4 mEq/dl and serum magnesium should be greater than 2 mg/dl prior to starting ibutilide infusion. The dose of ibutilide can be repeated once in 20 minutes if A-fib does not convert to NSR. The effects of this drug can last four to six hours after infusion, so monitoring for torsades des pointes should continue for that period (Fuster et al., 2011).

Thromboembolism Prevention

After it has been decided whether to pursue a rate control or a rhythm control strategy, the patient must be assessed for the risk of thromboembolic events and bleeding to determine if and what type of anticoagulation should be prescribed. Risk stratification for anticoagulation is guided by risk scores for both thrombus formation and bleeding.

Thromboembolic Risk Assessment

The CHADS$_2$ (**C**ongestive heart failure, **H**ypertension, **A**ge, **D**iabetic mellitus, **S**troke) score is a commonly used stratification tool to estimate the risk for thrombus formation in patients with A-fib (Lip, 2010). Medical conditions such as congestive heart failure, hypertension, age greater than 75 years, diabetes mellitus, and stroke or transient ischemic attack (TIA) history are assigned a point value. These conditions have been found to make patients with A-fib more susceptible to thrombus formation (Lip, 2010) (see Table 11-4).

On the basis of the CHADS$_2$ score, anticoagulation is recommended ranging from no treatment, low-dose or high-dose aspirin, or full-dose anticoagulation with low-molecular-weight heparin, warfarin, or one of the new direct thrombin inhibitors.

Bleeding Risk Assessment

Oncology nurses are very aware of the difficulty in managing the anticoagulation needs of patients with thrombocytopenia caused by the cancer itself or chemotherapeutic drugs. Prior to the start of anticoagulation, the patient's bleeding risk must be assessed, with a risk-benefit analysis performed to determine whether anticoagulation should be prescribed. It is often a difficult decision to make. Avoidance of bleeding complications such as an intracranial bleed or hemorrhagic event is weighed against the risk for an embolic stroke, pulmonary embolism, arterial embolism, or myocardial infarction. A commonly used scoring system for bleeding risk is the HAS-BLED tool (see Table 11-5) (Lip, Frison, Halperin, & Lane, 2011). If the HAS-BLED score is higher than the CHADS$_2$ score, anticoagulation is considered to be too much of a risk for bleeding, and anticoagulation is avoided.

Currently under study is a left atrial appendage occluder device designed to seal off the left atrial appendage and minimize this thromboembolic risk. The device is inserted via a percutaneous delivery system in the cardiac catheterization laboratory (Pappone, Vicedomini, Cremonesi, Zuffada, & Santinelli, 2011). The device has not completed clinical trials and so is not yet approved by the U.S. Food and Drug Administra-

Table 11-4. CHADS$_2$ Risk Score: Thromboembolic Risk for Patients With Atrial Fibrillation			
Calculating the Score		**Anticoagulation Recommendations**	
Risk Factor	**Points**	**CHADS$_2$ Risk Score**	**Recommended Anticoagulation***
Congestive heart failure	+1	**Low Risk** Score: "0" 1.9% risk VTE	None or aspirin 81 mg PO daily
Hypertension	+1	**Moderate Risk** Score: 1 2.8% risk VTE	Aspirin 325 mg PO daily, or warfarin (INR 2–3), or direct thrombin inhibitor
Age > 75 years	+1	**High Risk** Score: 2–6 4%–18% risk VTE	Warfarin (INR 2–3) or direct thrombin inhibitor
Diabetes mellitus	+1		
Stroke or transient ischemic attack history	+2		
CHADS$_2$ risk score	Sum of above		

INR—international normalized ratio; VTE—venous thromboembolism

*Side effects are bleeding and bruising for all treatment.

Note. Based on information from Lip, 2010.

tion (FDA), although it is available as part of a clinical trial (Hanna et al., 2004; Meier et al., 2003; Sievert et al., 2002).

Atrial Flutter

AFL is a better organized rhythm than A-fib. The ECG will show a discrete "sawtooth" pattern prior to QRS complexes (see Figure 11-5). AFL typically shows an atrial rate of 300 bpm and a ventricular rate of 150 bpm for a 2:1 block. The number of "sawtooth" waves between each QRS complex determines how many of the atrial flutter complexes are being blocked in the AV node. For example, three "sawtooth" waves between each QRS is termed a 3:1 block. This may be different from beat to beat, which would be labeled a variable block (Olgin & Zipes, 2012).

Pathophysiology and Classification

AFL occurs in many of the same situations as A-fib but is less common. It is classified as typical or atypical based on the rate and etiology of the flutter circuit. Typical AFL will display heart rates in the 240–340 bpm range compared with atypical AFL with heart rates in the 340–440 bpm range. The mechanism for the circuit in typical AFL can be clockwise or counterclockwise and travels through the tricuspid isthmus. This is the most common form. Atypical flutter is more prevalent in patients with repaired congenital heart defects. The circuit initiates and travels around scarring from previous surgical corrections of the congenital heart disease. It also can occur after A-fib ablation as a circuit pathway forms around the mitral valve isthmus. Atypical flutter is unusual in the normal heart (Olgin & Zipes, 2012).

Table 11-5. HAS-BLED Tool Risk Stratification Scoring for Bleeding With Anticoagulation

Risk Factor	Points	Anticoagulation Recommendation
Hypertension (SBP > 160 mg)	+1	No oral anticoagulation if HAS-BLED score is higher than CHADS$_2$ score.
Abnormal renal or liver function	+1 for each	
Stroke	+1	
Bleeding history	+1	
Labile INR (60% of time in therapeutic range	+1	
Elderly (≥ 65 years)	+1	
Drugs that may increase bleeding risk: ASA, steroids, NSAIDs or alcohol abuse (> 8 drinks/week)	+1 point for each	
HAS-BLED risk score	Sum of above	

ASA—aspirin; INR—international normalized ratio; NSAID—nonsteroidal anti-inflammatory drugs; SBP—systolic blood pressure

Note. Based on information from Lip et al., 2011.

Figure 11-5. Atrial Flutter With Block ("Sawtooth" Pattern)

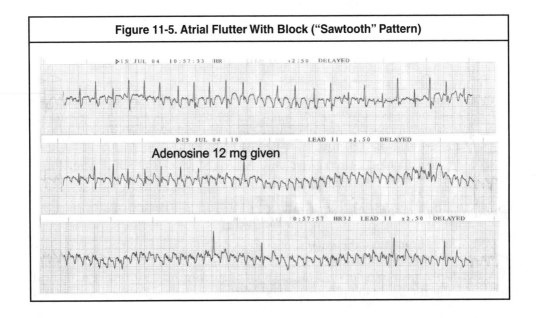

Adenosine 12 mg given

Risk Factors

Patients with cardiac conditions such as repaired or unrepaired congenital heart disease, left atrial enlargement, rheumatic heart disease (especially if the mitral valve is involved), or left or biventricular systolic failure are at risk for the development of AFL (Granada et al., 2000).

Medical Management and Nursing Considerations

Treatment for AFL is the same as for A-fib. Medications are used for rate control, and antiarrhythmics are used for rhythm control. Refer to the previous discussion on medical management and nursing considerations for patients with A-fib. Additional treatment includes ablative therapy to disrupt the circuit and "cure" the AFL substrate. A cardiologist who specializes in rhythm management (cardiac electrophysiologist) may help to guide treatment and perform ablative therapy for these patients. Catheter ablation is a common procedure used to disrupt the circuit and prevent AFL recurrences. However, patients actively undergoing cancer treatment can have comorbid complications such as thrombocytopenia that make it difficult to be able to offer ablative treatment. Patients require a minimum of six weeks of full-dose anticoagulation (low-molecular-weight heparin/warfarin) after ablation to prevent thromboembolic events as a result of thrombus forming at the site of the ablation where eschar has developed. Thrombocytopenia often limits the patient's ability to safely undergo anticoagulation because of bleeding complications, thus making the patient not an ideal candidate for the ablation. A six- to eight-week window when platelets can be maintained at a level of greater than 50,000 may be a time to consider ablation if medical therapy with rate control and antiarrhythmic medications is unsuccessful.

Supraventricular Tachycardia

An ECG finding of a narrow QRS complex tachycardia with a regular rate that starts and stops abruptly is most likely reentrant pathway supraventricular tachycardia (SVT) (see Figure 11-6).

Evaluation of the P wave is essential to determine the origin of the SVT. Different morphology (shapes) in the P waves is diagnostic for multifocal atrial tachycardia. The relationship of the P wave to the QRS complex (immediately after the QRS complex or buried in the QRS complex) is useful in diagnosing SVT. These atrial arrhythmias are different from A-fib and AFL because of their abrupt stop/start characteristic, rate, and pathophysiology. Heart rates can be in the 160–200 bpm range. Patients typical-

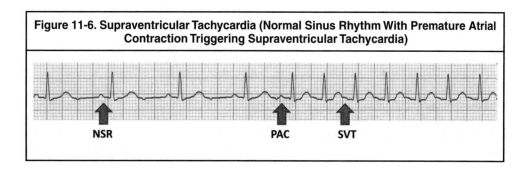

Figure 11-6. Supraventricular Tachycardia (Normal Sinus Rhythm With Premature Atrial Contraction Triggering Supraventricular Tachycardia)

NSR   PAC   SVT

ly complain of a "fluttering" sensation, palpitations, light-headedness, and sometimes syncope (Olgin & Zipes, 2012).

Pathophysiology

SVT is another impulse formation arrhythmia that is a congenital condition. AV node reentrant tachycardia and AV reentrant tachycardia are two such types. Wolff-Parkinson-White syndrome is another SVT reentrant tachycardia. Accessory pathways are found in or around the AV groove. An impulse conducts faster through this pathway than the NSR pathway, making a circuit that triggers repeated ventricular contractions.

Risk Factors

Most patients with SVT have a structurally normal heart. The patient is born with extra electrical tissue in the myocardium, causing a circuit through the AV node that conducts impulses at a rate faster than impulses from the SAN. Patients with congenital heart disease may be more prone to these dysrhythmias (Tanel et al., 1997).

Medical Management and Nursing Considerations

Treatment is aimed at breaking the circuit by slowing or pausing conduction through the AV node. This can be accomplished via stimulation of the vagus nerve. This stimulation is referred to as a *vagal maneuver* and can be accomplished with a Valsalva maneuver or carotid sinus massage.

Valsalva Maneuver

Patients can be taught to do a Valsalva maneuver (i.e., bearing down like when having a bowel movement) to try to stop the SVT. This maneuver increases intrathoracic pressure and affects the baroreceptors in the aorta, causing a reflex stimulation of the vagus nerve that then slows activity in the SAN and through the AV node. This disruption in the reentrant circuit can trigger conversion back to NSR (Miller & Zipes, 2012).

Carotid Sinus Massage

Carotid sinus massage similarly promotes activation of the vagus nerve with resultant slowing of impulses from the SAN and through the AV node. This maneuver is contraindicated in patients with a carotid bruit, previous stroke or TIA, myocardial infarction within the previous six months, or history of ventricular tachycardia. Failure to convert to NSR after either of these vagal maneuvers typically means a trip to the emergency department for IV medications to convert the rhythm to NSR (Miller & Zipes, 2012).

Medications

Adenosine is a potassium channel activator approved by the FDA for conversion of SVT to NSR. Before adenosine is given, continuous cardiac monitoring needs to be established. The nurse should teach patients that they may feel a strange sensation in their chest for a minute or less as the medication takes effect. Adenosine 6 mg is given as a rapid IV push followed by a saline flush to clear the drug from the IV line. If using a peripheral IV, the nurse should elevate the IV arm while administering the medication to foster the most rapid absorption and effect of the adenosine. The effects last only 5–10 seconds, as this medication rapidly metabolizes. A repeat dose of adenosine 12 mg rapid IV push with saline flush may be repeated in five minutes if the rhythm does not convert to NSR. A cardiac electrophysiologist may be consulted for treatment of these patients (Miller & Zipes, 2012).

Ablation

Catheter ablation is a common procedure used to permanently break the circuit and prevent SVT recurrences. The same thrombocytopenia issues are faced by these patients as in the previous discussion of ablative therapy in the AFL treatment section. Medical therapy is the same as those listed for A-fib and AFL in the previous sections. Cancer survivors are good candidates for ablation therapy (Miller & Zipes, 2012).

Sick Sinus Syndrome

The ECG finding for sick sinus syndrome will be alternation between tachycardia episodes and bradycardia episodes.

Pathophysiology

The sinus node is a collection of specialized electrical striated cardiac muscle cells that forms the heart's natural pacemaker. As a normal process of aging, the sinus node sometimes becomes diseased, causing episodes of severe bradycardia, or the inability to raise the heart rate to meet an increase in physical exertion. This severe bradycardia often alternates with tachycardia episodes that require rate control medications such as a beta-blocker. The patient may be taking a beta-blocker for the tachycardia and then have profound bradycardia episodes as well. Symptoms such as severe fatigue, light-headedness, and even syncope can occur with bradycardia (Olgin & Zipes, 2012).

Risk Factors

Any condition that causes disruption of the SAN can cause sick sinus syndrome. Myocardial infarction in the territory of the right coronary artery that supplies the SAN can cause this condition. Malignancy involving the heart is an uncommon cause. Fibrotic changes in the myocardium, such as those seen in amyloidosis, can affect the sinus node and cause sick sinus syndrome (Falk & Dubrey, 2010; James, 1977). Rate control medications such as beta-blockers, calcium channel blockers, digoxin, or antiarrhythmics such as amiodarone that are used to treat A-fib and AFL can alter the impulse formation in the sinus node and cause sick sinus syndrome.

Medical Treatment and Nursing Considerations

Sick sinus syndrome is a class I indication for a permanent pacemaker implant (see Chapter 13 for a full discussion on pacemakers). The pacemaker allows the patient to take a beta-blocker for rate control without experiencing the crippling symptoms of bradycardia. Nursing considerations include taking a careful history, as the diagnosis is based on the history and ECG findings of bradycardia. The most common complaints are fatigue, light-headedness or syncope, increasing dyspnea on exertion, or palpitations or tachycardia alternating with bradycardia. Athletes often have bradycardia but do not have these complaints, so they do not have sick sinus syndrome. Their bradycardia is due to physical conditioning, not pathology as seen in patients with sick sinus syndrome (Epstein et al., 2008; Vlay, 2009).

Atrioventricular Blocks

Classification

AVBs are classified as first-, second- (type I or II), or third-degree (complete) blocks (Olgin & Zipes, 2012). *First-degree AVB* is characterized on the ECG by a PR interval of 0.2 seconds or greater (see Figure 11-7). *Second-degree AVB, Mobitz type I (Wenckebach)* is characterized on the ECG as a sequence of prolonging PR intervals until a final P wave has a dropped QRS complex (nonconducted beat) before the sequence starts again (see Figure 11-8). The clinician should review the previous two to three beats after a dropped QRS complex to see if the PR interval increases. *Second-degree AVB type II* is characterized on ECG as a stable PR interval with intermittent dropped QRS complex following a P wave (see Figure 11-9). *Third-degree (complete) AVB* is characterized on the ECG as having no relationship between the P waves (atria) and QRS complexes (ventricle) (see Figure 11-10).

Pathophysiology

These dysrhythmias are part of normal aging but can be exacerbated with cancer treatments. Impulse conduction delays or "blocks" in the AV node can lead to first-, sec-

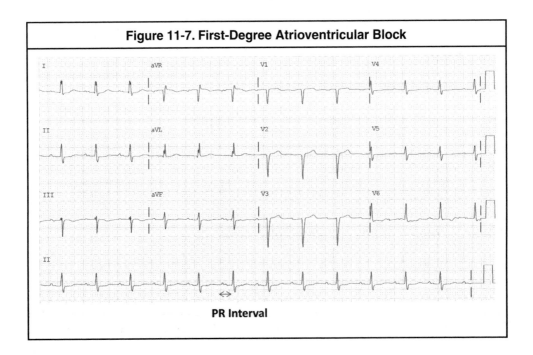

Figure 11-7. First-Degree Atrioventricular Block

PR Interval

ond-, and third-degree heart blocks. First-degree AVB indicates a block that is very high in the AV node and is not likely to be lethal. Second-degree heart block has two types: type 1 (Wenckebach) is stable and benign, whereas type II is considered unstable. Type II second-degree AVB has a conduction delay further down the AV nodal pathway and can progress to a complete heart block. Third-degree AVB indicates no connection in the AV node between the atria and the ventricles. The atria and ventricle are each beat-

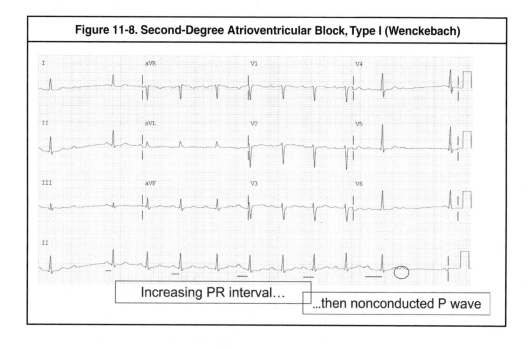

Figure 11-8. Second-Degree Atrioventricular Block, Type I (Wenckebach)

Increasing PR interval...

...then nonconducted P wave

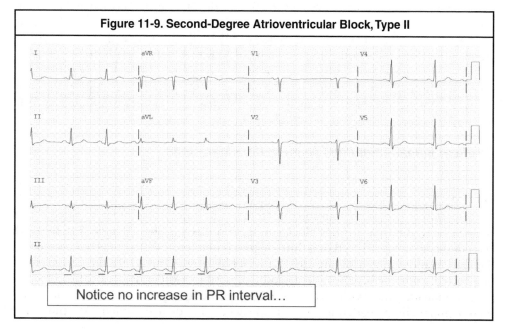

Figure 11-9. Second-Degree Atrioventricular Block, Type II

Notice no increase in PR interval...

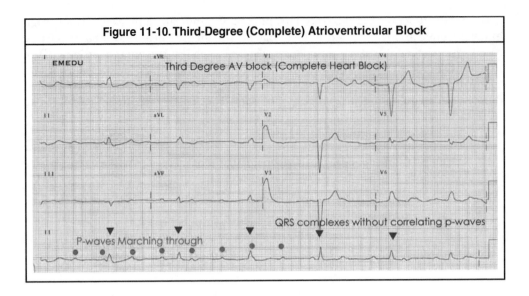

Figure 11-10. Third-Degree (Complete) Atrioventricular Block

ing with different pacemakers. This is a very unstable rhythm and a cardiac emergency (Olgin & Zipes, 2012).

Risk Factors

Patients with ischemic heart disease are at risk for developing an AVB (Gupta, Lichstein, & Chadda, 1976; Harpaz et al., 1999; Vijayaraman & Ellenbogen, 2011). Hypertrophic cardiomyopathy can predispose a patient to AVB. Development of AVB in a patient with myocarditis has a very poor prognostic outlook (Kleid, Kim, Brand, Eckles, & Gordon, 1972; Vijayaraman & Ellenbogen, 2011). AVB can occur in the setting of hyperkalemia and often corrects with correction of the electrolyte imbalance. Iatrogenic causes for AVB include cardiac surgery, especially involving the mitral valve (Berdajs et al., 2008) and aortic valve (Sanoudos & Reed, 1974; Vijayaraman & Ellenbogen, 2011). Medications may transiently induce complete AVB that resolves with discontinuation of the offending medication. Medications known to induce AVB include beta-blockers, calcium channel blockers, clonidine, digoxin, and amiodarone. Oncologic predispositions for AVB include infiltrative malignancies such as amyloidosis, lymphoma, and sarcoidosis. Cardiac tumors can cause AVB (Lim, Pak, & Kim, 2006).

Medical Management and Nursing Considerations

Treatment for AVB is directed toward avoiding any medications that may worsen the AVB. Medications such as digoxin, beta-blockers, calcium channel blockers that are dihydropyridines (i.e., verapamil and diltiazem), and clonidine should be avoided if possible because they may further block conduction through the AV node. Patients with a second-degree type II AVB or a third-degree (complete) AVB will need a pacemaker implant in addition to avoiding any AV nodal blocking agents. Once the pacemaker is implanted, these medications can again be prescribed (Miller & Zipes, 2012).

Symptomatic patients with AVB who are experiencing hypotension, chest pain, shortness of breath, light-headedness, or syncope need immediate treatment. Atropine 1 mg

IV push over one minute every five minutes up to a total of 2 mg is given to try to increase conduction through the AV node. The patient should be prepared for a temporary pacemaker placement (transvenous or transcutaneous) to stabilize the rhythm until a permanent pacemaker can be implanted. It is very important to avoid AV nodal blocking medications in these patients (Miller & Zipes, 2012).

Conclusion

Atrial dysrhythmias can have significant morbidity and mortality for patients with cancer. The oncology nurse's familiarity with the disease processes, treatment options, and prognoses can be a great aid in helping patients to understand their condition and be able to make informed decisions regarding their care.

References

Beheiry, S., Al-Ahmad, A., & Natale, A. (2011). Atrial fibrillation and flutter: Diagnosis and treatment. In A. Tsiperfal, L.K. Ottoboni, S. Beheiry, A. Al-Ahmad, A. Natale, & P. Wang (Eds.), *Cardiac arrhythmia management: A practical guide for nurses and allied professionals* (pp. 85–100). Chichester, West Sussex, UK: Wiley-Blackwell.

Berdajs, D., Schurr, U.P., Wagner, A., Seifert, B., Turina, M.I., & Genoni, M. (2008). Incidence and pathophysiology of atrioventricular block following mitral valve replacement and ring annuloplasty. *European Journal of Cardio-Thoracic Surgery, 34,* 55–61. doi:10.1016/j.ejcts.2008.03.051

Chugh, S.S., Blackshear, J.L., Shen, W.K., Hammill, S.C., & Gersh, B.J. (2001). Epidemiology and natural history of atrial fibrillation: Clinical implications. *Journal of the American College of Cardiology, 37,* 371–378. doi:10.1016/S0735-1097(00)01107-4

Ciriaco, P., Mazzone, P., Canneto, B., & Zannini, P. (2000). Supraventricular arrhythmia following lung resection for non-small cell lung cancer and its treatment with amiodarone. *European Journal of Cardio-Thoracic Surgery, 18,* 12–16. doi:10.1016/S1010-7940(00)00428-0

ECG interpretation made incredibly easy! (5th ed.). (2011). Philadelphia, PA: Wolters Kluwer/Lippincott Williams & Wilkins Health.

Epstein, A.E., DiMarco, J.P., Ellenbogen, K.A., Estes, N.A., 3rd, Freedman, R.A., Gettes, L.S., … Yancy, C.W. (2008). ACC/AHA/HRS 2008 Guidelines for Device-Based Therapy of Cardiac Rhythm Abnormalities: A report of the American College of Cardiology/American Heart Association Task Force on Practice Guidelines (Writing Committee to Revise the ACC/AHA/NASPE 2002 Guideline Update for Implantation of Cardiac Pacemakers and Antiarrhythmia Devices) developed in collaboration with the American Association for Thoracic Surgery and Society of Thoracic Surgeons. *Journal of the American College of Cardiology, 51*(21), e1–e62. doi:10.1016/j.jacc.2008.02.032

Falk, R.H., & Dubrey, S.W. (2010). Amyloid heart disease. In M.A. Gertz & S.V. Rajkumar (Eds.), *Amyloidosis: Diagnosis and treatment* (pp. 107–128). New York, NY: Humana Press. doi:10.1007/978-1-60761-631-3_8

Fuster, V., Rydén, L.E., Asinger, R.W., Cannom, D.S., Crijns, H.J., Frye, R.L., … Torbicki, A. (2001). ACC/AHA/ESC guidelines for the management of patients with atrial fibrillation: Executive summary: A report of the American College of Cardiology/American Heart Association Task Force on Practice Guidelines and the European Society of Cardiology Committee for Practice Guidelines and Policy Conferences (Committee to Develop Guidelines for the Management of Patients With Atrial Fibrillation) developed in collaboration with the North American Society of Pacing and Electrophysiology. *Circulation, 104,* 2118–2150.

Fuster, V., Rydén, L.E., Cannom, D.S., Crijns, H.J., Curtis, A.B., Ellenbogen, K.A., … Wann, L.S. (2011). 2011 ACCF/AHA/HRS focused updates incorporated into the ACC/AHA/ESC 2006 guidelines for the management of patients with atrial fibrillation: A report of the American College of Cardiology Foundation/American Heart Association Task Force on Practice Guidelines developed in partnership with the European Society of Cardiology and in collaboration with the European Heart Rhythm Association and the Heart Rhythm Society. *Journal of the American College of Cardiology, 57,* e101–e198. doi:10.1016/j.jacc.2010.09.013

Go, A.S., Hylek, E.M., Phillips, K.A., Chang, Y., Henault, L.E., Selby, J.V., & Singer, D.E. (2001). Prevalence of diagnosed atrial fibrillation in adults: National implications for rhythm management and stroke prevention: The AnTicoagulation and Risk Factors in Atrial Fibrillation (ATRIA) Study. *JAMA, 285,* 2370–2375. doi:10.1001/jama.285.18.2370

Granada, J., Uribe, W., Chyou, P.H., Maassen, K., Vierkant, R., Smith, P.N., ... Vidaillet, H. (2000). Incidence and predictors of atrial flutter in the general population. *Journal of the American College of Cardiology, 36,* 2242–2246. doi:10.1016/S0735-1097(00)00982-7

Gupta, P.K., Lichstein, E., & Chadda, K.D. (1976). Heart block complicating acute inferior wall myocardial infarction. *Chest, 69,* 599–604. doi:10.1378/chest.69.5.599

Hanna, I.R., Kolm, P., Martin, R., Reisman, M., Gray, W., & Block, P.C. (2004). Left atrial structure and function after percutaneous left atrial appendage transcatheter occlusion (PLAATO): Six-month echocardiographic follow-up. *Journal of the American College of Cardiology, 43,* 1868–1872. doi:10.1016/j.jacc.2003.12.050

Harpaz, D., Behar, S., Gottlieb, S., Boyko, V., Kishon, Y., & Eldar, M. (1999). Complete atrioventricular block complicating acute myocardial infarction in the thrombolytic era. SPRINT Study Group and the Israeli Thrombolytic Survey Group. Secondary Prevention Reinfarction Israeli Nifedipine Trial. *Journal of the American College of Cardiology, 34,* 1721–1728. doi:10.1016/S0735-1097(99)00431-3

Hidalgo, J.D., Krone, R., Rich, M.W., Blum, K., Adkins, D., Fan, M.Y., ... Khoury, H. (2004). Supraventricular tachyarrhythmias after hematopoietic stem cell transplantation: Incidence, risk factors and outcomes. *Bone Marrow Transplantation, 34,* 615–619. doi:10.1038/sj.bmt.1704623

Hollings, D.D., Higgins, R.S.D., Faber, L.P., Warren, W.H., Liptay, M.J., Basu, S., & Kim, A.W. (2010). Age is a strong risk factor for atrial fibrillation after pulmonary lobectomy. *American Journal of Surgery, 199,* 558–561. doi:10.1016/j.amjsurg.2009.11.006

James, T.N. (1977). The sinus node. *American Journal of Cardiology, 40,* 965–986. doi:10.1016/0002-9149(77)90048-0

Kleid, J.J., Kim, E.S., Brand, B., Eckles, S., & Gordon, G.M. (1972). Heart block complicating acute bacterial endocarditis. *Chest, 61,* 301–303. doi:10.1378/chest.61.3.301

Lim, H.E., Pak, H.N., & Kim, Y.H. (2006). Acute myocarditis associated with cardiac amyloidosis manifesting as transient complete atrioventricular block and slow ventricular tachycardia. *International Journal of Cardiology, 109,* 395–397. doi:10.1016/j.ijcard.2005.05.043

Lip, G.Y.H. (2010). Anticoagulation therapy and the risk of stroke in patients with atrial fibrillation at 'moderate risk' [CHADS$_2$ score=1]: Simplifying stroke risk assessment and thromboprophylaxis in real-life clinical practice. *Thrombosis and Haemostasis, 103,* 683–685. doi:10.1160/TH10-01-0038

Lip, G.Y.H., Frison, L., Halperin, J.L., & Lane, D.A. (2011). Comparative validation of a novel risk score for predicting bleeding risk in anticoagulated patients with atrial fibrillation: The HAS-BLED (Hypertension, Abnormal Renal/Liver Function, Stroke, Bleeding History or Predisposition, Labile INR, Elderly, Drugs/Alcohol Concomitantly) score. *Journal of the American College of Cardiology, 57,* 173–180. doi:10.1016/j.jacc.2010.09.024

Ma, J.-Y., Wang, Y., Zhao, Y.-F., Wu, Z., Liu, L.-X., Kou, Y.-L., & Yang, J.J. (2006). Atrial fibrillation after surgery for esophageal carcinoma: Clinical and prognostic significance. *World Journal of Gastroenterology, 12,* 449–452.

Meier, B., Palacios, I., Windecker, S., Rotter, M., Cao, Q.L., Keane, D., ... Hijazi, Z.M. (2003). Transcatheter left atrial appendage occlusion with Amplatzer devices to obviate anticoagulation in patients with atrial fibrillation. *Catheterization and Cardiovascular Interventions, 60,* 417–422. doi:10.1002/ccd.10660

Menard, O., Martinet, Y., & Lamy, P. (1991). Cisplatin-induced atrial fibrillation. *Journal of Clinical Oncology, 9,* 192–193.

Miller, J.M., & Zipes, D.P. (2012). Therapy for cardiac arrhythmias. In R.O. Bonow, D.L. Mann, D.P. Zipes, & P. Libby (Eds.), *Braunwald's heart disease: A textbook of cardiovascular medicine* (9th ed., pp. 771–823). Philadelphia, PA: Saunders.

Montella, L., Caraglia, M., Addeo, R., Costanzo, R., Faiola, V., Abbruzzese, A., & Del Prete, S. (2005). Atrial fibrillation following chemotherapy for stage IIIE diffuse large B-cell gastric lymphoma in a patient with myotonic dystrophy (Steinert's disease). *Annals of Hematology, 84,* 192–193. doi:10.1007/s00277-004-0867-6

Murthy, S.C., Law, S., Whooley, B.P., Alexandrou, A., Chu, K.-M., & Wong, J. (2003). Atrial fibrillation after esophagectomy is a marker for postoperative morbidity and mortality. *Journal of Thoracic and Cardiovascular Surgery, 126,* 1162–1167. doi:10.1016/S0022-5223(03)00974-7

Olgin, J., & Zipes, D.P. (2012). Therapy for cardiac arrhythmias. In R.O. Bonow, D.L. Mann, D.P. Zipes, & P. Libby (Eds.), *Braunwald's heart disease: A textbook of cardiovascular medicine* (9th ed., pp. 710–743). Philadelphia, PA: Elsevier Saunders.

Olivieri, A., Corvatta, L., Montanari, M., Brunori, M., Offidani, M., Ferretti, G.F., ... Leoni, P. (1998). Paroxysmal atrial fibrillation after high-dose melphalan in five patients autotransplanted with blood progenitor cells. *Bone Marrow Transplantation, 21,* 1049–1053. doi:10.1038/sj.bmt.1701217

Olshansky, B., Rosenfeld, L.E., Warner, A.L., Solomon, A.J., O'Neill, G., Sharma, A., ... Greene, H.L. (2004). The Atrial Fibrillation Follow-up Investigation of Rhythm Management (AFFIRM) study: Approaches to control rate in atrial fibrillation. *Journal of the American College of Cardiology, 43,* 1201–1208. doi:10.1016/j.jacc.2003.11.032

Onaitis, M., D'Amico, T., Zhao, Y., O'Brien, S., & Harpole, D. (2010). Risk factors for atrial fibrillation after lung cancer surgery: Analysis of the Society of Thoracic Surgeons general thoracic surgery database. *Annals of Thoracic Surgery, 90,* 368–374. doi:10.1016/j.athoracsur.2010.03.100

Palma, M., Mancuso, A., Grifalchi, F., Lugini, A., Pizzardi, N., & Cortesi, E. (2002). Atrial fibrillation during adjuvant chemotherapy with docetaxel: A case report. *Tumori, 88,* 527–529.

Pappone, C., Vicedomini, G., Cremonesi, A., Zuffada, F., & Santinelli, V. (2011). Device-based left atrial appendage closure. *Circulation: Arrhythmia and Electrophysiology, 4,* 418–419. doi:10.1161/CIRCEP.111.962423

Roselli, E.E., Murthy, S.C., Rice, T.W., Houghtaling, P.L., Pierce, C.D., Karchmer, D.P., & Blackstone, E.H. (2005). Atrial fibrillation complicating lung cancer resection. *Journal of Thoracic and Cardiovascular Surgery, 130,* 438–444. doi:10.1016/j.jtcvs.2005.02.010

Sanoudos, G., & Reed, G.E. (1974). Late heart block in aortic valve replacement. *Journal of Cardiovascular Surgery, 15,* 475–478.

Sievert, H., Lesh, M.D., Trepels, T., Omran, H., Bartorelli, A., Della Bella, P., ... Scherer, D. (2002). Percutaneous left atrial appendage transcatheter occlusion to prevent stroke in high-risk patients with atrial fibrillation: Early clinical experience. *Circulation, 105,* 1887–1889. doi:10.1161/01.CIR.0000015698.54752.6D

Siu, C.-W., Tung, H.-M., Chu, K.-W., Jim, M.-H., Lau, C.-P., & Tse, H.-F. (2005). Prevalence and predictors of new-onset atrial fibrillation after elective surgery for colorectal cancer. *Pacing and Clinical Electrophysiology, 28*(Suppl. 1), S120–S123. doi:10.1111/j.1540-8159.2005.00024.x

Tanel, R.E., Walsh, E.P., Triedman, J.K., Epstein, M.R., Bergau, D.M., & Saul, J.P. (1997). Five-year experience with radiofrequency catheter ablation: Implications for management of arrhythmias in pediatric and young adult patients. *Journal of Pediatrics, 131,* 878–887. doi:10.1016/S0022-3476(97)70037-4

Tavil, Y., Arslan, U., Okyay, K., Sen, N., & Boyaci, B. (2007). Atrial fibrillation induced by gemcitabine treatment in a 65-year-old man. [Case reports]. *Onkologie, 30,* 253–255. doi:10.1159/000100930

van Diepen, S., Bakal, J.A., McAlister, F.A., & Ezekowitz, J.A. (2011). Mortality and readmission of patients with heart failure, atrial fibrillation, or coronary artery disease undergoing noncardiac surgery: An analysis of 38,047 patients. *Circulation, 124,* 289–296. doi:10.1161/CIRCULATIONAHA.110.011130

Vijayaraman, P., & Ellenbogen, K.A. (2011). Bradyarrhythmias and pacemakers. In V. Fuster, R.A. Walsh, & R.A. Harrington (Eds.), *Hurst's the heart* (13th ed., pp. 1025–1057). New York, NY: McGraw-Hill Medical.

Vlay, S.C. (2009). The ACC/AHA/HRS 2008 guidelines for device-based therapy of cardiac rhythm abnormalities: Their relevance to the cardiologist, internist and family physician. *Journal of Invasive Cardiology, 21,* 234–237.

Wann, L.S., Curtis, A.B., Ellenbogen, K.A., Estes, N.A., 3rd, Ezekowitz, M.D., Jackman, W.M., ... Tracy, C.M. (2011a). 2011 ACCF/AHA/HRS focused update on the management of patients with atrial fibrillation (update on dabigatran): A report of the American College of Cardiology Foundation/American Heart Association Task Force on practice guidelines. *Journal of the American College of Cardiology, 57,* 1330–1337. doi:10.1016/j.jacc.2011.01.010

Wann, L.S., Curtis, A.B., January, C.T., Ellenbogen, K.A., Lowe, J.E., Estes, N.A., 3rd., ... Yancy, C.W. (2011b). 2011 ACCF/AHA/HRS focused update on the management of patients with atrial fibrillation (updating the 2006 guideline): A report of the American College of Cardiology Foundation/American Heart Association Task Force on Practice Guidelines. *Circulation, 123,* 104–123. doi:10.1161/CIR.0b013e3181fa3cf4

CHAPTER 12

QT Prolongation and Antineoplastic Agents

Tara Lech, PharmD, BCPS

Introduction

QT prolongation is an abnormality in the conduction system of the heart that can put patients at risk for ventricular arrhythmias (i.e., torsades de pointes [TdP], syncope, and sudden death) (Brell, 2010). Patients with cancer may be at particularly high risk because of comorbid disease states, possible hepatic or renal dysfunction, and electrolyte disturbances as a result of malnourishment, nausea and vomiting, or diarrhea, as well as increase in use of concomitant QT-prolonging medications such as antiemetics, quinolone or macrolide antibiotics, and azole antifungals (Fadol & Lech, 2011; Strevel, Ing, & Siu, 2007; Yeh & Bickford, 2009). Although QT prolongation can be congenital or acquired, this chapter will focus on the latter, targeting the incidence, pathophysiology, diagnosis, and management of drug-induced QT prolongation.

Incidence

The incidence of QT prolongation in the general population is largely unknown. This leaves clinicians to rely on reports of incidence, risk factors, and clinically significant drug interactions described in epidemiologic studies, case reports, drug development trials, and postmarketing surveillance (Brell, 2010). One notable study was a retrospective cohort trial conducted by the Centers for Education and Research on Therapeutics in which the authors reported that of 4.8 million patients followed, 4.4 million filled prescriptions for QT-prolonging medications. Furthermore, of those 4.8 million patients, 9.4% were prescribed either two or more QT-prolonging medications or an agent that decreased the clearance of these drugs. Twenty-two percent of the patients were also noted to be 65 years of age or older (Curtis et al., 2003).

When considering the potential risks of QT prolongation in patients with cancer, an important note is that many of these patients possess multiple predisposing risk factors, leaving them at increasingly higher risk. Some of the major concerns in this population include preexisting cardiovascular disease, the use of multiple QT-prolonging agents, and frequent electrolyte abnormalities. Figure 12-1 provides a more detailed list of other possible risks (Crouch, Limon, & Cassano, 2003; Gupta, Lawrence, Krishnan, Kavinsky, & Trohman, 2007).

Diagnosis

To determine if the QT interval is prolonged, it is important to know how the measurement is made. The QT interval is defined by measuring the distance between the start of the QRS complex and the end of the T wave on a standard electrocardiogram (ECG) (see Figure 12-2) (Al-Khatib, LaPointe, Kramer, & Califf, 2003). A normal QT interval is generally 440 milliseconds (ms) or less and is considered prolonged if it becomes greater than 450 ms in men or 470 ms in women; arrhythmias are most often associated with values 500 ms or greater (see Table 12-1) (Yeh & Bickford, 2009).

Unfortunately, the QT interval alone cannot be used to determine the severity of proarrhythmia because the risk varies from drug to drug and patient to patient. It therefore is important to screen patients for preexisting risk factors, as the extent of QT prolongation and the risk of TdP with any given drug may not be linearly related to the dose or its plasma concentration (Li, Esterly, Pohl, Scott, & McBride, 2010). Individual patient and metabolic factors also contribute heavily to the risk. Additionally, because this relationship is so multifactorial, it is important to remember that occasionally TdP can occur without any significant prolongation of the QT interval.

Nurses should also keep in mind that the QT interval is also influenced by heart rate. To correct for this, the RR interval (the time interval from the peak of one

---

Figure 12-1. Predisposing Risk Factors for QT Prolongation

- Altered nutrition (anorexia nervosa, starvation diets, alcoholism)
- Bradycardia (< 50 beats/min)
- Cardiovascular disease (heart failure, previous myocardial infarction, cardiomyopathy)
- Cerebrovascular disease (intracranial and subarachnoid hemorrhage, stroke, intracranial trauma)
- Congenital long QT syndrome
- Electrolyte disturbances
  - Hypokalemia
  - Hypomagnesemia
  - Hypocalcemia
- Female sex
- Hypothermia
- Hypothyroidism
- Ion channel polymorphisms
- Multiple QTc-prolonging drugs
- Older age (> 65 years)
- Prolonged QTc (> 450 ms) at baseline
- Recent conversion from atrial fibrillation

Note. Based on information from Crouch et al., 2003; Li et al., 2010; Slama, 2005.

Figure 12-2. Schematic Representation of Normal Electrocardiogram

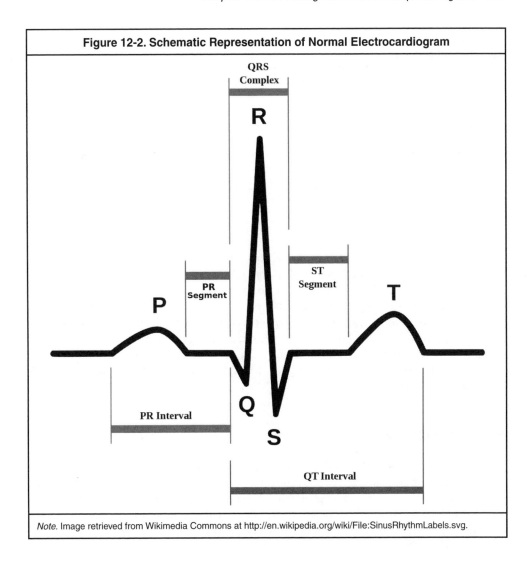

QRS complex to the peak of the next) preceding the QT interval should be measured. Several formulas can be used to correct the QT (QTc) interval for this effect of heart rate, but none is perfect. Two of the more common formulas are the Bazett ($QTc = QT/RR^{1/2}$) and the Fridericia ($QTc = QT/RR^{1/3}$) (Li et al., 2010). Calculations are usually done by computer, and the values are reported on the ECG as either the QTc_b or QTc_f, respectively. Other factors influencing the duration of the QT interval include sympathetic and vagal activity, medications, genetic abnormalities, electrolyte disorders, and cardiac or metabolic diseases. The relationship between the QT interval and the heart rate is different for every individual (Al-Khatib et al., 2003; Schwartz, 2005). Although the rate correction formulas are useful clinically, they may not be accurate enough, especially when assessing the minor changes of the QT interval induced by drugs. The suggested QTc values using the Bazett formula for diagnosing QT prolongation are outlined in Table 12-1 (Al-Khatib et al., 2003; Li et al., 2010).

Table 12-1. QTc Values for Normal and Prolonged QT Interval After Correction With the Bazett Formula

	QTc Values by Age Group and Sex (ms)		
	1–15 Years	Adult Males	Adult Females
Normal	< 440	< 430	< 450
Borderline	440–460	430–450	450–470
Prolonged (top 1%)	> 460	> 450	> 470

Note. Based on information from Yeh & Bickford, 2009.

The clinical diagnosis of QTc prolongation is based solely on the ECG reading. Established guidelines can aid the practitioner in determining which patients are at highest risk for developing cardiac events, but no definitive values have been identified. As stated earlier, a normal QTc interval is 440 ms or less, and prolonged is greater than 450 and 470 ms in men and women, respectively. Clinicians should pay particular attention to increases in the QTc 60 ms or greater, as changes can put patients at risk for developing arrhythmias and TdP. If the patient becomes symptomatic, the offending agents should be discontinued immediately (Al-Khatib et al., 2003; Vorchheimer, 2005; Yeh & Bickford, 2009).

Pathophysiology

The exact mechanism behind QT prolongation associated with many of the newer targeted cancer therapies remains unknown. However, when discussing drug-induced QT prolongation, it is generally understood that it is due in part to either the blockade of the delayed rectifier potassium currents or prolonged depolarization of the calcium or sodium currents, all of which contribute to the medication's proarrhythmic effect (Strevel et al., 2007).

Medications That Cause QT Prolongation

Many classes of anticancer therapies can cause marked prolongation of the QT interval (see Table 12-2) (Becker & Yeung, 2010; Fadol & Lech, 2011; Strevel et al., 2007). Oncology nurses must be aware of these therapies and understand that cumulative or total daily dose, drug formulations, prior exposures, and electrolyte abnormalities can all predispose patients to the proarrhythmic effects of these treatments. Nurses also should conduct a routine pretreatment evaluation and medication screening whenever a new QT-prolonging agent is initiated (see Figure 12-3). Baseline ECG should be performed to evaluate the QTc prior to therapy, and patients at high risk for QTc prolongation should be identified. Electrolyte abnormalities should be aggressively corrected, paying particular attention to patients receiving diuretics, and concomitant medications that can prolong the QT should be identified (see Table 12-3) (Al-Khatib et al., 2003; Strevel et al., 2007; Viskin, 1999).

Patients with renal insufficiency, hepatic dysfunction, congenital QT abnormalities, or a known family history of sudden cardiac death also are considered high risk (Vorchheimer, 2005). Because of the high morbidity and mortality rates associated with TdP, nurses must be aware of all the risk factors and report any new symptoms of palpitations, syncope, or pre-syncope to the primary healthcare providers (Ederhy et al., 2009).

Table 12-2. Anticancer Agents That Can Cause QT Prolongation		
Medication	**Incidence**	**Comments**
Histone deacetylase inhibitors		
Vorinostat	3.5%–6%	Not likely dose dependent
Romidepsin	Unreported[a]	Not likely dose dependent
Miscellaneous		
Arsenic	26%–93%	High rate of torsades de pointes associated with prolonged QT
Small-molecule tyrosine kinase inhibitors		
Lapatinib	16%	High frequency of QT prolongation
Vandetanib	14%	
Nilotinib	1%–10%	Multiple drug-drug interactions; extreme caution should be used with CYP3A4 inhibitors or inducers.[b]
Pazopanib	< 2%	
Dasatinib	< 1%–3%	
Sunitinib	< 0.1%	

[a] The exact incidence of QT prolongation with romidepsin has not been reported. However, the package insert lists QT prolongation as a risk and advises practitioners to ensure that potassium and magnesium are within the normal range before administration.

[b] Common CYP3A4 inhibitors: amiodarone, ritonavir, clarithromycin, erythromycin, ketoconazole, itraconazole, verapamil, diltiazem. Common CYP3A4 inducers: carbamazepine, phenytoin, phenobarbital, rifampin, efavirenz.

Note. Based on information from Clinical Pharmacology, 2010; Thomson Reuters Micromedex, 2011; Yeh & Bickford, 2009.

Figure 12-3. Preventive Strategies for Nurses

- Obtain and maintain an accurate health and medication history.
- Obtain a baseline electrocardiogram prior to starting any new QT-prolonging medications.
- Check patient laboratory values prior to drug administration (try to target potassium > 4 mEq/L and magnesium > 2 mg/dl).
- Consult with primary or cardiology healthcare providers and pharmacists before starting any new medications, over-the-counter products, and alternative or natural supplements.
- Keep informed about drugs (and combinations of drugs) that prolong the QT and inhibit the metabolism or elimination of QT-prolonging drugs.
- Alert healthcare providers of any reports of palpitations, syncope, or near-syncopal episodes.

Note. Based on information from Ederhy et al., 2009.

Table 12-3. QT-Prolonging Medications Commonly Used in Patients With Cancer

Class	Medications	Comments
Analgesics		
Opioid	Methadone, buprenorphine	QT prolongation occurs in up to 30% of patients using methadone.
Antiarrhythmics		
Class Ia	Procainamide, quinidine, disopyramide	–
Class III	Amiodarone, dofetilide, dronedarone, ibutilide, sotalol	Amiodarone is associated with a low incidence of torsades de pointes (TdP) despite high frequency of QT prolongation.
Antidepressants		
Tricyclic antidepressants	Amitriptyline, desipramine, imipramine	–
Selective serotonin reuptake inhibitors	Sertraline, fluoxetine, paroxetine	–
Antiemetics		
5-HT$_3$ antagonists	Ondansetron, granisetron	Risk decreases quickly after discontinuation.
Antifungals		
Azoles	Voriconazole, posaconazole, ketoconazole, itraconazole fluconazole	Not dose dependent. Azoles are unlikely to cause TdP in the absence of predisposing risk factors.
Antimicrobials		
Fluoroquinolones	Moxifloxacin, levofloxacin, ciprofloxacin	Onset is delayed.
Macrolides	Clarithromycin, erythromycin	High risk of drug-drug interactions that could lead to worsening QT prolongation.
Miscellaneous	Trimethoprim-sulfamethoxazole	Rare; mainly due to the trimethoprim component.
Antipsychotics		
Typical	Haloperidol, droperidol, chlorpromazine, pimozide, thioridazine	Effects are worse when concomitant electrolyte disturbances are present.
Atypical	Ziprasidone, olanzapine, risperidone	–

Note. Based on information from Arizona Center for Education on Research and Therapeutics, 2012; Becker & Yeung, 2010; Gupta et al., 2007.

Torsades de Pointes

Definition

TdP, which literally means "twisting about the points," is a rare but specific type of polymorphic ventricular tachycardia that can be the result of a prolonged QT interval. On ECG it resembles a twisted ribbon because of the morphology of the QRS complexes, which rotate upward and downward around the baseline axis (see Figure 12-4) (Gupta et al., 2007).

Management

Although TdP is rare, it is the main complication associated with QTc prolongation. It is important for nurses to recognize this polymorphic ventricular tachycardia, as it can have life-threatening consequences if not treated properly (see Table 12-4). Initial treatment of all patients should include a 2 g IV bolus of magnesium sulfate regardless of serum magnesium levels. This often is followed by a continuous infusion of magnesium sulfate at a rate of 2–4 mg/min (Viskin, 1999). Potassium levels should also be corrected and maintained in the high-normal range, targeting a potassium level greater than 4.5 mmol/dl (Viskin, 1999). Nurses should also immediately discontinue or hold any offending medications and any other therapy that may interact with the QT-prolonging agents to cause prolonged metabolism or increased concentrations of these drugs (Yeh & Bickford, 2009). If these measures do not result in terminating the arrhythmia, practitioners may also try to shorten the QT interval by increasing the heart rate. This can be achieved either through the use of overdrive transvenous temporary pacing or through the use of medications such as iso-

Figure 12-4. 12-Lead Electrocardiogram Showing Torsades de Pointes

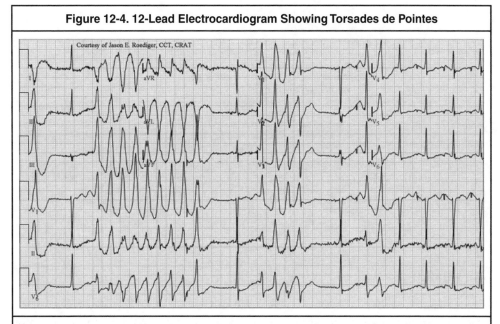

Note. Image courtesy of Jason E. Roediger, CCT, CRAT, retrieved from WikiMedia Commons at commons.wikimedia.org/wiki/file:Torsades_de_Pointes_tdp.png. Used under the Creative Commons Attribution-Share Alike 3.0 Unported license: http://creativecommons.org/licenses/by-sa/3.0/deed.en.

Table 12-4. Management of Torsades de Pointes		
Intervention	**Dose**	**Comments**
Pharmacologic		
Magnesium sulfate	2 g slow IV bolus initially; can be repeated. May follow with a continuous infusion at 2–4 mg/min.	May cause hypotension. Can be given regardless of serum magnesium level.
Potassium chloride	Give supplementation as needed to maintain potassium level above 4.5 mEq. Keep in mind institutional policies for replacement through peripheral and central lines. Oral supplementation may also be given.	Central line is preferred for IV administration. Caution regarding extravasation.
Lidocaine	1–1.5 mg/kg loading dose. If response is seen, may start maintenance infusion at 2–4 mg/min. After 30–60 minutes, a 50 mg bolus is repeated.	Being used as an antiarrhythmic, not as an anesthetic. May cause some central nervous system side effects (drowsiness, dizziness, confusion). Caution regarding bradycardia and hypotension.
Isoproterenol	Dosing ranges from 0.5–5 mcg/min in adults. Titrate to maintain heart rate > 90 beats per minute or until ventricular ectopy is suppressed.	Nonselective beta 1 and beta 2 agonist. May cause hypotension.
Nonpharmacologic		
Temporary ventricular pacing	Insert pacing electrode and target the minimal heart rate required to terminate ventricular ectopy.	–
Defibrillation	Deliver unsynchronized direct cardioversion shock if patient loses consciousness and torsades de pointes deteriorates into ventricular fibrillation.	–

Note. Based on information from Fadol & Lech, 2011; Viskin, 1999.

proterenol that act as a beta-receptor agonist to help speed up the heart. Isoproterenol is usually started at 2 mcg/min in adults and titrated to achieve a heart rate greater than 90 beats per minute if pacing is not available. If the patient becomes unstable at any point or if TdP deteriorates into polymorphic ventricular fibrillation, unsynchronized defibrillation is indicated (Fadol & Lech, 2011; Viskin, 1999; Yeh & Bickford, 2009).

Conclusion

Many patients with cancer will experience some degree of QT prolongation during the course of their treatment. Although most patients will remain asymptomatic, it is important to remember that TdP is a fatal but preventable side effect that can occur. It is important for nurses to screen each patient on a daily basis to look for potential risks such as drug-drug interactions, changes in dosing, and electrolyte abnormalities that could influence the severity of the patient's symptoms. A proactive approach will allow for early recognition of potential problems, which will translate into better outcomes for patients.

References

Al-Khatib, S.M., LaPointe, N.M., Kramer, J.M., & Califf, R.M. (2003). What clinicians should know about the QT interval. *JAMA, 289,* 2120–2127. doi:10.1001/jama.289.16.2120

Arizona Center for Education on Research and Therapeutics. (2012). QT drug lists by risk groups. Retrieved from http://www.azcert.org/medical-pros/drug-lists/drug-lists.cfm

Becker, T.K., & Yeung, S.-C.J. (2010). Drug-induced QT interval prolongation in cancer patients. *Oncology Reviews, 4,* 223–232. doi:10.1007/s12156-010-0058-8

Brell, J.M. (2010). Prolonged QTc interval in cancer therapeutic drug development: Defining arrhythmic risk in malignancy. *Progress in Cardiovascular Diseases, 53,* 164–172. doi:10.1016/j.pcad.2010.05.005

Clinical Pharmacology. (2010). Online database. Retrieved from http://www.clinicalpharmacology.com

Crouch, M.A., Limon, L., & Cassano, A.T. (2003). Clinical relevance and management of drug-related QT interval prolongation. *Pharmacotherapy, 23,* 881–908. doi:10.1592/phco.23.7.881.32730

Curtis, L.H., Østbye, T., Sendersky, V., Hutchison, S., LaPointe, N.M.A., Al-Khatib, S.M., ... Schulman, K.A. (2003). Prescription of QT-prolonging drugs in a cohort of about 5 million outpatients. *American Journal of Medicine, 114,* 135–141. doi:10.1016/S0002-9343(02)01455-9

Ederhy, S., Cohen, A., Dufaitre, G., Izzedine, H., Massard, C., Meuleman, C., ... Soria, J.C. (2009). QT interval prolongation among patients treated with angiogenesis inhibitors. *Targeted Oncology, 4,* 89–97. doi:10.1007/s11523-009-0111-3

Fadol, A., & Lech, T. (2011). Cardiovascular adverse events associated with cancer therapy. *Journal of the Advanced Practitioner in Oncology, 2,* 229–242.

Gupta, A., Lawrence, A.T., Krishnan, K., Kavinsky, C.J., & Trohman, R.G. (2007). Current concepts in the mechanisms and management of drug-induced QT prolongation and torsade de pointes. *American Heart Journal, 153,* 891–899. doi:10.1016/j.ahj.2007.01.040

Li, E.C., Esterly, J.S., Pohl, S., Scott, S.D., & McBride, B.F. (2010). Drug-induced QT-interval prolongation: Considerations for clinicians. *Pharmacotherapy, 30,* 684–701. doi:10.1592/phco.30.7.684

Schwartz, P.J. (2005). Management of long QT syndrome. *Nature Clinical Practice: Cardiovascular Medicine, 2,* 346–351. doi:10.1038/ncpcardio0239

Slama, T.G. (2005, June). Minimizing the risk for QT interval prolongation. *Journal of Family Practice, Supplement,* S15–S17.

Strevel, E.L., Ing, D.J., & Siu, L.L. (2007). Molecularly targeted oncology therapeutics and prolongation of the QT interval. *Journal of Clinical Oncology, 25,* 3362–3371. doi:10.1200/JCO.2006.09.6925

Thomson Reuters Micromedex. (2011). Retrieved from http://www.micromedex.com

Viskin, S. (1999). Torsades de pointes. *Current Treatment Options in Cardiovascular Medicine, 1,* 187–195. doi:10.1007/s11936-999-0022-8

Vorchheimer, D.A. (2005, June). What is QT interval prolongation? *Journal of Family Practice, Supplement,* S4–S7.

Yeh, E.T., & Bickford, C.L. (2009). Cardiovascular complications of cancer therapy: Incidence, pathogenesis, diagnosis, and management. *Journal of the American College of Cardiology, 53,* 2231–2247. doi:10.1016/j.jacc.2009.02.050

CHAPTER 13

Ventricular Dysrhythmias and Cardiac Implantable Electronic Devices

Sheryl W. Murphy, RN, BSN, MSN, FNP, and Darla Labasse, RN, BSN, BBA

Introduction

Ventricular dysrhythmias such as premature ventricular contractions (PVCs), ventricular tachycardia (VT), torsades de pointes (TdP), and ventricular fibrillation (V-fib) can cause sudden cardiac death in the general population, accounting for more annual deaths per year than cancer (Roger et al., 2011). Cancer therapies may trigger ventricular dysrhythmias or contribute to electrolyte disturbances, further increasing the risk for sudden cardiac death. Rapid recognition of these dysrhythmias is crucial for the prevention and treatment of sudden cardiac arrest, allowing for early activation of basic cardiac life support (BCLS) or advanced cardiac life support (ACLS) skills to offer the best chance of patient survival. As technology advances in the treatment of ventricular dysrhythmias, more and more patients with cancer have cardiac implantable electronic devices (CIEDs) such as an implantable cardioverter defibrillator (ICD), a cardiac pacemaker, or a cardiac resynchronization therapy (CRT) device. This chapter will review the pathophysiology, risk factors, medical and pharmacologic therapy, and nursing considerations for ventricular dysrhythmias. CIED components, pacemaker programming, ICD therapy, CRT, interpretation of a CIED interrogation report, effects of magnets on CIEDs, perioperative considerations, electromagnetic interference, radiation, central line placement, and nursing considerations for patients with CIEDs will be explored.

Premature Ventricular Contractions

A PVC is characterized on electrocardiogram (ECG) as a wide QRS complex with no preceding P wave, in contrast to a normal sinus complex that has a P wave prior to each QRS complex (see Figure 13-1) (Olgin & Zipes, 2012).

Pathophysiology

PVCs are early beats originating from ventricular ectopic foci that cause depolarization of the ventricles prior to sinus node depolarization (Olgin & Zipes, 2012). PVCs can happen in many different patterns. They can be single, isolated complexes with the same appearance, which are referred to as *uniform PVCs*. PVCs occurring in an every-other-beat pattern are called *ventricular bigeminy* (see Figure 13-1). PVCs that happen sequentially without a sinus beat in between are called *couplets* (two PVCs in a row). A pattern with more than three PVCs in a row but less than 30 seconds of PVCs in a row is called *nonsustained ventricular tachycardia* (see Figure 13-2) (Olgin & Zipes, 2012).

A compensatory pause can follow a PVC depending on its timing in the cardiac cycle (Olgin & Zipes, 2012). This is due to the premature beat coming early in the cardiac cycle, which causes a peripheral pulse to be too weak to be felt. For example, a patient with ventricular bigeminy may have an apical pulse of 80 beats per minute (bpm) heard on auscultation and at the same time have a palpated radial pulse of 40 bpm.

Risk Factors

Determining the etiology of PVCs is crucial in deciding whether the condition is benign or lethal, potentially leading to further rhythm disturbances such as VT, TdP, or V-fib (Rho & Page, 2008). Cardiac ischemia, acute congestive heart failure, electrolyte imbalances, and digitalis toxicity are some nononcology conditions that can cause PVCs (Rho & Page, 2008). 5-fluorouracil is a chemotherapeutic agent that can cause PVCs (Yilmaz et al., 2007).

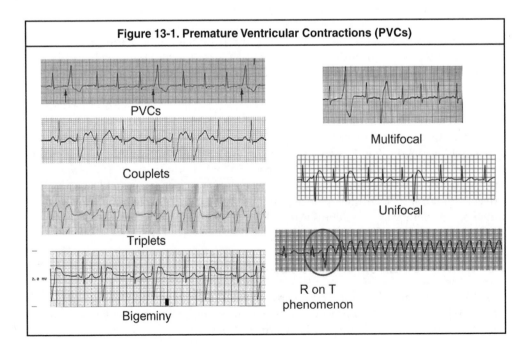

Figure 13-1. Premature Ventricular Contractions (PVCs)

PVCs

Couplets

Triplets

Bigeminy

Multifocal

Unifocal

R on T
phenomenon

Figure 13-2. Nonsustained Ventricular Tachycardia

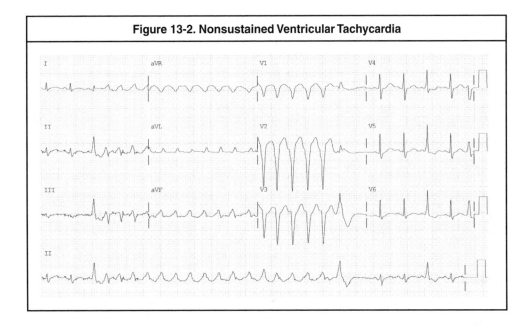

Symptoms

Palpitations are the most frequent complaint for patients with PVCs. Light-headedness or syncope is a more worrisome symptom when accompanied by PVCs. A patient with asymptomatic PVCs and without structural heart disease (no coronary artery disease, cardiomyopathy, or valvular heart disease) is considered to have benign PVCs. A patient with structural heart disease and asymptomatic PVCs can potentially have lethal PVCs. A symptomatic patient with structural heart disease that is having lethal PVCs requires treatment sooner rather than later (Rho & Page, 2008).

Assessment

Assessing patients with cancer for any of the aforementioned conditions is crucial in determining nursing interventions and anticipated treatment plans. Does the patient have symptoms of angina or congestive heart failure? Is there an electrolyte abnormality such as hypokalemia, hyperkalemia, or hypomagnesemia? Is the patient taking a digitalis preparation? If so, is there a medication compliance issue in which the patient may be forgetful and taking too much digitalis? Is the patient complaining of seeing yellow rings around lights (a common complaint with digitalis toxicity)? Is there renal impairment (elevated serum creatinine level) that may predispose the patient to digitalis toxicity because of decreased renal metabolism and clearance of the drug? Is the left ventricular ejection fraction (LVEF) normal? Is there any structural heart disease (valve abnormalities, heart blocks)?

Medical Management and Nursing Considerations

Asymptomatic PVCs without structural heart disease do not require treatment (Rho & Page, 2008). Symptomatic PVCs may require low-dose beta-blocker medication for suppression and alleviation of the palpitations (Rho & Page, 2008). Pure beta-blockers such as metoprolol, atenolol, and propanolol are commonly prescribed at low doses because they have a stronger chronotropic effect that slows the heart rate and may suppress the PVCs. Beta-blockers that also have some alpha blockade, such as labetalol, carvedilol, and nebivolol, are not commonly prescribed to treat symptomatic PVCs because they have a more pronounced blood pressure effect than a rate-slowing effect.

Nursing considerations should focus on monitoring for side effects of medications. The nurse should monitor for hypotension or bradycardia that could be causing lightheadedness, dizziness, or syncope and clarify the order if there are no hold parameters for these medicines. The initial workup should include a stress test to determine whether there is any ischemic component to the PVCs and an echocardiogram to look for structural abnormalities of the heart. The patient may have an order to wear a Holter monitor for 24–48 hours to enable the medical provider to determine how frequently the PVCs are happening and to correlate any symptoms with the PVCs (Rho & Page, 2008).

Ventricular Tachycardia

VT is characterized on the ECG by a sequential, wide complex QRS pattern that occurs in a fast and regular pattern, with no P wave preceding the QRS complex, at a rate of 100–250 bpm (see Figure 13-3).

Pathophysiology

As noted by Morganti and Hongo (2011), "VT is defined as a ventricular arrhythmia with three or more consecutive complexes in duration greater than 100 bpm" (pp. 127–128). This is an unstable rhythm that requires immediate assessment and intervention because it can quickly disintegrate into a lethal V-fib (Rho & Page, 2008). It propagates

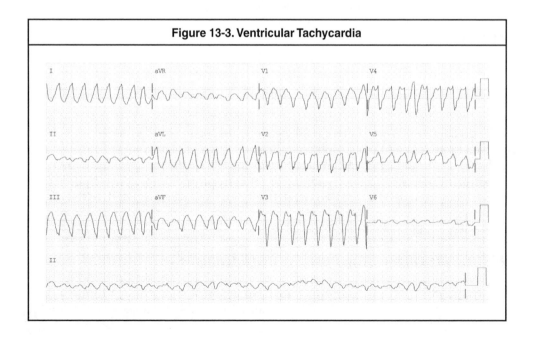

Figure 13-3. Ventricular Tachycardia

from an ectopic focus that may be a single site or multiple sites causing the wide complex tachycardia (Olgin & Zipes, 2012). Myocardial cells deprived of oxygen become ischemic and initiate VT as a signal that something is wrong (Rho & Page, 2008). VT can arise from the zone of tissue between healthy myocardial tissue and ischemic myocardial tissue such as that found in scar tissue after a myocardial infarction (MI) (Olgin & Zipes, 2012). VT can also be caused by an accessory pathway such as in Wolff-Parkinson-White syndrome (Rho & Page, 2008).

Risk Factors

The most common cause of VT is myocardial ischemia. The risk for VT is highest for the first 24 hours after an MI because of myocardial ischemia (Rho & Page, 2008). However, VT occurring later after an MI is more worrisome, as it tends to be more recurrent and associated with myocardial scarring after the MI. These patients have an ICD implanted for primary prevention of sudden cardiac death due to VT or V-fib. In a post-MI patient who has a syncopal event, VT is very likely to be the cause of the syncope (Rho & Page, 2008).

Nononcology conditions that can precipitate VT include cardiomyopathy (LVEF less than 35%), electrolyte imbalances, digitalis toxicity, antiarrhythmic drugs, psychotropic drugs, right ventricular dysplasia, and valvular heart disease, especially mitral regurgitation (Olgin & Zipes, 2012). Reentrant, congenital accessory pathway conditions such as Wolff-Parkinson-White syndrome also can cause VT (Rho & Page, 2008).

Chemotherapy agents such as interleukin, doxorubicin (Rudzinski, Ciesielczyk, Religa, Bednarkiewicz, & Krzeminska-Pakula, 2007), rituximab (Arai, Tadokoro, & Mitani, 2005), trastuzumab (Ferguson, Clarke, & Herity, 2006), and thalidomide (Ballanti et al., 2007) have been reported to have a proarrhythmic effect causing VT. Primary cardiac tumors can cause refractory VT but are quite rare (Gualis, Castaño, Gómez-Plana, Martin, & Alonso, 2010).

Syncope or near-syncope is the most common symptom in VT. Patients also may complain of palpitations just prior to the syncopal event. The symptoms may be so severe as to cause seizure-like activity with the syncope. This hemodynamic collapse is due to cerebral hypoperfusion causing an inability of the atria or ventricles to fill during the tachycardia. Some patients do not lose consciousness and may complain only of palpitations. Ischemia complaints such as angina or acute MI symptoms can precede VT (Rho & Page, 2008).

Assessment

The patient should be assessed for any of the aforementioned conditions to determine the risk for having VT. Asking the patient about ischemia symptoms can help to determine the risk for VT, TdP, or V-fib (see Chapter 5). Some patients can tolerate VT or TdP with minimal symptoms and no cardiovascular collapse (Rho & Page, 2008). It is not unusual for a patient to walk into the infusion or radiation suite for therapy and have a heart rate of 150 bpm or greater. ECG or cardiac monitoring will help to determine the rhythm.

The patient should be assessed for electrolyte imbalances that can increase the likelihood of these dysrhythmias. Serum potassium at 4–5 mEq/L and serum magnesium at 2–3 mg/dl are the targets for electrolyte replacement. This can be quite challenging with the gastrointestinal upsets caused by chemotherapy and radiation. Hypoxemia and metabolic imbalances also can contribute to the development of VT.

Medical Management and Nursing Considerations

Treatment for VT/V-fib is per the ACLS guidelines. Cardioversion is indicated for any unstable signs and symptoms such as hypotension, chest pain, shortness of breath, syncope, or diaphoresis associated with the VT episode (Olgin & Zipes, 2012).

Medications can be used to treat patients with stable VT (Craig & Day, 2011). First-line medical therapy is amiodarone 150 mg IV bolus over 10 minutes. The amiodarone IV infusion is continued at a rate of 1 mg/min for 6 hours, then 0.5 mg/min for 18 hours (Craig & Day, 2011). The infusion may be continued past these parameters depending on the patient's condition. Nursing consideration is to ensure continuous cardiac telemetry monitoring. Stop the infusion for heart rate less than 60 bpm and notify the physician. Liver function test results should be monitored for acute toxicity, and discontinuation of the infusion may be required for a tripling of transaminase levels (aspartate transaminase/alanine aminotransferase). Amiodarone is not usually prescribed for VT/V-fib suppression because of its ineffectiveness in preventing these rhythm disturbances (AVID Investigators, 1995). A patient with unstable VT will require immediate direct current cardioversion followed by IV amiodarone 150 mg bolus and continuous infusion at 1 mg/min for 6 hours followed by 0.5 mg/min for 18 hours. Consider sedation prior to cardioversion if the patient is awake and alert. These patients may have an ICD implanted for primary prevention of sudden cardiac death (Olgin & Zipes, 2012).

VT arising from myocardial scar tissue following MI can sometimes be treated with catheter ablation of the critical foci in the cardiac catheterization laboratory (Olgin & Zipes, 2012).

Intracardiac mapping of the VT foci is done via transvenous catheters. Once the ectopic foci are mapped, radiofrequency energy bursts are delivered to disrupt cell membranes, causing destruction of cells responsible for the reentrant pathway around the scar tissue that is causing the VT. The procedure has a relatively low morbidity and mortality rate in experienced, high-volume centers and is commonly performed as an outpatient procedure. Catheter ablation will require a minimum of six weeks of full-dose anticoagulation postablation because of the eschar formed during the ablation and the resulting potential for thrombus formation. Unfortunately, many patients with cancer are severely thrombocytopenic with bleeding risks and are not able to undergo six weeks of full-dose anticoagulation. In these situations, timing is crucial to find a window between treatments to perform the ablation when cell counts and platelet counts will most likely be stable.

Torsades de Pointes

In TdP, the ECG tracing will show a wide complex tachycardia with an alternating axis where the QRS complexes change from upright to inverted to upright, alternating back and forth, which is called *electrical alternans* (see Figure 13-4).

Pathophysiology

TdP is a type of rapid, polymorphic VT almost always associated with a prolonged QT interval (usually greater than 500 ms as a corrected QT interval) (Cubeddu, 2003).

Figure 13-4. Torsades de Pointes

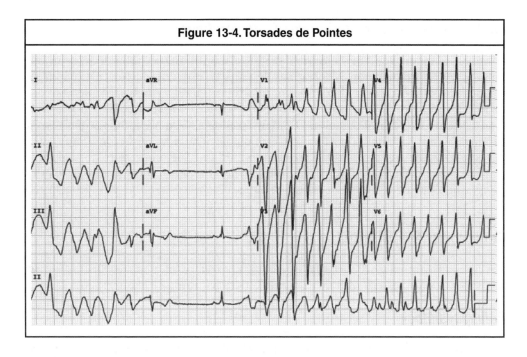

Medication interactions can cause this QT prolongation, or it can be caused by congenital heart disease. TdP also can occur with a sudden slowing in the heartbeat, such as that which may occur with a compensatory pause after a PVC.

Risk Factors

Chemotherapeutic agents such as 5-fluorouracil, cyclophosphamide, and tamoxifen have the potential to cause QT prolongation and make patients with cancer more susceptible to TdP (Kuittinen et al., 2010; Stewart, Pavlakis, & Ward, 2010). Antiarrhythmic agents such as amiodarone, sotalol, and dofetilide can be proarrhythmic, which can precipitate TdP (see Chapter 12).

Symptoms

Patients may have the same symptoms as with VT and can be either asymptomatic or very symptomatic. See the previous discussion of symptoms of VT.

Assessment

Frequent monitoring of the QT-corrected interval should be performed via ECG tracing while any of the aforementioned chemotherapeutic agents are active. All concurrent medications must be reviewed for QT prolongation as a known side effect. Efforts are aimed at ordering medications that are not as likely to prolong the QT interval. Antiarrhythmic drugs, fluoroquinolones, and antiemetic drugs are frequently prescribed drugs in patients with cancer that may have an additive QT prolongation effect, putting the patient at increased risk for the development of TdP (for a full discussion, see Chapter 12).

Medical Management and Nursing Considerations

Initial treatment for TdP is to immediately discontinue the offending agent that caused the QT prolongation. Medications that may be ordered to treat TdP include IV magnesium sulfate 2 g over 10 minutes or lidocaine 100 mg IV bolus followed by continuous infusion for 24 hours. Amiodarone is not usually ordered because it may provoke TdP due to QT prolongation. Overdrive pacing can be used if the patient has a pacemaker or if an external pacemaker is available. The device is set to a rate faster than the TdP rate and then slowed down to "break" the TdP and restore normal sinus rhythm. Direct-current cardioversion is the first-line therapy if there is any circulatory compromise during a TdP event (Olgin & Zipes, 2012).

Ventricular Fibrillation

V-fib is a rhythm disturbance that is lethal if not treated immediately. Its ECG characteristic is a wavy pattern with no discernible QRS pattern (see Figure 13-5).

Pathophysiology

V-fib is complete circulatory collapse and is fatal unless treated immediately. There is no organized ventricular depolarization, so the patient becomes pulseless. Defibrillation is the only successful treatment (Rho & Page, 2008).

Risk Factors

Conditions that may predispose patients with cancer to a V-fib arrest include hypoxemia, acute MI, and electrolyte or metabolic disturbances (Olgin & Zipes, 2012). VT

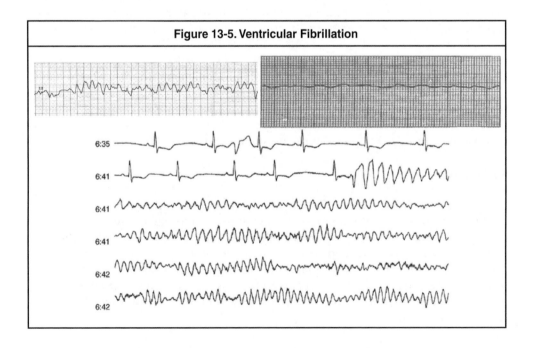

Figure 13-5. Ventricular Fibrillation

or TdP can degenerate to V-fib. This rhythm causes circulatory collapse, and BCLS and ACLS measures must be initiated to save the patient's life. Patients with Wolff-Parkinson-White syndrome can develop V-fib from the accessory pathway being stimulated. Cardiomyopathy is a known risk factor for V-fib arrest and is a primary prevention reason for an ICD implant (Olgin & Zipes, 2012).

Symptoms

Unresponsiveness is the first symptom that a bystander will see. The patient may have angina prior to the V-fib arrest (Rho & Page, 2008).

Assessment

Any unresponsive patient must be presumed to have suffered a V-fib arrest, and full BCLS and ACLS assessments should be initiated. Airway, breathing, and circulation must be assessed and optimized for a successful resuscitation.

Medical Management and Nursing Considerations

Defibrillation is the treatment most likely to successfully convert the rhythm back to a normal sinus rhythm (Olgin & Zipes, 2012). Metabolic and electrolyte disturbances may need to be corrected for the defibrillation to be successful. Antiarrhythmic agents and catecholamines may make defibrillation more successful (Craig & Day, 2011). Patients who survive a V-fib arrest in the early stages of an MI generally have a good prognosis. Correction of the ischemia via angioplasty and percutaneous stent deployment is the treatment of choice for acute MI with V-fib arrest (Rho & Page, 2011). V-fib occurring in the absence of one of the aforementioned conditions is more likely to be recurrent (Rho & Page, 2008). Congenital heart diseases such as Brugada syndrome, hypertrophic cardiomyopathy, and Wolff-Parkinson-White syndrome may predispose the patient to a V-fib arrest. Patients with an LVEF of 35% or less after three months of aggressive medical heart failure management are at heightened risk for a V-fib arrest and qualify for a primary prevention ICD (Moss, 2003; Reiffel, 2005).

Cardiovascular Implantable Electronic Devices

Device Components

It is important to know which CIED is implanted and how the device is programmed. A cardiac pacemaker is used to keep the heart from beating too slowly. These devices are commonly implanted to treat conditions such as atrioventricular blocks and sick sinus syndrome (Vijayaraman & Ellenbogen, 2008). A patient is considered to be pacemaker dependent if the heart rate without pacemaker beats (i.e., intrinsic heartbeat) is less than 30 bpm. ICDs treat fast, potentially lethal heart rhythms such as VT or V-fib (Vijayaraman & Ellenbogen, 2008). CIEDs comprise a pulse generator (the computer for the device) implanted in a surgically created pocket in the subcutaneous tissue below the clavicle and on top of the muscle layer. The generator (see Figure 13-6) has connected leads that are implanted in the endomyocardium to send electrical impulses to regulate the heartbeat (Vijayaraman & Ellenbogen, 2008).

Figure 13-6. Pacemaker and Implantable Cardioverter Defibrillator Pulse Generator

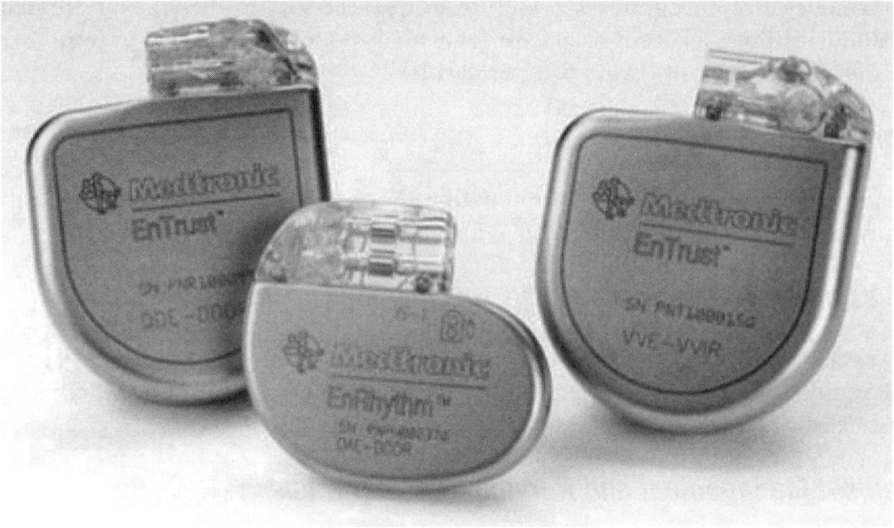

Note. Photo courtesy of Medtronic, Inc. Used with permission.

At implant, a lead is inserted through the subclavian vein and passed though the superior vena cava to the right atrium, through the tricuspid valve to the right ventricle. It is anchored in the endomyocardium with either an active or passive fixation device that is manipulated by the operator at the access site, thus avoiding sternotomy (Vijayaraman & Ellenbogen, 2008). One, two, or three leads may be seen on the patient's chest x-ray. If there is one lead, it usually is implanted in the right ventricle. Rarely one lead is implanted in the right atrium; however, this is a much more common practice in European countries. Most common is a two-lead implantation with leads in the right atrium and right ventricle, often referred to as a *dual-chamber implant* (Vijayaraman & Ellenbogen, 2008). CRT requires implantation of three leads (Olgin & Zipes, 2012). The dual-chamber implant will be seen in the right atrium and the right ventricle, along with the third lead implanted in the left ventricle via the coronary sinus as an epicardial lead. Figure 13-7 shows lead implant positions.

Pacemaker Programming

Programming of the pacemaker involves choosing a pacing mode, which tells the pacemaker how the CIED should perform, and a pacing rate, which is how fast it should pace. The Heart Rhythm Society (formerly the North American Society of Pacing and Electrophysiology) and the British Pacing and Electrophysiology Group designed a simple pacemaker code system to communicate both mode and rate (Vijayaraman & Ellenbogen, 2008). A pacing mode of DDD or VVI is frequently used. This pacing mode identifies which chambers (atria, ventricle, or both) are programmed for pacing, which chambers (atria, ventricle, or both) are programmed for sensing, and how sensing affects pacing. Figure 13-8 presents the code and its interpretation.

Take an example of a patient programmed to a pacing mode of DDD at 60 bpm to see how this chart works (Chiu-Man, Nygren, & De Souza, 2011). The first letter in our example "DDD" shows that it is a dual-chamber device because "D" indicates atria and ventricle. Looking at the table, the first column tells where the device is programmed to pace. <u>D</u> indicates the device will pace in both the atria and the ventricle. If it were

Figure 13-7. Cardiac Implantable Electronic Device Lead Placement

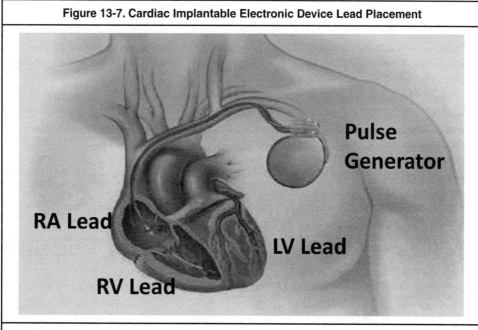

LV—left ventricular; RA—right atrial; RV—right ventricular

Note. Copyright © 2011 Boston Scientific Corporation or its affiliates. All rights reserved. Used with permission.

Figure 13-8. The NASPE/BPEG Generic (NBG) Pacemaker Code (Revised 2000)

I	II	III	IV	V
Chamber(s) Paced	Chamber(s) Sensed	Response to Sensing	Rate Modulation	Multisite Pacing
O = None A = Atrium V = Ventricle D = Dual (A + V) S = Single (A or V)	O = None A = Atrium V = Ventricle D = Dual (A + V) S = Single (A or V)	O = None T = Triggered I = Inhibited D = Dual (T + I)	O = None R = Rate modulation	O = None A = Atrium V = Ventricle D = Dual (A + V)

BPEG—British Pacing and Electrophysiology Group; NASPE—North American Society of Pacing and Electrophysiology

Note. From *CorePace, Single and Dual Chamber Pacemaker Timing,* Module 6, slide 4. Reprinted with permission from Medtronic, Inc. Retrieved from https://wwwp.medtronic.com/mdtConnectPortal/dynamicarea/corepace/2007080926

set to pace in the ventricle only and not the atria, the first letter would be a "V," such as VVI. The second letter tells where the pacemaker is programmed to sense or "look for" an intrinsic beat so that it does not send an impulse when the heart's own pacemaker system is working. The second letter in our example "DDD" indicates that it is looking for a native heartbeat, or sensing in both the atria and ventricle. The lead either sees a native heartbeat or not and sends this signal back to the pulse generator. The computer in the pulse generator will send a pacing impulse through the same lead to cause a heartbeat to happen if none was sensed. If there is an intrinsic heartbeat, it will not send an electrical impulse. The third column in the example "DDD" identifies what the computer will do if it sees a heart rate of more than or less than the set rate of 60 bpm. The "D" means that it will trigger an electrical impulse to pace in whichever chamber the first letter is programmed to pace if it senses a heart rate of less than 60 bpm. In the example "DDD," the device will send an electrical impulse down both the atrial and ventricular leads to cause them to depolarize and make a heartbeat. Likewise, if the heart rate is more than 60 bpm, the generator will inhibit or not send an electrical impulse down the atrial or ventricular lead, thereby letting the heart conduct an intrinsic heartbeat. In the example DDD at 60 bpm, the generator will sense for intrinsic heartbeats in both the atria and ventricle. It will either trigger a paced beat or inhibit a paced beat, depending on what it senses from the natural heartbeats, and send an electrical impulse to pace the atria and the ventricle.

Rate response is a programmable feature that allows the pacemaker to increase or decrease the pacing rate according to changes in patient activity (Vijayaraman & Ellenbogen, 2008). This is the fourth letter in the pacing mode and is indicated with an "R" (or its absence). The heart has a normal chronotropic response to exercise or physical activity, which means that the heartbeat increases naturally to meet the increased myocardial oxygen demand when, for example, a person walks up a flight of stairs. Patients with sick sinus syndrome lose this normal chronotropic response to exercise. The rate response feature attempts to mimic this natural response to physical activity. That is why a patient may have a heart rate higher than the programmed base rate. The example of the patient with a DDD at 60 bpm pacing mode does not have rate response programmed. DDDR at 60 bpm indicates rate response programming is turned on for the patient. Nurses may see a patient with rate response programming being paced at 90 bpm and think something is wrong. However, they should look at the pacing mode and see if the rate response is programmed before concluding that the pacemaker is not functioning correctly. The pacing rate can increase to the upper rate limit (usually 110–130 bpm), which is also programmable in dual-chamber devices (Chiu-Man et al., 2011). So if the patient with a pacemaker has a heart rate of 140 bpm, it cannot be the pacemaker because that is faster than the programmed upper rate limit, which is the fastest the pacemaker is programmed to pace. Therefore, it must be an intrinsic rhythm. Some devices have a sleep mode or rest rate that allows the pacemaker to pace at lower than the programmed base rate of 60 bpm during certain hours, usually while the patient is sleeping. Night nurses may encounter this feature.

Implantable Cardioverter Defibrillators

ICDs treat fast rhythms such as VT or V-fib with antitachycardia pacing and/or shock therapy (Olgin & Zipes, 2012). All ICDs have a pacemaker as part of their computer for two reasons. One is that many patients need both defibrillation and pacing, and hence these functions are combined into one device. Second, defibrillation therapy can stun the heart muscle and cause it to not beat. The pacemaker is there to remind the heart to resume beating. Antitachycardia pacing is painless therapy for VT that includes rapid pacing by the device to slow down the rate to normal rhythm (Swerdlow, Hayes, & Zipes, 2012). It can be likened to a runaway horse: a second rider races up to the horse, grabs its reigns, and slows it down. Antitachycardia pacing does the same thing. Through overdrive pacing, the device paces the heart at or just a little faster than the VT rate and then slows it down, with overdrive pacing converting the rhythm to normal sinus rhythm. Some devices are programmed with antitachycardia pacing therapy first, followed by shock therapy if unsuccessful (Swerdlow et al., 2012). The patient usually does not feel antitachycardia pacing therapy; however, shock therapy can be very uncomfortable. A patient can have a syncopal episode prior to shock therapy because of a lack of cerebral perfusion. For this reason, if an ICD patient has a syncopal episode, the device needs to be checked for a VT or V-fib event.

Cardiac Resynchronization Therapy Device

CRT is a treatment for heart failure. In heart failure, the left ventricle dilates. As the left ventricle dilates, its contractility is reduced, causing a drop in LVEF, which is a pathophysiologic finding in heart failure (Swerdlow et al., 2011). This dilated left ventricle can cause dysynchrony between the left ventricle and the right ventricle, leading to worsening heart failure (Bourassa, Khairy, & Roy, 2011). CRT offers the ability to resynchronize the left and right ventricles with the goal of increasing the LVEF and relieving heart failure symptoms (Badhwar & Lee, 2008). CRT utilizes a third lead that is an epicardial lead inserted through the coronary sinus and anchored on the outer surface of the left ventricle. The CRT generator times its pacing of the right and left ventricles to try to resynchronize their contractions. CRT can be a pacemaker alone or in combination with a defibrillator.

Interpretation of a Device Interrogation Report

All three of the previously described devices (pacemaker, ICD, and CRT) will generate an interrogation report when the device is checked. Reading this can be intimidating at first. Systematically looking for the following information allows understanding of how the CIED is programmed to perform. Most of the information can be found on the first page of the device interrogation sheet. A typical CIED interrogation summary will show the device model and manufacturer at the top of the page, date of implant and battery status, pacing mode, lower and upper rate limits, antitachycardia pacing or shock therapy programming, percentage of time pacing, any VT or V-fib episodes since the last check, and any supraventricular tachycardia/atrial fibrillation episodes since the last check.

Cardiovascular Implantable Electronic Device Response to Magnets

Most pacemakers have a magnet mode. Placing a magnet over the generator will cause it to pace at a predetermined rate in an asynchronous mode (i.e., it does not sense for an intrinsic heartbeat but paces regardless) (Cohan, Kusumoto, & Goldschlager, 2008). Magnet mode behavior differs for each manufacturer and model, so it is important to know how the patient's generator will respond to a magnet. Taping or holding a magnet directly over a pacemaker generator will activate the magnet mode. This mode is used in surgery or procedures in which the possibility of electrical interference from other tools (such as Bovie equipment) may cause the pacemaker to not sense appropriately. In general, the magnet rates are as follows: Boston Scientific, 100 bpm; Medtronic, 85 bpm; and St. Jude Medical, 98.6 bpm. Biotronik devices do not have a magnet mode. When the magnet is removed, the normal programmed values are restored (Cohan et al., 2008).

Placing a magnet over an ICD does not cause asynchronous pacing as seen with a pacemaker. Normally, placing a magnet over an ICD temporarily disables tachycardia therapy so that the device will not deliver antitachycardia pacing or shock should the patient have a VT or V-fib episode (Cohan et al., 2008). A magnet taped over an ICD generator will cause the device to ignore electrical interference from outside sources such as Bovie equipment during a surgical procedure. Any time a magnet is taped over an ICD, cardiac monitoring must be continuous. If a VT or V-fib episode happens, the magnet should be removed from the ICD and the generator will deliver antitachycardia pacing or shock as programmed.

Perioperative Considerations

Oncology nurses should ensure that the CIED team sees the patient in the preoperative period in order to provide recommendations regarding the intra- and postoperative management of the device. Essential information that should be provided about the patient's CIED during the perioperative management period includes

- The type of surgery/procedure and location of the CIED in relation to the surgery or procedure
- Date of last CIED interrogation: pacemaker within the last 12 months and an ICD within the last 6 months in stable patients (Crossley et al., 2011)
- Type of device (pacemaker, ICD, CRT), manufacturer, and model
- Indication for implant (determine the need for pacing, arrhythmia therapy, or heart failure management)
- Battery longevity (recommended to be at least six months' longevity; if not, could have increased sensitivity for damage from electromagnetic interference) (Crossley et al., 2011)
- Basic programming (pacing mode, lower rate limit, rate response/programmed therapy)
- Underlying rhythm (know if the patient is pacemaker dependent)
- The device's response to a magnet
- Pacing thresholds (should be recorded to verify adequate safety margin).

Electromagnetic Interference and Cardiovascular Implantable Electronic Devices

Electromagnetic interference is noncardiac electrical signals that the CIED senses that can affect the device's function (Cohan et al., 2008). Electromagnetic interference can be generated from electrical tools and heavy industrial equipment. In the hospital setting, it often is seen during the perioperative period and during procedures such as electrocautery and magnetic resonance imaging or with the use of transcutaneous electrical nerve stimulation units or any electronic device used on a patient (Hongo & Goldschlager, 2008).

Electromagnetic interference can cause inappropriate pacing inhibition by causing oversensing in which the pulse generator senses what it believes is an intrinsic heartbeat but is actually electromagnetic interference, so it inhibits the pacing, thus resulting in underpacing (Cohan et al., 2008). With an ICD, such incorrect sensing could lead to inappropriate therapy (shock) if the pulse generator thinks the electromagnetic interference is VT or V-fib and delivers therapy. Damage at the lead and tissue interface could cause an increase of pacing thresholds or loss of capture. Pulse generator damage or an electrical reset mode can occur. These are CIED emergencies in which the device is unstable and requires immediate replacement. This often is seen in radiation damage or post-cardioversion damage to the generator (Crossley et al., 2011).

Bipolar and Monopolar Electrosurgery and Cardiovascular Implantable Electronic Devices

When possible, bipolar electrosurgery should be used because it appears to have minimal chance for causing an adverse interaction. However, because bipolar electrosurgery is used for coagulation and not dissection, it is used less often in the operating room (OR) setting. Monopolar electrosurgery is the most common source of electromagnetic interference in the OR setting (Crossley et al., 2011). Given this fact, the following are some recommendations to consider.

- Keep the distance between the electrocautery current path (area between Bovie tip and grounding pad) and the pulse generator/leads greater than 6 inches apart (Crossley et al., 2011).
- Use a short burst of electrosurgery, 1–2 seconds every 10 seconds (Boston Scientific Corp., 2008; St. Jude Medical, 2008).
- Surgery in close proximity to the CIED should be performed using bipolar electrosurgery when possible (Boston Scientific Corp., 2008; St. Jude Medical, 2008).
- The electrosurgery return electrode pad should be placed so that the current path avoids the CIED (Boston Scientific Corp., 2008; St. Jude Medical, 2008).
- Consider reprogramming the ICD to disable tachyarrhythmia detection or taping a magnet over the ICD to inhibit therapy (Boston Scientific Corp., 2008; St. Jude Medical, 2011). If electrosurgery will be performed below the umbilicus and the CIED is placed in the upper chest, place the return electrode on the lower body, such as on the thigh or in the gluteal area.
- Consider reprogramming pacemaker-dependent patients with an ICD to asynchronous pacing (St. Jude Medical, 2008).
- Have a magnet available in all cases in which reprogramming was not performed.
- If a pacemaker reset occurs in Medtronic, Boston Scientific, St. Jude Medical, or Biotronik devices, they will resort to VVI pacing between 65 and 70 bpm. Be aware of a possible reset by a change in pacing. If a reset has occurred, contact the manufacturer's technical support.
- Consider taping a magnet over pacemaker-dependent patients to produce asynchronous pacing (Boston Scientific Corp., 2008; St. Jude Medical, 2008).
- Perform continuous cardiac monitoring of patients in whom ICDs are deactivated (Crossley et al., 2011). Emergent ACLS equipment and trained personnel must be available.

Central Venous Access

Use caution when placing central lines, especially if the leads have been inserted within the past three months (Crossley et al., 2011). If the leads were placed less than six weeks ago, do not attempt central venous access because of an increased risk for lead dislodgment. If absolutely necessary, the healthcare provider may consider placing central lines under fluoroscopy.

Radiation and Cardiovascular Implantable Electronic Devices

Many variables in the radiation environment can affect cardiac pacemakers and their resulting behavior. Because of this, it is difficult to develop a set of recommendations (Marbach, Sontag, Van Dyk, & Wolbarst, 1994). Diagnostic radiation rarely interferes with pacemaker or ICD function, but rare instances of oversensing and electrical resets have occurred (Crossley et al., 2011). However, significant damage can result from therapeutic radiation (Crossley et al., 2011; Solan, Solan, Bednarz, & Goodkin, 2004). Malfunction could be transient interference or permanent interference. In transient interference, the pacemaker returns to normal operation when the source of interference is removed. Permanent interference can result in either total malfunction or erratic behavior unless the device is reprogrammed or replaced (Marbach et al., 1994).

Pacemaker failure has been seen at cumulative radiation doses of 10–30 gray (Gy), and functional changes have been observed with 2–10 Gy (Marbach et al., 1994). Hudson, Coulshed, D'Souza, and Baker (2010) stated that radiation-induced device malfunction is rare; however, they recommended a conservative approach to minimize the risk of harm to the patient. Early changes in pacemaker parameters could signal a failure (Marbach et al., 1994).

Each oncology department needs to formulate its own policy about how to manage patients with a pacemaker or ICD. Things to consider are the cumulative dose received by the device, effects of backscatter, dose rate, fractionation, and potential electromagnetic interference (Hudson et al., 2010).

The Radiation Therapy Committee of the American Association of Physicists in Medicine formed Task Group 34 to determine the effects of radiation on implanted pacemakers (it did not address defibrillators) and formulate a set of guidelines for management (Marbach et al., 1994). These guidelines were published in 1994 and are still being followed by some oncology departments (Solan et al., 2004). Solan et al. (2004) presented guidelines using a more universal approach to streamline delivery of radiation therapy to patients. The Heart Rhythm Society generated a consensus from experts to provide guidance to healthcare professionals who care for patients with pacemakers and defibrillators. The following is a compiled list of their guidelines and recommendations.

- Identify patients with cardiac devices and obtain device details (Hudson et al., 2010; Solan et al., 2004).
- Refer to the cardiologist to determine whether the patient is pacemaker dependent (Hudson et al., 2010; Solan et al., 2004).
- The cardiologist should provide deactivation instructions for ICDs and full baseline interrogation of the pacemaker or ICD (Solan et al., 2004).
- The absorbed dose to be received by the pacemaker should be estimated before treatment (Crossley et al., 2011; Marbach et al., 1994).
- Shielding should be discussed in all cases (Crossley et al., 2011).
- The pacemaker or ICD should not be placed in the direct therapy beam (Crossley et al., 2011; Gelblum & Amols, 2009; Marbach et al., 1994). Keep the maximum pacemaker dose to less than 2 Gy and maximum ICD dose to less than 1 Gy (Hud-

son et al., 2010). The accumulated radiation dose should not exceed 5 Gy (Crossley et al., 2011; Hudson et al., 2010). Consider moving the device to another location if it is in the radiation field (Crossley et al., 2011; Gelblum & Amols, 2009; Solan et al., 2004).

- Test with low-energy beams (less than 10 mV) (Gelblum & Amols, 2009; Hudson et al., 2010).
- Keep the ICD as far from the treatment field as possible (Gelblum & Amols, 2009).
- Discuss each patient's care with the cardiologist or electrophysiologist to determine optimal practice based on the manufacturer and type of device (Gelblum & Amols, 2009).
- Do not treat with betatron (Marbach et al., 1994; Solan et al., 2004).
- Interrogate device before and after initial fraction and again with some frequency as determined with the electrophysiologist (Gelblum & Amols, 2009). If the estimated dose to the pacemaker might exceed 2 Gy, possibly check the device at the start of each week of therapy (Marbach et al., 1994).
- Estimate the cumulative ionizing radiation dose to the generator from the proposed treatment, and move the generator for doses estimated to be greater than 2 Gy for pacemakers and greater than 1 Gy for ICDs (Solan et al., 2004).
- Measure the dose at first treatment and compare with pretreatment estimate to keep within dose limits (Hudson et al., 2010; Solan et al., 2004).
- Patient should be observed on a monitor during all treatments (Solan et al., 2004). The treating physician should observe the patient during initial portal filming and first treatment. All patients should have pulse and blood pressure measurements before and after each treatment. Pacemaker-dependent patients should have continuous ECG monitoring (Hudson et al., 2010) during the first treatment and a weekly pacemaker/ICD check by the cardiologist (Solan et al., 2004). Monitoring should be performed by trained personnel who can respond to any arrhythmic event (Hudson et al., 2010). Monitoring of patients with an ICD should begin when therapy is disabled and continue until therapy is enabled after the treatment session (Hudson et al., 2010).
- The cardiologist may advise using a magnet to deactivate the ICD during treatment (Solan et al., 2004).
- Device checks are advised after each session, at least weekly (Hudson et al., 2010).
- After completion of radiation therapy, the cardiologist should complete a full interrogation of the pacemaker or ICD (Solan et al., 2004).
- If photon beam energy exceeds 10 mV, it may be necessary to evaluate the device after each treatment (Crossley et al., 2011). Electrical reset has not been reported with electron beam therapy (Crossley et al., 2011).

Table 13-1 will be a useful reference for oncology nurses to use when caring for patients with a CIED undergoing radiation therapy.

Conclusion

Oncology nurses play a preventive as well as a treatment role in patients with ventricular dysrhythmias and a CIED. Familiarity with these issues will guide nurses in anticipating care plans for individualized care. Oncology nurses can anticipate problems with these patients and intervene sooner rather than later to avoid any unfortunate incidents.

Table 13-1. Recommendations by Device Companies in Relation to Therapeutic Radiation

Concern/ Recommendations	Medtronic	Boston Scientific	St. Jude Medical
Precautions with pacemakers (PMs)	If inhibition occurs and patient can tolerate: Program asynchronous pacing or place magnet over PM.	If inhibition occurs, consider programming asynchronous pacing or placing magnet over device.	If inhibition occurs, consider programming device to asynchronous pacing or placing magnet over device. For rate-adaptive devices, if the sensor is ON, radiation may cause the device to pace up to the maximum sensor rate. May be programmed to Passage or OFF.
	Remove magnet or program device to original setting after each radiation treatment.		
Precautions with implantable cardioverter defibrillators (ICDs)	Suspend tachyarrhythmia detection by placing magnet over device, or disable through programmer.	Deactivate tachytherapy by placing magnet over device, or disable through programmer.	Deactivate tachyarrhythmia detection by placing magnet over device, or disable through programmer.
	Remove magnet or program device to original setting after each radiation treatment.		
Shielding/precaution to reduce scatter	Conventional x-ray shielding during radiation therapy does not protect the device from the effects of the neutrons.	Emphasize maximum shielding—both internal shielding on the radiation equipment and external shielding for the patient. Also include beam focus, energy level selection, and treatment field design.	Coning the radiation field to avoid the pacer region helps to reduce overall received dosage.
Moving device location	Move device to alternate location if it is not possible to avoid the device with the radiation beam.	Consider moving the device to a different location if the beam is aimed at the implanted device.	If ionizing radiation is required in the vicinity of the implanted device, may be necessary to move the device to another location.

(Continued on next page)

Table 13-1. Recommendations by Device Companies in Relation to Therapeutic Radiation *(Continued)*

Concern/ Recommendations	Medtronic	Boston Scientific	St. Jude Medical
Accumulated dose of radiation	Consider accumulated dose to the device from previous exposures for patients undergoing multiple courses of radiation treatment. Average dose rates at the device of less than 1 cGy/min (centigray per minute) are unlikely to produce device interference. Increasing the distance between the device and the beam decreases the risk of interference.	Accumulated effects of radiation in sufficient doses can permanently degrade performance below device specifications. Device exposure to radiation more often than once a day increases the likelihood that the device will revert to safety mode or cause permanent damage.	Damage can occur to device circuits with cumulative doses of radiation. Risk of effects on device operation increases with increasing cumulative radiation exposure.
Radiation thresholds for PMs	Device tolerance for PM is 500 cGy. Minor radiation damage at accumulated dosages over 500 cGy. If dose is greater than 500 cGy, device should be monitored after each treatment and considered for replacement.	No single dose limit can be specified due to variations. Manufacturer refers to study recommending maximum total dose of 2 Gy.	No exact threshold for damage has been determined. Permanent damage is rare.
Radiation thresholds for ICD	Dose limits: • 100 cGy: AT500, GEM, InSync, Jewel, Micro Jewel, Onyx • 300 cGy: Concerto, Virtuoso • 500 cGy: Concerto II, Consulta, Entrust, InSync Marquis, InSync Maximo, InSync II Protect, InSync Sentry, Intrinsic, Marquis, Maximo, Secura, Virtuoso II	No single dose limit can be specified due to variations.	No exact threshold for damage has been determined. Permanent damage is rare.

(Continued on next page)

Table 13-1. Recommendations by Device Companies in Relation to Therapeutic Radiation *(Continued)*

Concern/ Recommendations	Medtronic	Boston Scientific	St. Jude Medical
Effects	Damage to a device may not be immediately apparent. Device reset may be delayed for several days due to memory errors. Electron beams that do not produce neutrons do not cause electrical reset. Pacing leads or extenders will not be damaged by radiation.	Effects of radiation exposure on implanted devices may remain undetected until some time following exposure. Malfunction caused by radiation may not be discovered until a device feature is activated several months later.	Interactions or failure from exposure to radiation therapy is random.
Monitoring	Device marker channels can be monitored for interference during the initial therapy. If no interference in the marker channel, it is unlikely to occur with future treatments as long as no change in therapy.	Cardiologist or electrophysiologist will determine the extent, timing, and frequency of evaluations. For example, pacemaker-dependent patients may require continuous cardiac monitoring during every therapy session.	Electrocardiogram (ECG) monitoring is advisable during therapeutic radiation treatment. During the initial sessions, the clinician can determine if there is any interaction between the device and radiation equipment and can then decide if subsequent ECG monitoring during each therapy session is necessary. If device-related symptoms occur during radiation therapy, the pacemaker or ICD should be interrogated. Monitor and record the cumulative radiation dosage to which the device has been exposed. Pacemaker-dependent patients should have a detailed evaluation of the pacing system once or twice during the course of treatment. A change in capture or sensing threshold may reflect an early problem with the pacing system.

(Continued on next page)

Table 13-1. Recommendations by Device Companies in Relation to Therapeutic Radiation *(Continued)*

Concern/ Recommendations	Medtronic	Boston Scientific	St. Jude Medical
Evaluation for a reset	Use a magnet to check whether an electrical reset has occurred. ICD: Place magnet over device and listen for patient alert tone. If no tone or steady tone, no reset has occurred. If high or low tone, then an electrical reset occurred and the device must be checked. PM: Place magnet over device; pacing at rate of 65 bpm indicates that a reset has occurred.	–	–
Follow-up	Device evaluation is recommended when all therapies are complete.	Evaluation of device function should take place following radiation treatment. Continue to monitor device closely weeks or months following radiation therapy.	Detailed evaluation of device should take place following completion of the course of therapeutic radiation. For patients with an ICD, induction testing should be considered to evaluate the high-voltage functions of the device.

Note. Based on information from Boston Scientific Corp., 2008; Medtronic, Inc., 2008; St. Jude Medical, 2011.

References

Arai, Y., Tadokoro, J., & Mitani, K. (2005). Ventricular tachycardia associated with infusion of rituximab in mantle cell lymphoma. *American Journal of Hematology, 78*, 317–318. doi:10.1002/ajh.20303

AVID Investigators. (1995). Antiarrhythmics versus implantable defibrillators (AVID)—Rationale, design, and methods. *American Journal of Cardiology, 75*, 470–475.

Badhwar, N., & Lee, B.K. (2008). Cardiac resynchronization therapy for congestive heart failure. In F.M. Kusumoto & N.F. Goldschlager (Eds.), *Cardiac pacing for the clinician* (2nd ed., pp. 429–452). New York, NY: Springer Science + Business Medical, LLC.

Ballanti, S., Mastrodicasa, E., Bolli, N., Lotti, F., Capolsini, I., Berchicci, L., … Tabilio, A. (2007). Sustained ventricular tachycardia in a thalidomide-treated patient with primary plasma-cell leukemia. *Nature Clinical Practice Oncology, 4*, 722–725. doi:10.1038/ncponc1008

Boston Scientific Corp. (2008). *Electrocautery and implantable device systems.* Natick, MA: Author.

Bourassa, M.G., Khairy, P., & Roy, D. (2011). An early proof-of-concept of cardiac resynchronization therapy. *World Journal of Cardiology, 3*, 374–376. doi:10.4330/wjc.v3.i12.374

Chiu-Man, C.H., Nygren, A., & De Souza, L. (2011). Pacemaker timing cycles, programming, and troubleshooting. In A. Tsiperfal, L.K. Ottoboni, S. Beheiry, A. Al-Ahmad, A. Natale, & P. Wang

(Eds.), *Cardiac arrhythmia management: A practical guide for nurses and allied professionals* (pp. 181–230). Chichester, West Sussex, UK: Wiley-Blackwell.

Cohan, L., Kusumoto, F., & Goldschlager, N.F. (2008). Environmental effects on cardiac pacing systems. In F.M. Kusumoto & N.F. Goldschlager (Eds.), *Cardiac pacing for the clinician* (2nd ed., pp. 595–618). New York, NY: Springer Science + Business Medical, LLC.

Craig, K.J., & Day, M.P. (2011). Are you up to date on the latest BLS and ACLS guidelines? *Nursing, 41*(5), 40–44.

Crossley, G.H., Poole, J.E., Rozner, M.A., Asirvatham, S.J., Cheng, A., Chung, M.K., ... Thompson, A. (2011). The Heart Rhythm Society (HRS)/American Society of Anesthesiologists (ASA) expert consensus statement on the perioperative management of patients with implantable defibrillators, pacemakers and arrhythmia monitors: Facilities and patient management. *Heart Rhythm, 8,* 1114–1154. doi:10.1016/j.hrthm.2010.12.023

Cubeddu, L.X. (2003). QT prolongation and fatal arrhythmias: A review of clinical implications and effects of drugs. *American Journal of Therapeutics, 10,* 452–457.

Ferguson, C., Clarke, J., & Herity, N.A. (2006). Ventricular tachycardia associated with trastuzumab. *New England Journal of Medicine, 354,* 648–649. doi:10.1056/NEJMc052708

Gelblum, D.Y., & Amols, H. (2009). Implanted cardiac defibrillator care in radiation oncology patient population. *International Journal of Radiation Oncology, Biology, Physics, 73,* 1525–1531. doi:10.1016/j.ijrobp.2008.06.1903

Gualis, J., Castaño, M., Gómez-Plana, J., Martin, C., & Alonso, D. (2010). Surgical treatment of giant intramural left ventricular fibroma in an adult patient with refractory ventricular tachycardia. *Journal of Cardiac Surgery, 25,* 656–658. doi:10.1111/j.1540-8191.2010.01105.x

Hongo, R.H., & Goldschlager, N.F. (2008). Cardiac pacing in the critical care setting. In F.M. Kusumoto & N.F. Goldschlager (Eds.), *Cardiac pacing for the clinician* (2nd ed., pp. 565–592). New York, NY: Springer Science + Business Medical, LLC.

Hudson, F., Coulshed, D., D'Souza, E., & Baker, C. (2010). Effect of radiation therapy on the latest generation of pacemakers and implantable cardioverter defibrillators: A systematic review. *Journal of Medical Imaging and Radiation Oncology, 54,* 53–61. doi:10.1111/j.1754-9485.2010.02138.x

Kuittinen, T., Jantunen, E., Vanninen, E., Mussalo, H., Nousiainen, T., & Hartikainen, J. (2010). Late potentials and QT dispersion after high-dose chemotherapy in patients with non-Hodgkin lymphoma. *Clinical Physiology and Functional Imaging, 30,* 175–180. doi:10.1111/j.1475-097X.2009.00920.x

Marbach, J.R., Sontag, M.R., Van Dyk, J., & Wolbarst, A.B. (1994). Management of radiation oncology patients with implanted cardiac pacemakers: Report of AAPM Task Group No. 34. American Association of Physicists in Medicine. *Medical Physics, 21,* 85–90. doi:10.1118/1.597259

Medtronic, Inc. (2008). CorePace: Single and dual chamber pacemaker timing. Retrieved from http://connect.medtronic.com

Morganti, K., & Hongo, R. (2011). Ventricular tachycardia in structurally normal hearts. In A. Tsiperfal, L.K. Ottoboni, S. Beheiry, A. Al-Ahmad, A. Natale, & P. Wang (Eds.), *Cardiac arrhythmia management: A practical guide for nurses and allied professionals* (pp. 127–138). Chichester, West Sussex, UK: Wiley-Blackwell.

Moss, A.J. (2003). MADIT-I and MADIT-II. *Journal of Cardiovascular Electrophysiology, 14*(Suppl. 9), S96–S98. doi:10.1046/j.1540-8167.14.s9.5.x

Olgin, J., & Zipes, D.P. (2012). Specific arrhythmias: Diagnosis and treatment. In R.O. Bonow, D.L. Mann, D.P. Zipes, & P. Libby (Eds.), *Braunwald's heart disease: A textbook of cardiovascular medicine* (9th ed., pp. 771–823). St. Louis, MO: Elsevier Saunders.

Reiffel, J.A. (2005). Drug and drug-device therapy in heart failure patients in the post-COMET and SCD-HeFT era. *Journal of Cardiovascular Pharmacology and Therapeutics, 10*(Suppl. 1), S45–S58. doi:10.1177/10742484050100i406

Rho, R.W., & Page, R.L. (2008). Ventricular arrhythmias. In V. Fuster, R.A. O'Rourke, R. Walsh, & P. Poole-Wilson (Eds.), *Hurst's the heart* (12th ed., pp. 1003–1019). New York, NY: McGraw-Hill Medical.

Roger, V.L., Go, A.S., Lloyd-Jones, D.M., Adams, R.J., Berry, J.D., Brown, T.M., ... Wylie-Rosett, J. (2011). Heart disease and stroke statistics—2011 update: A report from the American Heart Association. *Circulation, 123*(4), e18–e209. doi:10.1161/CIR.0b013e3182009701

Rudzinski, T., Ciesielczyk, M., Religa, W., Bednarkiewicz, Z., & Krzeminska-Pakula, M. (2007). Doxorubicin-induced ventricular arrhythmia treated by implantation of an automatic cardioverter-defibrillator. *Europace, 9,* 278–280. doi:10.1093/europace/eum033

Solan, A.N., Solan, M.J., Bednarz, G., & Goodkin, M.B. (2004). Treatment of patients with cardiac pacemakers and implantable cardioverter-defibrillators during radiotherapy. *International Journal of Radiation Oncology, Biology, Physics, 59,* 897–904. doi:10.1016/j.ijrobp.2004.02.038

St. Jude Medical. (2008). *Effects of electrocautery on St. Jude Medical implantable cardiac pacemakers.* Sylmar, CA: St. Jude Medical Technical Services.

St. Jude Medical. (2011). *Effects of electrocautery on St. Jude Medical implantable cardioverter defibrillators.* Sylmar, CA: St. Jude Medical Technical Services.

Stewart, T., Pavlakis, N., & Ward, M. (2010). Cardiotoxicity with 5-fluorouracil and capecitabine: More than just vasospastic angina. *Internal Medicine Journal, 40,* 303–307. doi:10.1111/j.1445-5994.2009.02144.x

Swerdlow, C.D., Hayes, D.L., & Zipes, D.P. (2012). Pacemakers and implantable cardioverter defibrillators. In In R. Bonow, D. Mann, D. Zipes, & P. Libby (Eds.), *Braunwald's heart disease: A textbook of cardiovascular medicine* (9th ed., pp. 745–764). St. Louis, MO: Saunders.

Tsiperfal, A., Ottoboni, L.K., Beheiry, S., Al-Ahmad, A., Natale, A., & Wang, P. (Eds.). (2011). *Cardiac arrhythmia management: A practical guide for nurses and allied professionals.* Chichester, West Sussex, UK: Wiley-Blackwell.

Vijayaraman, P., & Ellenbogen, K.A. (2008). Bradyarrhythmias and pacemakers. In V. Fuster, R.A. O'Rourke, R. Walsh, & P. Poole-Wilson (Eds.), *Hurst's the heart* (12th ed., pp. 1020–1054). New York, NY: McGraw-Hill Medical.

Yilmaz, U., Oztop, I., Ciloglu, A., Okan, T., Tekin, U., Yaren, A., ... Kirimli, O. (2007). 5-fluorouracil increases the number and complexity of premature complexes in the heart: A prospective study using ambulatory ECG monitoring. *International Journal of Clinical Practice, 61,* 795. doi:10.1111/j.1742-1241.2007.01323.x

Cardiovascular Evaluation of Patients With Cancer Prior to Chemotherapy and Surgery

Sue Buzzurro, RN, MS, FNP-BC

Introduction

Patients with cancer who are undergoing chemotherapy and cancer surgery have an increased risk of developing cardiovascular complications, and the risk is higher with a known history of cardiac disease. Besides malignant neoplastic diseases, patients often have pathologic processes affecting the cardiovascular system. Chemotherapeutic agents, radiation therapy, and molecular targeted therapies are all approaches that can injure the cardiovascular system through their effects on the heart function as well as in the periphery (Albini et al., 2009). These agents often interfere with blood flow and hemodynamic pressures and cause thrombotic events, which are increased in patients with cancer because of a hypercoagulable state. The prechemotherapy evaluation and preoperative management of patients with cancer can be complex. Although patients with cancer are similar in many ways to those without cancer, the direct and indirect (systemic) effects of the cancer and the side effects of cancer therapy can influence preoperative evaluation and management. This chapter will discuss the importance of cardiovascular evaluation of patients with cancer prior to chemotherapy and surgery, cardiac risk factors, indications for diagnostic testing, and preoperative management of anticoagulation.

Epidemiology

The prevalence of cardiovascular disease increases with age, and the number of people older than 65 years in the United States is estimated to increase 25%–35% over the next 30 years (American College of Cardiology [ACC] Foundation & American Heart Association [AHA], 2009). This will be the same age group who will undergo the largest number of surgical procedures. Thus, the number of noncardiac surgical procedures performed in older adults will increase from the current 6 million to nearly 12 million per year; these procedures have been associated with significant perioperative cardiovascular morbidity and mortality (Fleisher et al., 2007).

Prechemotherapy Evaluation

Cardiovascular assessment and early identification of patients who are at risk for cardiotoxicity should be a primary goal of oncologists prior to administration of chemotherapy. Prechemotherapy cardiac assessment will allow modification or selection of alternative antineoplastic therapeutic strategies for patients who are identified as being at high cardiac risk, who might then be treated with either a different or less-cardiotoxic agent. Some of the common risk factors are hypertension, arrhythmias, pericardial disease, thromboembolism, and previous exposure to chemotherapy and radiation (Hong, Iimura, Sumida, & Eager, 2010). The development of combination, adjuvant, and targeted chemotherapies has resulted in increased cardiac side effects and toxicity (Monsuez, Charniot, Vignat, & Artigou, 2010). Drugs such as anthracyclines, which are potent antineoplastic drugs used in the treatment of solid and hematologic cancers, are associated with slow progressive deterioration of cardiac function for years after treatment cessation (Elliott, 2006). The cardiovascular effects of the most commonly used chemotherapeutic agents are outlined in Table 14-1.

Preoperative Cardiac Evaluation for Noncardiac Surgery

Cardiovascular complications are the major cause of perioperative morbidity and mortality related to the presence of an underlying coronary artery disease. Patients undergoing noncardiac surgery are potentially at risk for major perioperative cardiac events (cardiac death, nonfatal myocardial infarction [MI], and nonfatal cardiac arrest). Surgery, with its associated trauma, anesthesia and analgesia, intubation and extubation, pain, hypothermia, bleeding, anemia, and fasting, is analogous to an extreme stress test. These factors tend to initiate inflammatory, hypercoagulable, stress, and hypoxic states, which are associated with perioperative elevations in troponin levels, arterial thrombosis, and mortality (Mahla et al., 2000). Patients who experience MI after noncardiac surgery have a hospital mortality rate of 15%–25% (Kumar et al., 2001). On the contrary, patients who have a cardiac arrest after noncardiac surgery have a hospital mortality rate of 65% (Sprung et al., 2003).

Preoperative risk assessment is an important step in reducing perioperative morbidity and mortality in patients undergoing noncardiac surgery. The purpose of preoperative cardiovascular evaluation is not to give cardiac clearance or to "clear" patients for the proposed surgical procedures, but rather to perform an evaluation of the patient's current cardiac status; make recommendations concerning the evaluation and findings and management, and identify the potential risk of cardiac problems that could arise over the entire perioperative period; and provide a clinical risk profile that the patient, primary physician, anesthesiologist, and surgeon can use in making treatment decisions. The primary goal of preoperative evaluation is to reduce perioperative morbidity and

Table 14-1. Cardiovascular Toxicity of Chemotherapeutic Agents	
Cardiotoxic Effects	**Chemotherapeutic Agents**
Congestive heart failure	Anthracyclines/anthraquinones Cyclophosphamide Trastuzumab and other monoclonal antibody–based tyrosine kinase inhibitors
Myocardial ischemia or thromboembolism	Antimetabolites (5-fluorouracil, capecitabine) Antimicrotubule agents (paclitaxel, docetaxel) Cisplatin Thalidomide
Hypertension	Bevacizumab Cisplatin Sunitinib, sorafenib
Cardiac tamponade and endomyocardial fibrosis	Busulfan
Hemorrhagic myocarditis (rare)	Cyclophosphamide (high-dose therapy)
Bradyrhythmias	Paclitaxel
Autonomic neuropathy	Vincristine
QT prolongation or torsades de pointes	Arsenic trioxide

Note. From "Cardiotoxicity of Chemotherapeutic Agents and Radiotherapy-Related Heart Disease: ESMO Clinical Practice Guidelines," by D. Bovelli, G. Plataniotis, and F. Riola, 2010, *Annals of Oncology, 21*(Suppl. 5), p. v278. doi:10.1093/annonc/mdq200. Copyright 2010 by the authors. Adapted with permission.

mortality. Major cardiac complications associated with surgery include MI, congestive heart failure (CHF), and arrhythmias (McCallion & Krenis, 1992).

The initial step in any preoperative evaluation is a thorough history and physical examination. The history and physical examination should focus on identifying any cardiac pathology and establishing severity and stability of the disease, as well as prior treatments. The extent to which cardiac evaluation should be performed on a patient undergoing surgery depends on risk factors as outlined by Cagirici, Nalbantgil, Cakan, and Turhan, 2005 (see Table 14-2).

The ACC/AHA 2007 perioperative guidelines specify four active cardiac conditions: (a) unstable coronary syndromes, (b) decompensated heart failure (New York Heart Association functional class IV; worsening or new-onset heart failure), (c) significant arrhythmias, and (d) severe valvular disease, for which an evaluation and treatment are required before noncardiac surgery (Fleisher et al., 2007) as outlined in Table 14-3.

Estimation of Cardiac Risk Prior to Noncardiac Surgery

The risk of perioperative complications depends on the condition of the patient prior to surgery, the prevalence of comorbidities, and the magnitude and duration of the surgical procedure (Poldermans, Hoeks, & Feringa, 2008). Several well-known indices of cardiac risk are routinely used when assessing a preoperative patient. Goldman et al.

(1977) developed the first preoperative cardiac risk index by looking at nine variables that increase the risk of perioperative cardiac complications: third heart sound or jugular venous distention; MI in the preceding six months; more than five premature ventricular contractions per minute documented at any time before surgery; rhythm other than sinus or presence of premature atrial contractions on electrocardiogram; age older than 70; intraperitoneal, intrathoracic, or aortic operation; emergency operation; valvular aortic stenosis; and poor general medical condition. In the preoperative assessment, each factor is added, and the greater the sum, the greater the risk of life-threatening cardiac events (MI, pulmonary edema, and ventricular tachycardia) or cardiac death.

Since 1977, multiple cardiac risk indices have been developed, as well as guidelines for preoperative cardiac evaluation. Detsky et al. (1986) modified the original Goldman criteria by adding unstable angina and pulmonary edema to the variables. A point scale is assigned to each variable; the points are then added to determine the patient's "class" and cardiac risk.

In 1996, ACC and AHA developed a guideline for preoperative cardiovascular evaluation for noncardiac surgery that incorporated clinical predictors and functional status into the risk assessment algorithm (Eagle et al., 1996). The guideline was updated in early 2002 with an emphasis on optimizing the assessment of cardiac risk without subjecting the patient to unnecessary intervention that would otherwise not be indicated (Eagle et al., 2002). Patients are stratified according to major, intermediate, or minor "clinical predictors" of increased cardiac risk. Patients who have had coronary revascularization within five years or a favorable result on coronary angiography or cardiac stress testing within two years may proceed to surgery without further cardiac evaluation.

Despite the availability of multiple cardiac risk indices, no particular ideal method exists for assessing cardiac risks before surgery. Cardiologists are commonly asked about the exact percentage of cardiac risk for a certain patient undergoing a surgical procedure. The answer is complex and almost impossible to be given, mainly considering only the currently available cardiac risk indices. One should always remember that the purpose of the preoperative assessment is not to provide medical authorization for surgery or to provide percentages of risk. The preoperative assessment aims to analyze the patient's current physical status, provide recommendations, and establish a clinical

---

Table 14-2. Cardiac Risk Factors That May Determine Postoperative Outcome

Risk Factor	Definition
Smoking	Current tobacco use
Hypertension	Blood pressure ≥ 140/90 mm Hg
Hyperlipidemia	≥ 240 mg/dl total serum cholesterol or ≥ 150 mg/dl serum triglyceride
Advanced age	≥ 70 years
Diabetes mellitus	≥ 120 mg/dl serum glucose level
History of cardiac disease	Coronary artery or heart valve disease, congestive heart failure, or exertional chest pain

Note. From "A New Algorithm for Preoperative Cardiac Assessment in Patients Undergoing Pulmonary Resection," by U. Cagirici, S. Nalbantgil, A. Cakan, and K. Turhan, 2005, *Texas Heart Institute Journal, 32,* p. 160. Copyright 2005 by Texas Heart Institute, Houston. Adapted with permission.

Table 14-3. Active Cardiac Conditions for Which Patients Should Undergo Evaluation and Treatment Before Noncardiac Surgery

Condition	Examples
Unstable coronary syndromes	Unstable or severe angina (CCS class III or IV) Recent MI
Decompensated HF (NYHA functional class IV; worsening or new-onset HF)	–
Significant arrhythmias	High-grade atrioventricular block Mobitz II atrioventricular block Third-degree atrioventricular heart block Symptomatic ventricular arrhythmias Supraventricular arrhythmias (including atrial fibrillation) with uncontrolled ventricular rate (HR greater than 100 bpm at rest) Symptomatic bradycardia Newly recognized ventricular tachycardia
Severe valvular disease	Severe aortic stenosis (mean pressure gradient greater than 40 mm Hg, aortic valve area less than 1.0 cm², or symptomatic) Symptomatic mitral stenosis (progressive dyspnea on exertion, exertional presyncope, or HF)

bpm—beats per minute; CCS—Canadian Cardiovascular Society; HF—heart failure; HR—heart rate; MI—myocardial infarction; NYHA—New York Heart Association

Note. From "ACC/AHA 2007 Guidelines on Perioperative Cardiovascular Evaluation and Care for Noncardiac Surgery: Executive Summary," by L.A. Fleisher, J.A. Beckman, K.A. Brown, H. Calkins, E.L. Chaikof, K.E. Fleischmann, ... C.W. Yancy, 2007, *Journal of the American College of Cardiology, 50,* p. 1714. doi:10.1016/j.jacc.2007.09.001. Copyright 2007 by the American College of Cardiology Foundation and the American Heart Association, Inc. Reprinted with permission.

---

profile of the cardiac risk that will assist the patient, clinician, surgeon, and anesthesiologist to better decide upon therapeutic management (Eagle et al., 1996).

In 2007, the ACC/AHA guidelines recommended a stepwise approach to perioperative cardiac assessment and evaluation. Based on clinical findings, further cardiac testing may be recommended or surgery may be delayed in high-risk patients (see Figure 14-1).

Preoperative Diagnostic Modalities

Patients with significant cardiac risk factors scheduled to undergo noncardiac surgery or receive chemotherapy and who are considered to be at high risk for developing cardiac complications should undergo pretreatment cardiac assessment. Several noninvasive diagnostic tests such as electrocardiography (ECG), echocardiography, multigated acquisition (MUGA) scan scintigraphy, and cardiac magnetic resonance imaging (MRI) may be used for baseline cardiac assessment.

Electrocardiography

ECG is a convenient and inexpensive method to screen for conduction disturbances and signs of cardiomyopathy. Several chemotherapeutics can induce cardiac problems that might lead to changes in an ECG, such as repolarization abnormalities and prolongation of the corrected QT interval. Cardiomyopathy may be manifested by low QRS

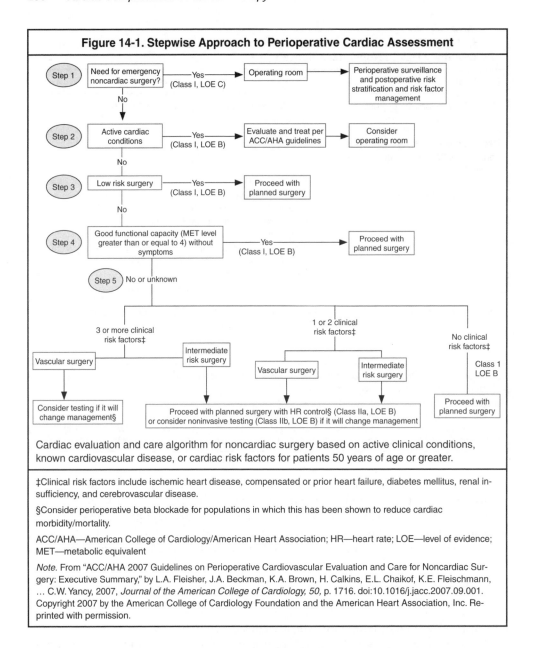

Figure 14-1. Stepwise Approach to Perioperative Cardiac Assessment

Cardiac evaluation and care algorithm for noncardiac surgery based on active clinical conditions, known cardiovascular disease, or cardiac risk factors for patients 50 years of age or greater.

‡Clinical risk factors include ischemic heart disease, compensated or prior heart failure, diabetes mellitus, renal insufficiency, and cerebrovascular disease.

§Consider perioperative beta blockade for populations in which this has been shown to reduce cardiac morbidity/mortality.

ACC/AHA—American College of Cardiology/American Heart Association; HR—heart rate; LOE—level of evidence; MET—metabolic equivalent

Note. From "ACC/AHA 2007 Guidelines on Perioperative Cardiovascular Evaluation and Care for Noncardiac Surgery: Executive Summary," by L.A. Fleisher, J.A. Beckman, K.A. Brown, H. Calkins, E.L. Chaikof, K.E. Fleischmann, ... C.W. Yancy, 2007, *Journal of the American College of Cardiology, 50,* p. 1716. doi:10.1016/j.jacc.2007.09.001. Copyright 2007 by the American College of Cardiology Foundation and the American Heart Association, Inc. Reprinted with permission.

voltages on an ECG (Jannazzo, Hoffman, & Lutz, 2008). The advantages of ECG are easy availability with no side effects. The disadvantages of using ECG for monitoring chemotherapy-induced cardiotoxicity include (a) information on left ventricular function is lacking, (b) the timing of ECG changes during development of cardiotoxicity is unknown, and (c) ECG changes may also indicate adverse effects of other medication such as digoxin.

Echocardiography

Echocardiogram is the most frequently used diagnostic modality and is an effective approach to monitor cardiac function and its impairment by chemotherapy. The procedure allows assessment of systolic and diastolic cardiac function. Diastolic measurements are the most sensitive to early changes in cardiac function (Altena, Perik, van Veldhuisen, de Vries, & Gietema, 2009). Left ventricular ejection fraction (LVEF) is one of the most important predictors of cardiac function, and patients with substantially reduced ejection fractions typically have poorer prognoses (Albini et al., 2009).

Echocardiography has advantages and disadvantages. The procedure is noninvasive, with no undue side effects, and both the systolic and diastolic function can be measured, including tissue velocity imaging and strain and strain rate, which allows for early detection of subclinical changes. The disadvantage is the preload dependence of ventricular filling and right atrial pressure and dependence on the expertise and interpretation of echocardiographer.

Multigated Acquisition Scan

This is the gold standard for assessing LVEF. MUGA scan is the most widely accepted method to assess patients' LVEF during cancer treatment (Jannazzo et al., 2008). No guidelines are currently available that specify which is preferred. Although MUGA scan is a reliable and widely used method for assessment of LVEF, it is insensitive for detecting subtle changes in cardiac function. Therefore, it has limited value for early detection of cardiotoxicity. MUGA scan has the advantage of the reliability in calculation of LVEF with low intraindividual and interobserver variation. However, the test provides limited information on diastolic function, and patients are exposed to radiation with the procedure.

Magnetic Resonance Imaging

This diagnostic modality is a reliable and reproducible method to assess cardiac structural features, including the coronary arteries and pericardium, and enables consistent calculation of LVEF. MRI combined with late gadolinium contrast enhancement can detect subtle areas of irreversibly damaged myocardium (Bandettini & Arai, 2008). The advantages of cardiac MRI are that it provides detailed information of anatomy with high resolution and contrast, it does not expose the patient to radiation, the calculation of LVEF is reliable, and the combination with late gadolinium enhancement provides detailed information on myocardial function. The disadvantages are its availability, cost, and contraindication in patients with metal implants.

Preoperative Management of Anticoagulation

Anticoagulant therapy that includes aspirin, clopidogrel (Plavix®), warfarin (Coumadin®), or dabigatran (Pradaxa®) is associated with increased bleeding during noncardiac surgery. In some patients, the risk is outweighed by the benefit of anticoagulant therapy and the drug therapy should be maintained or modified. Conversely, in patients with low risk of thrombosis, therapy should be stopped to minimize bleeding complications.

Aspirin

Aspirin irreversibly inhibits platelet cyclooxygenase, which may increase intraoperative blood loss and hemorrhagic complications (Connelly & Panush, 1991). However, the same effect can help to prevent perioperative cardiovascular complications. The optimal perioperative management of patients who are taking aspirin is uncertain, and significant practice variation exists. The decision to continue or withhold aspirin should reflect a balance of the consequences of perioperative hemorrhage versus the risk of perioperative vascular complications. Patients who are at high risk for perioperative vascular complications and in whom perioperative hemorrhage would result in minimal morbidity should continue aspirin. This includes patients on maintenance aspirin therapy who have coronary stents or who are undergoing coronary artery bypass graft or peripheral arterial surgery (Dacey et al., 2000). Aspirin should be withheld prior to surgical procedures in which perioperative hemorrhage could be catastrophic (e.g., central nervous system surgery) or impact surgical outcome. If the decision is made to stop aspirin, 7–10 days should elapse before surgery is undertaken (Douketis et al., 2008). The 2008 American College of Chest Physicians (ACCP) guidelines on antithrombotic therapy recommended resuming aspirin approximately 24 hours (or the next morning) after surgery when there is adequate hemostasis (Douketis et al., 2008).

Clopidogrel

Antiplatelet therapy is mandatory for patients after coronary artery stent placement, as platelets play a major role in thrombus formation after coronary artery stenting. Coronary artery stents are associated with a very high risk of thrombosis (Van Brabandt, 2007). Clopidogrel combined with aspirin is the commonly prescribed regimen. The loading dose of clopidogrel is 300 mg, followed by 75 mg daily, and the recommended duration of anticoagulation varies depending on the type of stent—bare metal or drug-eluting. See Chapter 5 for the recommended duration of anticoagulation for the different types of stents.

If clopidogrel has to be discontinued, "bridge" the patient to surgery by using a short-acting antiplatelet agent with a glycoprotein IIb/IIIa inhibitor or an antithrombin, and restart clopidogrel as soon as possible after surgery in collaboration with the surgeon.

Warfarin

The management of patients treated with warfarin who require interruption of anticoagulation for surgery or other invasive procedures can be problematic. Once warfarin is held, it takes several days for the international normalized ratio (INR) to fall below 2.0, when it is considered safe for surgical procedure. Following surgery and after warfarin is restarted, it takes about three to four days for the INR to rise above 2.0. It is therefore estimated that if warfarin is withheld for four days before surgery and is restarted as soon as possible afterward, patients would have a subtherapeutic INR for approximately two days before and two days after surgery (Kearon & Hirsh, 1997). In patients with an INR between 2.0 and 3.0 who are undergoing elective surgery that requires temporary cessation of anticoagulation, warfarin should be withheld for approximately three to four days to allow the INR to fall to 1.5–2.0 before surgery (White, McKittrick, Hutchinson, & Twitchell, 1995). Warfarin should be withheld for approximately five days if the surgeon feels it is necessary to reduce the INR to a lower or normal level in order to reduce the risk of bleeding (e.g., less than 1.5).

The risk of a short period of under-anticoagulation is uncertain, especially because randomized studies have not been conducted of heparin versus placebo bridging among warfarin-treated patients who need procedures. Because of the lack of evidence-based information indicating those patients in whom bridging anticoagulation is or is not warranted, considerable variation exists in the use of this modality (Jaffer et al., 2010) (see Table 14-4).

Dabigatran

Dabigatran is an orally active direct thrombin inhibitor that has been used for the prevention and treatment of venous and arterial thromboembolic disorders (e.g., prevention of venous thromboembolism after total knee or total hip arthroplasty, treatment of acute venous thromboembolism, prevention of stroke in atrial fibrillation) (Eriksson et al., 2007). The manufacturer recommends stopping dabigatran one to two days before elective surgery for patients who have normal renal function and a low risk of bleeding and three to five days before surgery for patients who have a creatinine clearance of 50 ml/min or less. Before major surgery or placement of a spinal or epidural catheter, the manufacturer (Boehringer Ingelheim Pharmaceuticals, 2012) recommends that dabigatran be held even longer.

Anticoagulation in Special Situations

Atrial Fibrillation

Patients with atrial fibrillation have an increased risk of stroke and thromboembolic complications, a risk that is substantially reduced with anticoagulation therapy. It may be necessary to discontinue anticoagulation a few to several days before surgery. Bridging anticoagulation with either low-molecular-weight or unfractionated heparin may be indicated depending on the thromboembolic risk assessment. The annual stroke risk

Table 14-4. Recommendations for Bridge Therapy Protocol Based on Expert Opinion

Day	Recommendations
–7	Stop aspirin therapy and check international normalized ratio (INR).
–5 or –4	Stop warfarin therapy and check INR.
–3 or –2	Start low-molecular-weight heparin (LMWH) once or twice daily.
–1	Last dose of LMWH 12–24 hours before procedure. Check INR; if 1.5 or higher, give vitamin K (1 mg orally).
0 (day of surgery)	No LMWH. Assess hemostasis. Start regular warfarin dosage in evening.
1	Continue regular warfarin dosage. Restart LMWH therapeutic dosage (procedures with low risk of bleeding and/or patients or procedures with high risk of thrombosis) or LMWH prophylactic dosage (procedures with high risk of bleeding)
2	Check INR.
4 to 10	Check INR. Stop LMWH when INR is 2.0 or higher.

Note. Based on information from Jafri, 2004.

for each patient can be estimated based on the presence of risk factors (CHF, hypertension, age, diabetes mellitus, and history of stroke or transient ischemic attack). The stroke risk can be assessed using the validated $CHADS_2$ scoring system as shown in Figure 14-2 (Snow et al., 2003). Patients who have a $CHADS_2$ score of 3 or higher should receive bridge therapy, whereas in those with a $CHADS_2$ score of 2 or lower, bridging is not recommended. If surgery is emergent, the effect of warfarin can be reversed by parenteral vitamin K or fresh frozen plasma.

Mechanical Prosthetic Heart Valves

Anticoagulant therapy is required in patients with a mechanical prosthetic heart valve to prevent stroke and systemic embolism and to prevent valve thrombosis, which is associated with a 15% mortality rate (Martinell et al., 1991). The optimal approach to anticoagulation during noncardiac operations in patients with mechanical valves is uncertain. No large, well-designed prospective studies have been conducted to provide reliable estimates of the risk of thromboembolism in patients with a mechanical heart valve who have interruption of warfarin and receive bridging anticoagulant therapy. Based on the available evidence, a classification scheme that stratifies patients with a mechanical heart valve according to thromboembolic risk and a suggested anticoagulation management strategy for each risk category is summarized in Table 14-5 (Douketis, 2002).

Figure 14-2. $CHADS_2$ Scoring System		
C	Congestive heart failure	1
H	Hypertension	1
A	Age > 75 years	1
D	Diabetes	1
S_2	Stroke or transient ischemic attack	2
Annual Stroke Risk		
$CHADS_2$ Score	**Stroke Risk (%)**	
0	1.9	
1	2.8	
2	4	
3	5.9	
4	8.5	
5	12.5	
6	18.2	
Note. Based on information from Snow et al., 2003.		

Table 14-5. Perioperative Anticoagulant Management in Patients With a Mechanical Prosthetic Heart Valve

Thromboembolism Risk Category	Patient Characteristics	Suggested Anticoagulant Management
High risk	Recent (within one month) stroke or transient Ischemic attack Any mitral valve Caged-ball or tilting-disc aortic valve	Bridging anticoagulant therapy is strongly recommended.
Moderate risk	Bileaflet aortic valve and two or more stroke risk factors	Bridging anticoagulant therapy should be considered.
Low risk	Bileaflet aortic valve and fewer than two stroke risk factors	Bridging anticoagulant therapy is optional.

Note. From "Perioperative Anticoagulation Management in Patients Who Are Receiving Oral Anticoagulant Therapy: A Practical Guide for Clinicians," by J.D. Douketis, 2002, *Thrombosis Research, 108*, p. 5. doi:10.1016/S0049-3848 (02)00387-0. Copyright 2002 by Elsevier Science Ltd. Reprinted with permission.

In patients with mechanical aortic valve prosthesis and no other risk factors for thromboembolism, warfarin therapy can safely be discontinued three to four days before surgery (Vongpatanasin, Hillis, & Lange, 1996). No bridging anticoagulation is usually necessary. The 2008 ACCP guidelines suggest no bridging or low-dose subcutaneous low-molecular-weight heparin in this setting (Douketis et al., 2008). Warfarin anticoagulation is reinstituted immediately after surgery because it will take a few days for the INR to reach a therapeutic level.

Coronary Stents and Perioperative Major Adverse Cardiac Events

Noncardiac surgery performed in patients who have had recent coronary stenting exposes them to an increased risk of major cardiac events in the perioperative period, especially if the oral anticoagulation therapy is interrupted. Stent thrombosis is a catastrophic complication that can occur in patients receiving either bare metal or drug-eluting stents during perioperative period. Both types of stents can easily thrombose, especially if surgery is performed early after stenting and if dual antiplatelet therapy is discontinued. To minimize perioperative stent thrombosis, the recommended treatment is to continue dual antiplatelet therapy during and after surgery. Patients with a coronary stent present a significant risk regardless of the type of noncardiac surgery undertaken. Delaying elective noncardiac surgery after coronary stenting allows the stents to endothelialize.

Drug-Eluting Stents

Drug-eluting stents were designed by coating a standard coronary stent with a thin polymer containing a substance that inhibits smooth muscle proliferation and neointimal hyperplasia within the stented segment (Costa & Simon, 2005). The mechanism of obstruction of drug-eluting stents is different from that of bare metal stents. In drug-eluting stents, the stent struts remain uncovered and therefore are prone to thrombosis. The optimal delay after implantation of a drug-eluting stent before noncardiac surgery remains unknown but is likely to be more than 12 months, particularly if antiplatelet therapy must be discontinued for the surgical procedure. The ACC/AHA guidelines recommend that patients who have been treated with drug-eluting stents should have elective surgical procedures with significant risk of bleeding deferred up to one year. In emergent noncardiac surgery that requires stopping clopidogrel, the guidelines recommend continuing aspirin therapy if possible and restarting clopidogrel as soon as possible. In patients with cancer who have had a drug-eluting stent in place for less than 12 months who need urgent major surgical intervention, the surgical oncologist and cardiologist should determine the risks versus the benefits of surgery.

Bare Metal Stents

The incidence of major cardiac events was found to be lowest when noncardiac surgery was performed more than 90 days after percutaneous coronary intervention (PCI) with bare metal stents. According to the ACC/AHA guidelines, elective noncardiac surgery should be delayed for four to six weeks after bare metal stent implantation to allow for at least partial endothelialization of the stent (Fleisher et al., 2007). The best data suggest that delaying surgery for six weeks may be even better than four weeks (Wilson et al., 2003). This is based on the assumption that a delay of six weeks will allow for a complete course of antiplatelet therapy and facilitate reendothelialization of the bare metal stent, thus decreasing the likelihood of potentially catastrophic stent thrombosis. Similar to with drug-eluting stents, clopidogrel and aspirin should be continued in the perioperative period, and therapy can be bridged with short-acting antiplatelet agent if clopidogrel and aspirin had to be discontinued. The exact timing for noncardiac surgery after PCI with stents implantation is unknown; however, recommendations are summarized in Figure 14-3.

Conclusion

Increased knowledge about the cardiotoxicity of various chemotherapeutic agents is prompting researchers to explore alternative chemotherapies, look for ways to identify who is most at risk for cardiac toxicity, and find ways to prevent cardiovascular damage.

A baseline cardiovascular assessment and examination along with careful cardiovascular management would not only prevent adverse events from antineoplastic drugs but also could be used to exclude their use in potentially high-risk individuals. The preoperative evaluation of patients with cancer should include obtaining a thorough history and clinical examination. If the patient has significant cardiac disease that requires treatment, and surgery can be delayed, the patient's underlying cardiac disease should be treated as in a nonoperative setting. For patients with low-risk cardiac disease, generally no further testing is necessary and the patient can proceed directly to surgery. For high-risk patients, further cardiac testing is highly recommended, and the types of cardiac diagnostic evaluation depend on the patient's underlying cardiac disease.

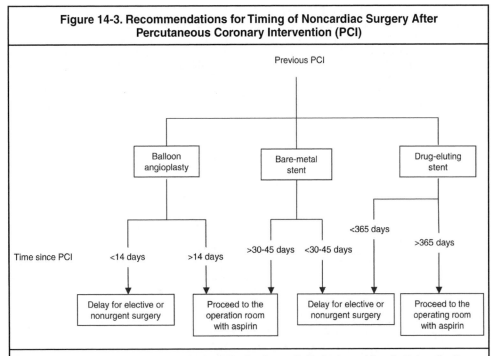

Figure 14-3. Recommendations for Timing of Noncardiac Surgery After Percutaneous Coronary Intervention (PCI)

Note. From "ACC/AHA 2007 Guidelines on Perioperative Cardiovascular Evaluation and Care for Noncardiac Surgery: Executive Summary," by L.A. Fleisher, J.A. Beckman, K.A. Brown, H. Calkins, E.L. Chaikof, K.E. Fleischmann, … C.W. Yancy, 2007, *Journal of the American College of Cardiology, 50,* p. 1720. doi:10.1016/j.jacc.2007.09.001. Copyright 2007 by the American College of Cardiology Foundation and the American Heart Association, Inc. Reprinted with permission.

References

Albini, A., Pennesi, G., Donatelli, F., Cammarota, R., De Flora, S., & Noonan, D.M. (2009). Cardiotoxicity of anticancer drugs: The need for cardio-oncology and cardio-oncological prevention. *Journal of the National Cancer Institute, 102,* 14–25. doi:10.1093/jnci/djp440

Altena, R., Perik, P.J., van Veldhuisen, D.J., de Vries, E.G., & Gietema, J.A. (2009). Cardiovascular toxicity caused by cancer treatment: Strategies for early detection. *Lancet Oncology, 10,* 391–399. doi:10.1016/S1470-2045(09)70042-7

American College of Cardiology & American Heart Association. (2007). Guidelines on perioperative cardiovascular evaluation and care for noncardiac surgery. *Circulation, 116,* e418–e500.

American College of Cardiology Foundation & American Heart Association. (2009). *Manual for ACCF/AHA guideline writing committees: Methodologies and policies.* Retrieved from http://www.acc.org/qualityandscience/clinical/manual/pdfs/methodology

Bandettini, W.P., & Arai, A.E. (2008). Advances in clinical applications of cardiovascular magnetic resonance imaging. *Heart, 94,* 1485–1495. doi:10.1136/hrt.2007.119016

Boehringer Ingelheim Pharmaceuticals. (2012). *Pradaxa® (dabigatran etexilate capsules)* [Prescribing information]. Ridgefield, CT: Author.

Cagirici, U., Nalbantgil, S., Cakan, A., & Turhan, K. (2005). A new algorithm for preoperative cardiac assessment in patients undergoing pulmonary resection. *Texas Heart Institute Journal, 32,* 159–162.

Connelly, C.S., & Panush, R.S. (1991). Should nonsteroidal anti-inflammatory drugs be stopped before elective surgery? *Archives of Internal Medicine, 151,* 1963–1966. doi:10.1001/archinte.1991.00400100049008

Costa, M.A., & Simon, D.I. (2005). Molecular basis of restenosis and drug-eluting stents. *Circulation, 111,* 2257–2273. doi:10.1161/01.CIR.0000163587.36485.A7

Dacey, L.J., Munoz, J.J., Johnson, E.R., Leavitt, B.J., Maloney, C.T., Morton, J.R., ... O'Connor, G.T. (2000). Effect of preoperative aspirin use on mortality in coronary artery bypass grafting patients. *Annals of Thoracic Surgery, 70,* 1986–1990. doi:10.1016/S0003-4975(00)02133-0

Detsky, A.S., Abrams, H.B., McLaughlin, J.R., Drucker, D.J., Sasson, Z., Johnston, N., ... Hilliard, J.R. (1986). Predicting cardiac complications in patients undergoing non-cardiac surgery. *Journal of General Internal Medicine, 1,* 211–219. doi:10.1007/BF02596184

Douketis, J.D. (2002). Perioperative anticoagulation management in patients who are receiving oral anticoagulant therapy: A practical guide for clinicians. *Thrombosis Research, 108,* 3–13. doi:10.1016/S0049-3848(02)00387-0

Douketis, J.D., Berger, P.B., Dunn, A.S., Jaffer, A.K., Spyropoulos, A.C., Becker, R.C., & Ansell, J. (2008). The perioperative management of antithrombotic therapy: American College of Chest Physicians evidence-based clinical practice guidelines (8th edition). *Chest, 133*(Suppl. 6), 299S–339S. doi:10.1378/chest.08-0675

Eagle, K.A., Berger, P.B., Calkins, H., Chaitman, B.R., Ewy, G.A., Fleischmann, K.E., ... Smith, S.C., Jr. (2002). ACC/AHA guideline update for perioperative cardiovascular evaluation for noncardiac surgery—Executive summary: A report of the American College of Cardiology/American Heart Association Task Force on Practice Guidelines (Committee to Update the 1996 Guidelines on Peri-operative Cardiovascular Evaluation for Non-cardiac Surgery). *Journal of the American College of Cardiology, 39,* 542–553. doi:10.1016/S0735-1097(01)01788-0

Eagle, K.A., Brundage, B.H., Chaitman, B.R., Ewy, G.A., Fleisher, L.A., Hertzer, N.R., ... Ryan, T.J. (1996). Guidelines for perioperative cardiovascular evaluation of the noncardiac surgery. Report of the American College of Cardiology/American Heart Association Task Force on Practice Guidelines. Committee on Perioperative Cardiovascular Evaluation for Noncardiac Surgery. *Circulation, 93,* 1278–1317.

Elliott, P. (2006). Pathogenesis of cardiotoxicity induced by anthracyclines. *Seminars in Oncology, 33*(3, Suppl. 8), S2–S7. doi:10.1053/j.seminoncol.2006.04.020

Eriksson, B.I., Dahl, O.E., Rosencher, N., Kurth, A.A., van Dijk, C.N., Frostick, S.P., ... Büller, H.R. (2007). Dabigatran etexilate versus enoxaparin for prevention of venous thromboembolism after total hip replacement: A randomised, double-blind, non-inferiority trial. *Lancet, 370,* 949–956. doi:10.1016/S0140-6736(07)61445-7

Fleisher, L.A., Beckman, J.A., Brown, K.A., Calkins, H., Chaikof, E.L., Fleischmann, K.E., ... Yancy, C.W. (2007). ACC/AHA 2007 guidelines on perioperative cardiovascular evaluation and care for noncardiac surgery: A report of the American College of Cardiology/American Heart Association Task Force on Practice Guidelines (Writing Committee to Revise the 2002 Guidelines on Perioperative Cardiovascular Evaluation for Noncardiac Surgery) developed in collaboration with the American Society of Echocardiography, American Society of Nuclear Cardiology, Heart Rhythm Society, Society of Cardiovascular Anesthesiologists, Society for Cardiovascular Angiography and Interventions, Society for Vascular Medicine and Biology, and Society for Vascular Surgery. *Journal of the American College of Cardiology, 50*(17), e159–e241. doi:10.1016/j.jacc.2007.09.003

Goldman, L., Caldera, D.L., Nussbaum, S.R., Southwick, F.S., Krogstad, D., Murray, B., ... Slater, E.E. (1977). Multifactorial index of cardiac risk in noncardiac surgical procedures. *New England Journal of Medicine, 297,* 845–850. doi:10.1056/NEJM197710202971601

Hong, R.A., Iimura, T., Sumida, K.N., & Eager, R.M. (2010). Cardio-oncology/onco-cardiology. *Clinical Cardiology, 33,* 733–737. doi:10.1002/clc.20823

Jaffer, A.K., Brotman, D.J., Bash, L.D., Mahmood, S.K., Lott, B., & White, R.H. (2010). Variations in perioperative warfarin management: Outcomes and practice patterns at nine hospitals. *American Journal of Medicine, 123,* 141–150. doi:10.1016/j.amjmed.2009.09.017

Jafri, S.M. (2004). Periprocedural thromboprophylaxis in patients receiving chronic anticoagulation therapy. *American Heart Journal, 147,* 3–15. doi:10.1016/j.ahj.2003.06.001

Jannazzo, A., Hoffman, J., & Lutz, M. (2008). Monitoring of anthracycline-induced cardiotoxicity. *Annals of Pharmacotherapy, 42,* 99–104. doi:10.1345/aph.1K359

Kearon, C., & Hirsh, J. (1997). Management of anticoagulation before and after elective surgery. *New England Journal of Medicine, 336,* 1506–1511. doi:10.1056/NEJM199705223362107

Kumar, R., McKinney, W.P., Raj, G., Heudebert, G.R., Heller, H.J., Koetting, M., & McIntire, D.D. (2001). Adverse cardiac events after surgery: Assessing risk in a veteran population. *Journal of General Internal Medicine, 16,* 507–518. doi:10.1046/j.1525-1497.2001.016008507.x

Mahla, E., Tiesenhausen, K., Rehak, P., Fruhwald, S., Pürstner, P., & Metzler, H. (2000). Perioperative myocardial cell injury: The relationship between troponin T and cortisol. *Journal of Clinical Anesthesia, 12,* 208–212. doi:10.1016/S0952-8180(00)00150-1

Martinell, J., Jiménez, A., Rábago, G., Artiz, V., Fraile, J., & Farré, J. (1991). Mechanical cardiac valve thrombosis: Is thrombectomy justified? *Circulation, 84*(Suppl. 5), III70–III75.

McCallion, J., & Krenis, L.J. (1992). Preoperative cardiac evaluation. *American Family Physician, 45,* 1723–1732.

Monsuez, J.J., Charniot, J.C., Vignat, N., & Artigou, J.Y. (2010). Cardiac side-effects of cancer chemotherapy. *International Journal of Cardiology, 144,* 3–15. doi:10.1016/j.ijcard.2010.03.003

Poldermans, D., Hoeks, S.E., & Feringa, H.H. (2008). Pre-operative risk assessment and risk reduction before surgery. *Journal of the American College of Cardiology, 51,* 1913–1924. doi:10.1016/j.jacc.2008.03.005

Snow, V., Weiss, K.B., LeFevre, M., McNamara, R., Bass, E., Green, L.A., … Mottur-Pilson, C. (2003). Management of newly detected atrial fibrillation: A clinical practice guideline from the American Academy of Family Physicians and the American College of Physicians. *Annals of Internal Medicine, 139,* 1009–1017.

Sprung, J., Warner, M.E., Contreras, M.G., Schroeder, D.R., Beighley, C.M., Wilson, G.A., & Warner, D.O. (2003). Predictors of survival following cardiac arrest in patients undergoing noncardiac surgery: A study of 518,294 patients at a tertiary referral center. *Anesthesiology, 99,* 259–269. doi:10.1097/00000542-200308000-00006

Van Brabandt, H. (2007). Stent thrombosis: Antiplatelets alone won't do the job. *BMJ, 334,* 57. doi:10.1186/bmj.39086.931019.1F

Vongpatanasin, W., Hillis, L.D., & Lange, R.A. (1996). Prosthetic heart valves. *New England Journal of Medicine, 335,* 407–416. doi:10.1056/NEJM199608083350607

White, R.H., McKittrick, T., Hutchinson, R., & Twitchell, J. (1995). Temporary discontinuation of warfarin therapy: Changes in the international normalized ratio. *Annals of Internal Medicine, 122,* 40–42.

Wilson, S.H., Fasseas, P., Orford, J.L., Lennon, R.J., Horlocker, T., Charnoff, N.E., … Berger, P.B. (2003). Clinical outcome of patients undergoing non-cardiac surgery in the two months following coronary stenting. *Journal of the American College of Cardiology, 42,* 234–240. doi:10.1016/S0735-1097(03)00622-3

Screening and Management of Cardiovascular Risk Factors in Cancer Survivors

Jessica S. Coviello, DNP, APRN, ANP-BC,
and M. Tish Knobf, PhD, RN, FAAN, AOCN®

Introduction

Overall survival and the quality of extended survival are key treatment outcomes for the 13.7 million cancer survivors living in the United States, representing approximately 4% of the total population. Patients with breast (22%), prostate (20%), colorectal (9%), and gynecologic cancers (8%) represent the greatest numbers of survivors (Siegel et al., 2012). As cancer survival rates have improved, competing causes of death have contributed to an increase in all-cause mortality (Chapman et al., 2008). Cardiovascular disease (CVD) has been reported as the most common cause of noncancer death among breast cancer survivors (Chapman et al., 2008; Hanrahan et al., 2007; Maurea et al., 2010). Increased CVD morbidity and mortality may be attributed to preexisting CVD in newly diagnosed patients with cancer, cardiotoxicity resulting in decreased ventricular function, and treatment effects that result in increased CVD risk factors such as dyslipidemia, hypertension (HTN), and central adiposity. Barriers to reducing or preventing cancer treatment–associated cardiovascular adverse effects include lack of routine screening to identify cardiac risk factors, failure to integrate preexisting cardiac risk factors into treatment planning, low diagnostic sensitivity for cardiac damage with standard echocardiography or radionuclide angiography, emerging novel targeted agents that affect the cardiovascular system, and lack of systematic evaluation of cardiac biomarkers that may identify subclinical disease (Albini et al., 2010; Jurcut et al., 2008; Peng, Pentassuglia, & Sawyer, 2010). No evidence-based standards exist for cardiovascular risk assessment before or after cancer therapy in adult cancer survivors despite a growing body of evidence that they are needed (Abu-Khalaf & Harris, 2009; Daher & Yeh, 2008; Khakoo & Yeh, 2007; Patnaik, Byers, DiGuiseppi, Dabelea, & Denberg, 2011). Identification of patients at risk for CVD because of personal susceptibility factors and cancer treatment would direct risk reduction and therapeutic interventions to reduce morbidity and mortality (Giordano & Hortobagyi, 2007; Granger, 2006).

This chapter will review the significance of CVD in midlife and older adults, describe common cardiovascular risk factors, discuss the complexity of CVD risk factors and cardiotoxicity, provide screening and surveillance recommendations for cardiovascular risk factors in patients with cancer, and suggest management approaches for patients with cardiovascular risk factors or cardiotoxicity.

Cardiovascular Risk Factors and Cardiovascular Disease in the General Population

An estimated 82,600,000 American adults (more than 1 in 3) have one or more types of CVD (Roger et al., 2012). CVD is simply defined as any condition that results from narrowed, stiffened, or blocked blood vessels that can lead to a heart attack or angina (both can also be referred to as *coronary artery disease* [CAD] or *coronary heart disease* [CHD]), stroke, or peripheral vascular disease.

Risk factors for CVD are classified into two groups: major risk factors and contributing risk factors. Major risk factors are those that have been shown to significantly increase the risk of CVD, such as HTN. Contributing risk factors (stress, anxiety, depression, metabolic syndrome [MetS]) are known to be associated with an increase in CVD, but their significance and prevalence are still under investigation. Major risk factors are defined as nonmodifiable (age, heredity, race, and gender) and those that can be modified or controlled with lifestyle modification and therapeutic treatment (smoking, dyslipidemia, HTN, obesity [especially excess belly fat], diabetes, and sedentary lifestyle). In addition, menopause, with a decrease in estrogen levels superimposed on the natural aging process, is an established CVD risk factor for women (Bittner, 2009).

CVD is a result of atherosclerosis, a complex, insidious process beginning in early childhood with the appearance of arterial fatty streaks. As one ages, the inner protective layer of the artery known as the endothelium becomes damaged, usually from causative risk factors. Three known causes of atherosclerotic damage include elevated lipids (low-density lipoproteins [LDLs] and triglycerides), HTN, and cigarette smoking. Fatty substances, cellular waste, calcium, and fibrin pass through the damaged endothelial wall of the vessel and are deposited in areas of vessel erosion. Deposition of these substances in a vessel begins to create lipid plaques with a fibrous covering, forming an atheroma. As atheromas increase in size, they create partial obstruction of blood flow. White blood cells, smooth muscle cells, and platelets aggregate to the site. The endothelium thickens as a result. The core of the plaque can become necrotic, hemorrhage, and calcify, thereby creating even more blockage. Fibrous plaque is most often found in the coronary, carotid, and popliteal arteries as well as the abdominal aorta.

Symptoms of decreased blood flow usually do not occur until blood flow is diminished by 75%. The occurrence of symptoms may depend on the extent of the development of collateral vessels, small arteries that connect two larger arteries or different segments of the artery. As blood flow diminishes, pressure within the artery may cause these smaller vessels to dilate, redirect, and improve flow. The ability to produce these small collateral vessels is variable among individuals and may be genetically dependent (Gaziano, 2008).

In recent years, scientific advances have highlighted the role of inflammation in the pathophysiologic process in atherosclerosis and assessment of cardiovascular risk, as measured by high-sensitivity cardiac C-reactive protein (hs-CRP) (Ridker, Buring, Rifai, & Cook, 2007). In the presence of inflammation, fibrous plaque can rupture, form a thrombus, and occlude an artery. An hs-CRP level of less than 1 mg/dl is associated with a low risk for developing CVD. A value of 1–3 mg/dl is a moderate risk, and a value of 3 mg/dl or greater is considered high risk. MetS, diabetes, smoking, and obesity are all associated with arterial inflammation and generally an increase in hs-CRP. There also is an interplay between hs-CRP and sleep-disordered breathing (Kenchaiah, Gaziano, & Vasan, 2004; Kenchaiah, Narula, & Vasan, 2004; McNicholas, 2009). Pharmacologic therapy with a statin, aspirin, and/or angiotensin-converting enzyme (ACE) inhibitor has been associated with a reduction of hs-CRP (Ridker et al., 2007).

CVD is more common and more severe in older patients. The risk of cardiovascular events increases as individuals get older, with age remaining one of the strongest predictors of disease. The majority of cardiovascular risk begins to emerge in the fourth and fifth decade of life with a gradual increase in vascular stiffness and a decrease in metabolic rate, which can lead to obesity, HTN, and insulin resistance.

Race and Ethnicity

CVD remains the leading cause of death in the United States, accounting for deaths in 39.6% of Hispanics, 36.2% of Caucasians, up to 34.8% of Asians, 33.6% of African Americans, and 24.9% of Native Americans. In Asian populations, death rates for CAD vary according to ethnic subgroups with the highest rates in Asian Indians, Hawaiians, and Guamanians (American Heart Associaton [AHA], 2010). African Americans are more likely than Caucasians to be obese and have HTN, diabetes, and peripheral vascular disease. They also have a higher CVD mortality rate than Caucasians and are at increased risk for premature death from CAD. Ethnic differences in all causes of CVD appear to be related to clustering of risk factors. The Dallas Heart Study showed that risk factors such as cigarette smoking, HTN, and diabetes were significantly more common among African Americans than Caucasians (Nguyen et al., 2011). This risk factor clustering has also been observed in Asian Indians who have a higher fasting insulin, reduced glucose uptake during hyperinsulinemia, higher LDL and triglycerides and lower high-density lipoprotein (HDL) levels than Caucasians (AHA, 2010; Ferdinand, 2006).

These racial and ethnic differences highlight the need for individual cardiovascular assessment in young adulthood so that risk factor reduction occurs early enough to reduce morbidity and mortality. Several recent studies have suggested the need to begin cardiovascular risk assessment and intervention as early as age 9, particularly with the increase in obesity in this country (Gidding, 2010). In both genders, lipids begin to change after the age of 20, providing the rationale behind the National Cholesterol Education Program's Adult Treatment Panel III (NCEP/ATP III) guideline recommending a baseline CVR assessment at age 20 (NCEP/ATP III, 2001).

Age

Age is a known risk factor for heart disease and is calculated in the Framingham risk equation during ATP III assessment. Until age 45, men tend to have higher total cholesterol levels than women, yet women tend to have higher HDL levels. Men in their 40s are four times more likely to die from heart disease than women the same age. After menopause, however, a woman's LDL level tends to rise while her HDL level decreases, and overall risk of heart disease increases with age (Stangl, Baumann, & Stangl, 2002). NCEP/ATP III guidelines recommend measuring lipid and lipoprotein levels at least once every five years (Grundy et al., 2004). Patients with abnormal levels should be treated and be reassessed yearly (Grundy et al., 2004; NCEP/ATP III, 2001).

The incidence of acute coronary syndrome is the highest in the fifth and sixth decades of life, with stroke occurring most often after age 55. This is particularly true in individuals with a strong family history of atherosclerotic disease and is one of the reasons why an early risk reduction program is recommended (Gaziano, 2008). The risk for peripheral vascular arterial disease is closely associated with smoking, which can cause up to a 10-fold increase in relative risk. In addition, cigarette smoking can have a direct toxic effect on heart cells. The immediate effect of tobacco smoke is the displacement of circulating oxygen to carbon monoxide, thereby reducing the oxygen-carrying power of the cells. For those with CAD, smoking can alter the angina threshold through a change in oxygen-carrying power. Angina can be induced with smoking in anemic patients, who already have a low oxygen-carrying power, by further reducing the oxygen capacity of the cells even in the absence of coronary disease. Smoking also promotes insulin resistance, diabetes, coronary artery spasm, increased cholesterol levels, and pulmonary diseases. Cigarette smoking now ranks fourth as a cardiovascular risk factor in this country, with obesity and inactivity ranking first and second. Smoking cessation reduces risk of a heart attack by 50%–75% within five years (AHA, 2010). Peripheral vascular disease is also associated with diabetes and is seen in 1 out of 3 diabetics (Norgren et al., 2007).

Anxiety and Depression

Depressive disorders are associated with increased cardiovascular morbidity and mortality (Wulsin & Singal, 2003), and depressed women may face an increased risk of stroke (Pan et al., 2011). Anxiety and depression in women with CVD are associated with poorer outcomes (Beckie, Fletcher, Beckstead, Schocken, & Evans, 2008; May et al., 2009; Székely et al., 2007; Todaro, Shen, Niaura, & Tilkemeier, 2005) with younger women (younger than 65) appearing more vulnerable.

The Nurses' Health Study has followed more than 80,000 women and reported that 22% of women age 54–74 have depression. High levels of anxiety also were associated with fatal cardiac events in this population (Albert, Chae, Rexrode, Manson, & Kawachi, 2010).

Both biologic and behavioral mechanisms have been proposed to explain the link between depression and CVD. The increase in morbidity and mortality is thought to be partially related to heart rate variability as a result of deregulation of autonomic nervous system control of the heart, particularly in those older than age 55 (Hamer, Molloy, & Stamatakis, 2008). Other theories include the increase in inflammation seen in both depression and anxiety as a possible factor for cardiovascular morbidity and mortality. In comparison with nondepressed individuals, depressed patients with cardiac disease frequently have higher levels of biomarkers that are predictive of cardiac events or promote atherosclerosis (e.g., C-reactive protein, interleukin-6). In a recent study, cigarette smoking, physical activity, alcohol intake, C-reactive protein, and HTN were independently associated with psychological distress (Hamer et al., 2008).

Even in individuals as young as 18 years of age, anxiety independently predicted subsequent coronary heart disease in men who were followed for occurrence of a heart attack over a 30-year period. Psychological stress, particularly family conflict and job loss, is associated with a higher CVD morbidity and mortality in men (Gallo et al., 2004; Kriegbaum, Christensen, Lund, Prescott, & Osler, 2008). The National Health and Nutrition Examination Survey (NHANES) I Study was the first to demonstrate that depression affects heart disease risk in women (Ferketich, Schwartzbaum, Frid, & Moeschberger, 2000). Elevated depressive symptoms are associated with worse prognosis in both men and women with known CVD, and more severe depression is associated with earlier and more severe cardiac events (Beckie et al., 2008).

Only recently have depression and anxiety been recognized as risk factors warranting inclusion in a cardiovascular risk assessment. These have specifically been included as part of AHA's new prevention guidelines for women (Mosca, Barrett-Connor, & Wenger, 2011). Screening is strongly recommended in both men and women as a basis for intervention.

Cardiovascular risk factors are strong predictors of CVD. The prevalence of having two or more risk factors in American adults is 37% (Roger et al., 2012). HTN, obesity, and type 2 diabetes are predominant risk factors in the American population with 76,400,000 individuals using antihypertensive agents or having a systolic blood pressure of 140 mm Hg or higher and/or diastolic pressure of 90 mm Hg or higher; 68% of Americans being overweight or obese; 27% of the population meeting the criteria for MetS; and 28% having a diagnosis of diabetes (Roger et al., 2012). More than 2,200 Americans die of CVD each day with an average of one death every 39 seconds. CVD claims more lives each year than cancer, lung disease, and accidents combined. These statistics highlight the need for assessing a population where cardiovascular risk is high even before cancer treatment begins.

Cardiovascular Disease Risk in the Diagnosis and Treatment of Women With Breast Cancer

Breast cancer is the most common cancer and has the most data of all cancers among women in the United States (American Cancer Society, 2012). Combined with improved survival outcomes for this disease, a substantial body of research about the cardiovascular sequelae of women diagnosed and treated for breast cancer has emerged. Similarly, CVD is common among mid-life and older women, with an estimated lifetime risk of 39% for a woman at age 50 (Berger, Jordan, Lloyd-Jones, & Blumenthal, 2010). Women newly diagnosed with breast or other cancers may be at risk for cardiac disease unrelated to their cancer treatments. Preexisting heart disease and presence of known cardiac risk factors such as HTN, diabetes, overweight/obesity, sedentary behavior, older age, ethnicity, and elevated lipid profile increase a woman's risk for CVD and may influence her susceptibility to cardiotoxicity (Khakoo & Yeh, 2008; Martin et al., 2009). Using breast cancer as illustrative of adverse cardiovascular outcomes, Jones, Haykowsky, Swartz, Douglas, and Mackey (2007) described a "multiple hit" hypothesis integrating the complex relationship of cardiovascular risk factors and receipt of cardiotoxic adjuvant chemotherapy with decreased cardiovascular reserve leading to an increased risk for preclinical or clinical CVD.

The presence of cardiovascular risk factors in women newly diagnosed with cancer has not been well documented. However, there is a growing body of literature on women with breast cancer, cardiovascular risk factors, and morbidity and mortality for cancer and noncancer causes.

Hypertension

HTN is the most common comorbidity in women newly diagnosed with breast cancer (Harlan et al., 2009). A higher percentage of men than women have HTN until the age of 45 years. The incidence between women and men is similar between 45–54 years but after the menopausal transition, a much higher percentage of women are diagnosed with HTN. It is a major risk factor for CAD and stroke and increases the risk of developing heart failure by threefold in women (Chobanian et al., 2003). HTN is thought to contribute to the risk for cardiotoxicity associated with anthracycline and trastuzumab therapy (Ewer & Ewer, 2010; Khakoo & Yeh, 2008; Martin et al., 2009) and is a common side effect of newer targeted therapies (Harbeck & Thomssen, 2011). Disparate outcomes for Caucasians versus ethnic minorities in cancer are well documented. In the United States, the prevalence of HTN in African Americans is higher than anywhere else in the world. Compared to Caucasians, HTN develops in African Americans at an earlier age with significantly higher average blood pressures. Recent data support genetic factors as a contributor (Taylor, Sun, Hunt, & Kardia, 2010). Besides being a major risk factor for heart attack and stroke, HTN promotes hypertrophy, myocardial fibrosis, and loss of contractility of the heart muscle and can potentiate pathophysiologic changes, referred to as *remodeling*, of the left ventricle, leading to heart failure. African Americans are also at greater risk for diabetes and obesity, further increasing the CVD risk. HTN is the leading cause of heart failure in women, unlike in men, where CAD is the major contributing factor (Mosca, Barrett-Connor, et al., 2011).

While cardiovascular risk is multifactorial, including genetic differences, comorbidities are significant influencing factors. Nearly half of African American women (45%) have some form of CVD, compared to 32% of Caucasian women, and HTN has been identified as an independent predictor of poorer survival outcomes among African American breast cancer survivors compared to Caucasian women (Braithwaite et al., 2009). Maintaining an adequate blood pressure of less than 130/85 mm Hg is a major goal for the nation (Healthy People 2020, 2012). In 2001, AHA and the American College of Cardiology changed the classification of heart failure from that of the New York Heart Association functional class to that of categories of prevention (Hunt et al., 2005). This guideline was updated in 2009 with stage A being the patient at risk for heart failure but without structural heart disease or symptoms of heart failure. This includes patients with HTN, diabetes, obesity, MetS, and atherosclerotic disease or patients with a family history of cardiomyopathy or previous use of cardiotoxins. Stage A is further defined in the guidelines as *pre–heart failure* to reinforce to the healthcare provider and the patient the risk and the opportunity for early intervention and risk reduction (Hunt et al., 2009). Screening for and managing HTN prior to cancer treatment is essential in minimizing cardiovascular complications and enhancing long-term survival outcomes.

Recommendations to maintain a healthy weight (or lose weight if indicated) and national physical activity guidelines of 30 minutes of moderate-intensity exercise most days of the week are essential components to patient management. Pharmacologic therapy is the primary therapeutic approach with a regimen of diuretics, beta-blockers, ACE inhibitors, and calcium channel blockers. Effective management of blood pressure to the goal of a normal blood pressure is the mainstay of HTN treatment and prevention of heart failure and stroke. Further information for the assessment and management of HTN can be found in Chapter 7.

Diabetes

The prevalence of diabetes in patients with cancer is 8%–18% (Nicolucci, 2010). Pre-existing diabetes in cancer survivors is associated with poorer survival (Erickson et al., 2011; Lipscombe, Goodwin, Zinman, McLaughlin, & Hux, 2008; Peairs et al., 2011). Diabetes mellitus is associated with a two- to fivefold increase in both CAD and heart failure. With every 1% increase in hemoglobin A1c, there is an 8%–16% increase in the risk of hospitalization and death due to heart failure (Iribarren et al., 2001). Atherosclerosis in diabetes results from a complex interplay among a number of risk factors including HTN, which is twice as common in people with diabetes or impaired glucose tolerance as in the general population. Atherosclerosis in people with diabetes tends to be accelerated, more severe, and more widespread. Because atherosclerosis damages both medium and large blood vessels, the term *macroangiopathy* is often used to indicate its presence in people with diabetes. It is a direct result of chronic hyperglycemia. Microangiopathy adversely affects capillary function, leading to a shortage of supply of oxygen and nutrients to the tissues and a leakage of proteins into the tissue spaces. Capillaries throughout the body are affected, but damage to the microcirculation of the eyes, kidneys, and nerves is responsible for the major clinical manifestations of retinopathy, nephropathy, neuropathy, and peripheral vascular disease. Microangiopathic complications of diabetes are the most readily preventable with good glycemic control. Endothelial dysfunction is an important component of both macroangiopathy and autonomic changes but also can appear early in the course of diabetes before the onset of detectable vascular disease. In addition, the outer layers of the vessel wall composed of muscle or elastic tissue can be damaged. This also can impair the regulation of the blood flow and may weaken the vessel wall. Other factors such as HTN and dyslipidemia also contribute to vessel wall decline. Damage to the autonomic nervous system can be a direct result of chronic hyperglycemia or can follow microangiopathy involving the small vessels, which supply blood to the nerves themselves, thereby causing a vicious circle of nerve and blood vessel damage. Damage to the nerve supply of the heart affects the regulation of the pulse rate. In the blood vessels, manifestations such as a fall in blood pressure on standing or exercising (orthostatic hypotension) can produce disabling symptoms and can affect measures aimed at treating HTN. Loss of the nerve supply to small blood vessels also can impair the regulation of blood flow. Women appear to be at greater risk for the development of diabetes, especially those who are overweight or obese and less physically active (Gaziano, 2008).

Overweight, obesity, and MetS contribute to insulin resistance in patients with cancer (Boyd, 2003), and there is a growing body of literature on the relationship of hyperinsulinemia, insulin resistance, and diabetes and poorer breast cancer outcomes (Goodwin et al., 2002; Goodwin, Ligibel, & Stambolic, 2009; Rose, Komninou, & Stephenson, 2004). MetS is a major cardiovascular risk factor (Eshtiaghi, Esteghamati, & Nakhjavani, 2010) defined by HTN, dyslipidemia, abdominal obesity, and glucose intolerance (see Table 15-1) (Collins et al., 2007). The criteria for the diagnosis of MetS include any

Table 15-1. AHA/NHLBI: The Metabolic Syndrome	
Diagnosis is established when three or more risk factors are present.	
Risk Factor	**Defining Level**
Waist circumference[a] • Men • Women	 > 102 cm (> 40 in) > 88 cm (> 35 in)
Triglycerides[b]	≥ 150 mg/dl
HDL-C[b] • Men • Women	 < 40 mg/dl < 50 mg/dl
Blood pressure[b]	≥ 130/≥ 85 mm Hg
Fasting glucose[b]	≥ 100 mg/dl

[a] Some U.S. adults of non-Asian origin with marginal increases should benefit from lifestyle changes. Lower cut-points (≥ 90 cm in men and ≥ 80 cm in women) are used for Asian Americans.

[b] Or on drug treatment for the risk factor

AHA—American Heart Association; HDL-C—high-density lipoprotein cholesterol; NHLBI—National Heart, Lung, and Blood Institute

three of the five risks as defined by NCEP/ATP III, the International Diabetes Foundation, and the World Health Organization (Lorenzo, Williams, Hunt, & Haffner, 2007). In addition, the menopausal transition appears to contribute to the risk of MetS (Coviello, LaClerque, & Knobf, in press). Abdominal obesity (visceral fat) and insulin resistance contribute to dyslipidemia, oxidative stress, inflammation, and altered coagulation, ultimately leading to atherosclerosis (Gaspard, 2009). MetS is associated with a fivefold increase in the risk of developing diabetes and a threefold increase in the risk of cardiovascular death (Gaspard, 2009).

The shared risk of hyperinsulinemia and diabetes to CVD and cancer underscores the need to include fasting insulin and glucose levels in risk assessment, especially in patients who are overweight or obese.

Overweight and Obesity

Being overweight (body mass index [BMI] 25–29.9 kg/m²) or obese (BMI greater than 30 kg/m²) is a risk factor for CVD and has been associated with increased risk of recurrence and lower survival rates in women with breast cancer (Chen et al., 2010; Kroenke, Chen, Rosner, & Holmes, 2005; Nichols et al., 2009). Weight gain can also be a significant contributor to preexisting HTN. Obesity and inactivity represent 80% of the CVD risk in the United States (Warren, Wilcox, Dowda, & Baruth, 2012). Obesity is a major risk factor for CVD and predisposes individuals to HTN, diabetes, MetS, CAD/CHD, and renal or heart failure. This predisposition is related to weight influencing blood glucose, lipid levels, and blood pressure. Direct mechanisms link visceral adiposity and the atherosclerotic process through the action of adipose-derived inflammation that sets the stage for insulin resistance and progressive loss of endothelial integrity and vascular tone, as well as increase in triglycerides. This allows for both plaque formation and rupture caused by plaque inflammation–induced instability. In addition, obesity increases preload and afterload—pressures that affect cardiac output and predispose to HTN.

Weight gain during and after treatment in women with breast cancer (McInnes & Knobf 2001; Irwin et al., 2005) is associated with increased fat mass, decreased lean muscle mass (Ingram & Brown, 2004), and central adiposity, all of which contribute to risk of MetS (Thomson et al., 2009, 2010). Elevation in the inflammatory marker hs-CRP and central obesity, both of which are considered significant cardiovascular risk factors, have been associated with the development of MetS in breast cancer survivors (Chen et al., 2009; Hamer, Chida, & Stamatakis, 2010). Monitoring weight and body composition, especially central adiposity, among breast cancer survivors is essential to target interventions (Demark-Wahnefried, Peterson, McBride, Lipkus, & Clipp, 2000).

Dyslipidemia

Blood lipid and lipoprotein lipid analysis includes the measurement of LDL, HDL, triglycerides, very low density lipoproteins, and total blood cholesterol. In both genders, lipids begin to change after the age of 20, providing the rationale behind the NCEP/ATP III. The guideline recommends a baseline CVR assessment at 20 years of age, and at least once every five years (Grundy et al., 2004). Patients with abnormal levels should be treated and be reassessed yearly (Grundy et al., 2004; NCEP/ATP III, 2001) (see ATP III Guidelines at a Glance: Quick Desk Reference at www.nhlbi.nih.gov/guidelines/cholesterol/atglance.htm).

Endocrine therapy for women with breast cancer includes selective estrogen receptor modulators (e.g., tamoxifen) and aromatase inhibitors (AIs). Tamoxifen appears to have beneficial estrogen-agonist effects on lipids, but the increased risk of thromboembolism and stroke negates the potential cardioprotective effects of a favorable lipid profile (Esteva & Hortobagyi, 2006; Lewis, 2007; Ng, Better, & Green, 2006). In contrast, AIs have been associated with hypercholesterolemia and an unfavorable HDL/LDL ratio (Esteva & Hortobagyi, 2006; Ligibel et al., 2010). Because low HDL and high cholesterol, LDL, and triglycerides are all known cardiovascular risks, it is important to obtain baseline screening data on newly diagnosed patients and to monitor survivors over time.

Menopause

Cardiovascular risk is affected by a change in ovarian function associated with menopause and aging (Bittner, 2009). Premenopausal women diagnosed with breast cancer are at risk for premature chemotherapy-induced menopause, and endocrine therapy with an AI for five years is commonly recommended for postmenopausal women with hormone receptor–positive breast cancer. The abrupt menopause induced by chemotherapy is due to direct toxicity to the ovaries, and AIs significantly reduce estrogen. Although the evidence linking decreased estrogen levels to cardiovascular risk is controversial, it is strongly suggested to monitor peri- and postmenopausal women (Ewer & Gluck, 2009; Matthews et al., 2009). Significant changes in cholesterol, triglyceride, LDL, HDL, and lipoprotein-a, or Lp(a), levels were reported in premenopausal women who experienced chemotherapy-induced menopause (Saarto, Blomquist, Ehnholm, Taskinen, & Elomaa, 1996).

Visceral fat varies inversely with estrogen levels. Visceral fat accumulation occurs in women when estrogen levels become sufficiently low (Bouchard, Després, & Mauriège, 1993). Body fat is not only an energy reservoir but also an endocrine organ. As visceral fat accumulates in response to lowering estrogen levels, hormones that control hunger also shift, with a resultant increase in hunger. The interplay of these intricate pathways is associated with insulin resistance and accumulation of visceral fat, which increases the risk of MetS. The combination of drug-induced menopause, effects of endocrine therapy, and weight gain among breast cancer survivors underscores the potential CVD risk unique to this population.

Older Age

Age-related organ system changes, a higher prevalence of cardiac risk factors, and physical inactivity predispose older women to higher rates of cardiotoxicity (Shenoy et al., 2011) (see Figure 15-1). In older women with breast cancer, the presence of cardiovascular risk factors significantly heightens the risk for cardiotoxicity with anthracyclines and/or trastuzumab. Despite the advances in cancer therapy, CVD has become the primary cause of death among breast cancer survivors, especially those with one or more comorbid conditions (Patnaik et al., 2011).

Cardiovascular Risk in Men

Treatments for prostate and testicular cancers have been shown to increase cardiovascular risk in men (Keating, O'Malley, & Smith, 2006; Levine et al., 2010; Redig &

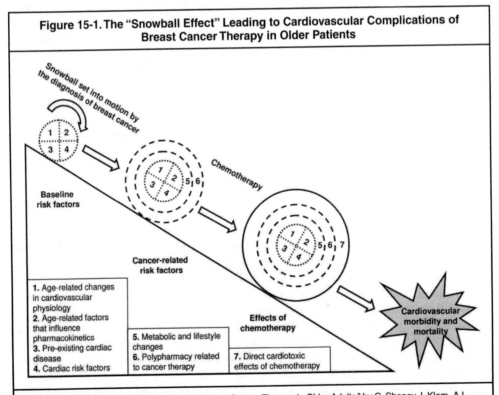

Figure 15-1. The "Snowball Effect" Leading to Cardiovascular Complications of Breast Cancer Therapy in Older Patients

Snowball set into motion by the diagnosis of breast cancer

Baseline risk factors

Cancer-related risk factors

Chemotherapy

Effects of chemotherapy

Cardiovascular morbidity and mortality

1. Age-related changes in cardiovascular physiology
2. Age-related factors that influence pharmacokinetics
3. Pre-existing cardiac disease
4. Cardiac risk factors
5. Metabolic and lifestyle changes
6. Polypharmacy related to cancer therapy
7. Direct cardiotoxic effects of chemotherapy

Note. From "Cardiovascular Complications of Breast Cancer Therapy in Older Adults," by C. Shenoy, I. Klem, A.L. Crowley, M.R. Patel, M.A. Winchester, C. Owusu, and G.G. Kimmick, 2011, *Oncologist, 16*, p. 1140. Copyright 2011 by AlphaMed Press. Reprinted with permission.

Munshi, 2010; Tsai, D'Amico, Sedetsky, Chen, & Carroll, 2007; van den Belt-Dusebout et al., 2006). A smoking history, HTN, and known CVD risk factors combined with radiation and chemotherapy have resulted in increased CVD in men (van den Belt-Dusebout et al., 2006).

Androgen suppression therapy has adversely affected CVD mortality, even in men with low-risk prostate cancer (Saigal et al., 2007; Tsai et al., 2007). Androgen therapy has also been associated with increased risk of CAD, myocardial infarction, and sudden cardiac death (Keating et al., 2006). Low testosterone levels, whether secondary to gonadal dysfunction or androgen suppression therapy, have been shown to contribute to increased total cholesterol and elevated LDL and triglycerides, known risk factors for CVD (Traish, Saad, & Guay, 2009). In addition, insulin resistance has been reported with androgen suppression therapy related to hyperglycemia and diabetes. Decreased testosterone levels precede detectable elevations of glucose, insulin, and hemoglobin A1c, indicating that testosterone decline may be an early indicator of incident diabetes (Traish et al., 2009). The link among visceral body fat, insulin resistance, MetS, and diabetes significantly increases cardiovascular risk (Braga-Basaria et al., 2006; Keating et al., 2006; Levine et al., 2010). In men with preexisting diabetes, use of androgen suppression therapy led to worsening of glycemic control as demonstrated by adverse changes in hemoglobin A1c and serum glucose levels (Derweesh et al., 2007). Preexisting cardiovascular risk factors superimposed on androgen therapy highlights the need for measuring pretreatment fasting glucose, serum insulin, and lipid and hs-CRP levels in men in order to monitor risk during and after therapy.

Cardiovascular Risk Identification and Management in Survivorship

Susceptibility to cardiac complications in cancer survivors is multifactorial and requires an understanding of the interplay of CVD risk, cardiotoxicity, and cancer outcomes in survivors. Identification of patients at risk for cardiac complications will direct risk reduction and therapeutic cardioprotective interventions to reduce morbidity and mortality. Despite the incidence of known CVD risks in the general population, compliance among providers to screen the general public for cardiovascular risk has been inconsistent (Cabana & Kim, 2003; Christian, Mills, Simpson, & Mosca, 2006; Mosca et al., 2005, 2007; Mosca, Benjamin et al., 2011) despite that more than 50% of men and nearly 40% of women will have CVD during their lifetime even if free of CVD at 50 years of age (Mosca et al., 2005). This underscores the importance of a baseline cardiovascular risk assessment prior to cancer therapy. Identification of risk will permit early intervention as well as guide the development of surveillance protocols (Daher & Yeh, 2008; Ewer, Swain, Cardinale, Fadol, & Suter, 2011; Khakoo & Yeh, 2008; Lenihan & Esteva, 2008; Levine et al., 2010; Maitland et al., 2010; Mouhayar & Salahudeen, 2011; Murray et al., 2010; Redig & Munshi, 2010; Tsimberidou, Minotti, & Cardinale, 2011).

Screening and Surveillance for Cardiac Risk

Screening for cardiovascular risk is a comprehensive assessment that includes medical and family history, weight, waist circumference, physical examination, and specific gynecologic history (e.g., history of birth control pills, hormone replacement therapy, menopause) for women. Laboratory tests include fasting cholesterol, HDL, LDL, triglycerides, Lp(a), hs-CRP, fasting serum insulin level, and glucose. Patients with diabetes should have a recent hemoglobin A1c.

Because psychological distress, commonly measured as anxiety and depression, affects outcomes in men and women with CVD and cancer, screening is strongly recommended as a basis for intervention (Hegel et al., 2008; Székely et al., 2007). Depression is estimated to occur in 20%–30% of women with breast cancer (Chen et al., 2010; Institute of Medicine, 2004; Knobf, 2007). Anxiety is prevalent before therapy and at the end of treatment as women transition away from the medical system to survivorship, thus supporting the need for assessment (Bender, Ergÿn, Rosenzweig, Cohen, & Sereika, 2005; Institute of Medicine, 2004; Lethborg, Kissane, Burns, & Snyder, 2000; Norris, Ljubsa, & Hegadoren, 2009).

An electrocardiogram is indicated and left ventricular function is assessed in all patients prior to cardiotoxic therapy and also in patients with long-standing HTN to detect left ventricular hypertrophy. The rationale for screening (see Tables 15-2 and 15-3) is to identify risk and provide data to target interventions, specifically class I lifestyle interventions for all risk groups (smoking cessation, healthy eating, regular physical activity, and weight management) and class II (i.e., therapy for high LDL, triglycerides) and pharmacologic interventions where indicated (Berger et al., 2010; Mosca et al., 2007; Mosca, Benjamin, et al., 2011).

The Framingham Risk Assessment for Coronary Heart Disease (FRACHD) is the gold standard to identify CHD risk in midlife and older adults according to the ATP III. This tool is designed to estimate risk in adults age 20 and older who do not have heart disease or diabetes. The tool is easy to use and is carried out using Framingham risk scoring. The risk factors included in the calculation are age, total cholesterol, HDL cholesterol, systolic blood pressure, treatment for HTN, and cigarette smoking. The Framingham risk score gives estimates for "hard CHD," which includes myocardial infarction and coronary death (see Figure 15-2). The FRACHD assigns high-, moderate-, or low-risk categories based on the score but falls short of identifying general cardiovascular risk. Over the past half-century since the original FRACHD, understanding of the biologic processes underlying atherosclerosis in women has markedly shifted to encompass the complex biology of hemostasis, changes in endothelial and vascular smooth muscle dysfunction, thrombosis formation, and inflammation. Women's risk for stroke and heart failure through middle and older age typically exceeds their risk of CHD, in contrast to the pattern seen in men, where CAD occurs earlier (Mosca, Benjamin, et al., 2011) (see Figure 15-3).

As the development of the Framingham tool progressed, the CHD markers were codified into global risk scores for assessment of general overall cardiovascular risk instead of CHD risk and coincided with this knowledge concerning the pathophysiology of atherosclerosis in women (Picard, Plu-Bureau, Neves-e Castro, & Gompel, 2008; Ridker et al., 2007). Along with this new knowledge of pathophysiologic changes and shift in focus to general cardiovascular risk, it was noted that patients who are 50 years of age or older may have a high lifetime risk amenable to risk factor reduction but may be considered to be at low risk because they have a low 10-year risk with the FRACHD. CVD risk, not just CHD risk, is supported by recent data indicating that 56% of adults, including 47.5 million women overall and 64% of women 60–79 years of age, have a 10-year risk for CHD of less than 10% but a *predicted lifetime risk for CVD* of 39% or greater. Among people free of CVD at age 50, more than 50% of men and nearly 40% of women will have CVD during their lifetime (D'Agostino et al., 2008). For this reason, the

Table 15-2. American Heart Association 2011 Cardiovascular Risk Categories	
Risk Status	**Criteria**
High risk[a]	• Established coronary heart disease • CVD • Peripheral arterial disease • Abdominal aortic aneurysm • End-stage or chronic renal disease • Diabetes mellitus • 10-year Framingham global risk > 20%

At risk	• > 1 major risk factor for CVD, including
	  – Cigarette smoking
	  – Atherogenic diet (a diet high in fat, low in fiber)
	  – Physical inactivity
	• Obesity with waist circumference > 35 inches for women or > 40 inches for men
	• Family history of premature CVD (< 55 years of age in male relatives and < 65 years of age in female relatives)
	• Hypertension (BP > 130/85 mm Hg or taking BP medications)
	• Dyslipidemia (HDL < 50 mg/dl, < 40 mg/dl for men)
	• Triglycerides > 150 mg/dl, LDL > 100 mg/dl
	• Evidence of subclinical vascular disease
	• Metabolic syndrome
	• Poor exercise capacity on treadmill test and/or abnormal heart rate recovery after stopping exercise

Optimal risk	• Framingham global risk < 10% and a healthy lifestyle, with
	  – No clinical CVD
	  – Total cholesterol < 200 mg/dl
	  – HDL ≥ 50 mg/dl in women and ≥ 40 mg/dl in men
	  – Fasting blood glucose < 100 mg/dl
	  – BMI < 25 kg/m²
	  – No tobacco use
	  – Physical activity at recommended levels
	  – DASH/Mediterranean-like diet

[a] For patients at high risk, implement class I and II recommendations.

BMI—body mass index; BP—blood pressure; CVD—cardiovascular disease; DASH—Dietary Approaches to Stop Hypertension; HDL—high-density lipoprotein; LDL—low-density lipoprotein

Note. Based on information from Mosca, Benjamin, et al., 2011.

Framingham CVD Risk Profile was developed (see Figure 15-2). As of the time of this publication, the ATP III guidelines are in the process of being revised.

Because the presence of a single risk factor at 50 years of age is associated with a substantially increased lifetime absolute risk for CVD or shorter duration of survival (Lloyd-Jones et al., 2006), the 2011 update to the American Heart Association's effectiveness-based guidelines for the prevention of CVD in women highlights the need to include preexisting HTN, diabetes, valve disease, arrhythmias, obesity, family history, and poor lifestyle habits, which all contribute to CVD (Mosca, Benjamin, et al., 2011). Incorporated into the risk assessment is the national guideline for establishing a lipid profile (Grundy et al., 2004; NCEP/ATP III, 2001). A lipid profile includes total cholesterol, HDL, LDL, and triglyceride levels and usually is drawn following a 10- to 12-hour fast.

Lp(a) is a genetic marker for CVD. Excess Lp(a) is the most common inherited lipid disorder in patients with premature CAD and affects about 25% of the population. Studies suggest that Lp(a) is a strong, independent predictor of CVD, particularly in women. Evidence has supported an independent role of Lp(a) in cor-

---

Table 15-3. Therapeutic Targets and Self-Care Interventions to Reduce Risk of Metabolic Syndrome Based on Prevention Guidelines

Therapeutic Target and Goals for Therapy	Recommendations
Abdominal obesity/visceral fat • Goal: waist circumference ≤ 35 inches, waist-to-hip ratio ≤ 0.80 Atherogenic diet • Goal: nonatherogenic diet	Balance of physical activity, calorie intake, formal behavioral program in order to • Reduce waist circumference to ≤ 35 inches • Reduce waist:hip ratio to ≤ 0.80 • Reduce weight by 7%–10% in order to achieve ideal body weight. Even small amounts of weight loss are associated with significant health benefits. Mediterranean/DASH diet patterns to include • Fruits and vegetables: ≥ 4.5 cups/day • Fish: twice a week • Whole grains: 3 servings/day • Nuts, legumes, seeds: ≥ 4 servings/week • Saturated fat: < 7% total energy intake • Cholesterol: < 150 mg/day • Limiting sugary drinks and desserts • Fiber content 25–30 g/day • No more than 6 oz red wine/day • No or limited trans fat • Sodium < 1,500 mg/day
Physical inactivity • Goal: regular–moderate activity 30–60 min/day. Most days of the week (5 days/week minimum). Accumulate 150 min/week of moderate-intensity exercise or 75 min/week of vigorous exercise, or a combination of moderate and vigorous intensity. Aerobic activity can be intermittent at no less than 10-minute intervals.	• Encourage 30–60 minutes of moderate-intensity aerobic activity on most days. • Supplement with an increase in daily lifestyle activities (gardening, taking the stairs, parking farther away from destinations). Higher exercise times can be achieved by accumulating exercise throughout the day. • Encourage strength training 2 days/week (using resistance bands, kettle bells, etc.). • Recommend a medically supervised program for patients with established high risk (history of heart failure, etc.).

Resources
- University of Maryland Medical Center health calculators: Calculators for waist-to-hip ratio and for carbohydrates, fat, protein, and calories: www.healthcalculators.org/calculators
- Go Red for Women: Free online 12-week nutrition and fitness program and step-by-step guide, with tool kit available in Spanish and English: www.goredforwomen.org/betteru/index.aspx
- National Heart, Lung, and Blood Institute's "Aim for a Healthy Weight": http://www.nhlbi.nih.gov/health/public/heart/obesity/aim_hwt.pdf
- Preventive Cardiovascular Nurses Association's *Living Guidelines for Women*, adapted from the American Heart Association's heart disease prevention guidelines for women (Mosca, Benjamin, et al., 2011): www.pcna.net/documents/Living_Guidelines_for_Women.pdf

Note. Based on information from Babio et al., 2009; Grundy et al., 2004; Inzucchi et al., 2012; Mosca, Benjamin, et al., 2011.

onary disease for men and women (Bennet et al., 2008; Clarke et al., 2009; Erqou et al., 2009).

In addition to the lipid profile, hs-CRP is recommended because of its association with MetS and CVD risk. In the Women's Health Study (Pelletier et al., 2009), levels of CRP were found to increase linearly as the number of MetS criteria increased (p-trend < 0.0001), from 0.68 mg/L for women who met none of the criteria to 5.75 mg/L for women who met all five criteria for MetS (see Table 15-1). In survival analyses, an elevated hs-CRP level was similarly predictive of MetS (three or more criteria present) and of a first cardiovascular event. Similar associations have been found in men (Braga-Basaria et al., 2006; Keating et al., 2006; Levine et al., 2010).

Figure 15-2. Framingham Point Scores (Coronary Heart Disease)

Age	Points
20–34	–7
35–39	–3
40–44	0
45–49	3
50–54	6
55–59	8
60–64	10
65–69	12
70–74	14
75–79	16

HDL (mg/dl)	Points
≥ 60	–1
50–59	0
40–49	4
< 40	2

Systolic BP (mm Hg)	If Untreated	If Treated
<120	0	0
120–129	1	3
130–139	2	4
140–159	3	5
≥ 160	4	6

Point Total	10-Year Risk (%)
< 9	< 1
9	1
10	1
11	1
12	1
13	2
14	2
15	3
16	4
17	5
18	6
19	8
20	11
21	14
22	17
23	22
24	27
≥ 25	≥ 30

	Age				
Total Cholesterol	20–39	40–49	50–59	60–69	70–79
< 160	0	0	0	0	0
160–199	4	3	2	1	1
200–239	8	6	4	2	1
240–279	11	8	5	3	2
≥ 280	13	10	7	4	2
	20–39	40–49	50–59	60–69	70–79
Nonsmoker	0	0	0	0	0
Smoker	9	7	4	2	1

Note. Data tables courtesy of the Framingham Heart Study and the National Heart, Lung, and Blood Institute.

Figure 15-3. Framingham Heart Study Estimate of Risk of General Cardiovascular Disease in Women

CVD Points

Points	Age	HDL	Total Cholesterol	SBP Not Treated	SBP Treated	Smoker	Diabetes
< −3				< 120			
−2		60+					
−1		50–59			< 120		
0	30–34	45–49	< 160	120–129		No	No
1		35–44	160–199	130–139			
2	35-39	<35		140–149	120–129		
3			200–239		130–139	Yes	
4	40–44		240–279	150–159			Yes
5	45–49		280+	160+	140–149		
6					150–159		
7	50–54				160+		
8	55–59						
9	60–64						
10	65–69						
11	70–74						
12	75+						

CVD Risk

Points	Risk	Points	Risk	Points	Risk
−2 or less	Below 1%	6	3.3%	14	11.7%
−1	1.0%	7	3.9%	15	13.7%
0	1.2%	8	4.5%	16	15.9%
1	1.5%	9	5.3%	17	18.5%
2	1.7%	10	6.3%	18	21.5%
3	2.0%	11	7.3%	19	24.8%
4	2.4%	12	8.6%	20	28.5%
5	2.8%	13	10.0%	21+	Above 30%

Heart Age/Vascular Age

Points	Heart Age	Points	Heart Age
Less than 1	Younger than 30	8	51
1	31	9	55
2	34	10	59
3	36	11	64
4	39	12	68
5	45	13	73
6	45	14	79
7	48	15+	Older than 80

CVD—cardiovascular disease; HDL—high-density lipoprotein; SBP—systolic blood pressure

Note. Data tables courtesy of the Framingham Heart Study and the National Heart, Lung, and Blood Institute.

Biomarkers as Potential Predictors of Cardiotoxicity

Two biomarkers, B-type natriuretic peptide (BNP, also known as brain natriuretic peptide) and troponin, have been proposed to identify myocardial injury that will predict subsequent ventricular dysfunction (Ewer & Ewer, 2010; Verma & Ewer, 2011). Increases in the plasma BNP concentration have been demonstrated in pediatric patients with cancer who are treated with anthracyclines (Hayakawa et al., 2001) and correlate with decreases in left ventricular mass (Germanakis et al., 2006). In patients with breast cancer, a correlation between plasma BNP concentration and decreases in left ventricular ejection fraction (LVEF) have been reported (Pichon et al., 2005). Although one study demonstrated no changes in plasma BNP concentration immediately (10 minutes) after trastuzumab infusion (Knobloch, Tepe, Lichtinghagen, Luck, & Vogt, 2008), insufficient data exist regarding the use of BNP concentrations to identify individuals at risk, and more research is needed.

Troponin may be the most sensitive biomarker to date for myocardial damage (Verma & Ewer, 2011; Zambelli et al., 2011). Four studies have been published regarding the use of serum troponin in the setting of chemotherapy: one was a study of patients receiving high-dose chemotherapy for hematologic malignancies (Auner et al., 2003), and three were of patients receiving high-dose chemotherapy primarily for advanced breast cancer (Cardinale et al., 2000, 2002, 2004). In the three breast cancer studies, troponin was measured soon after each dose of chemotherapy and at 12, 24, 36, and 72 hours later. These studies showed that 30%–33% of patients had an increase in serum troponin concentrations after chemotherapy; the highest rise was soon after chemotherapy administration, and troponin levels remained elevated at 72 hours in 10%–13% of the patients. Changes in left ventricular function were also monitored and found to be correlated with troponin levels. A significant pattern of elevated troponin and declines in LVEF occurred across all three studies (Cardinale et al., 2000, 2002, 2004). These investigators concluded that troponin had an 84% positive predictive value for cardiac toxicity and a 99% negative predictive value (Cardinale et al., 2004). A smaller rise in troponin and its persisted duration suggest more minor myocardial damage; however, even this level of damage appears to predict subsequent cardiac dysfunction (Auner et al., 2003; Cardinale et al., 2000). A recent study evaluating troponin in 251 women with breast cancer receiving trastuzumab reported that 14% of the patients had elevated troponin levels (Cardinale et al., 2010). Of the women in that study who developed cardiotoxicity, 62% of women had elevated troponin levels compared to 5% of women with normal levels. Prior anthracycline chemotherapy and a lower baseline LVEF increased the risk of cardiotoxicity, but elevated serum troponin predicted women at higher risk for cardiac toxicity and those who did not recover ventricular function. Whether troponin will be an equally sensitive marker of myocardial damage with standard-dose chemotherapy is unknown.

Neuregulin is the ligand for ErbB receptors (the target of trastuzumab). It is synthesized by vascular endothelial cells and released in response to a number of different stimuli (Kalinowski et al., 2010; Lemmens, Doggen, & De Keulenaer, 2007). Elevated serum levels of neuregulin have been shown to be associated with poor prognosis in patients with congestive heart failure (Ky et al., 2009). This finding has been proposed to be a result of the body's attempts to activate ErbB cardioprotection (by increasing synthesis and release of neuregulin) in the failing heart. In the setting of interrupted ErbB signaling by trastuzumab combined with subsequent cardiac injury (especially when compounded by additional cardiotoxic drugs such as anthracyclines), a similar mechanism of neuregulin release may occur. This released neuregulin therefore may serve as an early marker of cardiac injury in patients undergoing chemotherapy with these agents (Ky et al., 2009). Research is needed to define the role of neuregulin in the identification of patients who are at risk and for whom intervention is indicated.

Monitoring biomarkers during cancer treatment may be as important a component to determining overall cardiovascular risk as monitoring for HTN, diabetes, and obesity because their presence, whether alone or in combination, may affect left ventricular function and the incidence of heart failure over time. As cardiovascular risks predispose a patient to left ventricular dysfunction and heart failure, it would seem that the addition of cardiotoxic therapy can only support the "multiple hit" hypothesis (Jones et al., 2007). ("Multiple hit" refers to the additional cardiovascular risk associated with chemotherapy superimposed on preexisting risk.) A thorough pretreatment assessment combined with consistent surveillance and intervention may alter the increased risk for preclinical or clinical CVD.

Cardiovascular Surveillance Recommendations

Recommendations for cardiovascular screening and surveillance are based on the current state of the science as outlined in this and previous chapters addressing both cardiovascular risk and cancer treatment (see Figure 15-4).

Because radiation, anthracycline-based therapies, and trastuzumab are all associated with adverse cardiac outcomes, including heart failure, nurses should be cognizant of the potential for cardiovascular complications during long-term follow-up. Routine follow-up should continue indefinitely.

Management

AHA refers to ideal cardiovascular health as "the simple 7" (see http://mylifecheck .heart.org):
- Never smoked or has not smoked for more than one year
- BMI less than 25
- Physical activity of 150 min/week of moderate-intensity exercise or 75 min/week of vigorous-intensity exercise
- Total cholesterol less than 200 mg/dl
- Blood pressure less than 120/80 mm Hg
- Fasting glucose less than 100 mg/dl
- Diet that includes four of the six recommended components of a healthy diet (diet rich in fruits and vegetables, fiber, low sodium, low fat, limited intake of processed meats, increased intake of fish).

The achievement of ideal cardiovascular health is defined by the Healthy People 2020 health objectives for all Americans (Bambs et al., 2011; Yancy, 2011). Many risk factors associated with the development of CVD can be modified with healthy lifestyle interventions (see Table 15-3). A healthy diet, regular physical activity, smoking cessation, and maintenance of a healthy weight (or weight loss if indicated) can reduce the risk of CVD, cancer, and diabetes (Eyre, Kahn, & Robertson, 2004; Lloyd-Jones et al., 2006; Mosca, Benjamin, et al., 2011). A healthy diet is characterized by high fiber; daily consumption of five or more servings of vegetables and fruits; rich in legumes and fish; moderate in alcohol; low in red meat, processed meats, sodium

---

Figure 15-4. Assessment, Management, and Long-Term Surveillance

Assessment of Cardiovascular Risk
- Baseline data
- Medical and family history
- Symptoms of cardiovascular disease
- Physical examination including BP, waist circumference, weight, cardiovascular and pulmonary assessment
- Laboratory tests including lipids, lipoproteins, Lp(a), hs-CRP, fasting serum insulin level, glucose
- Framingham General Risk Profile if no diabetes or cardiovascular disease. If diabetes and/or documented cardiovascular disease, secondary prevention measures should be instituted. This would include an LDL target of 70 mg/dl or less.
- Depression screening
- Menopausal status
- ECG and evaluation of LV function

Management Goals
- Referral to cardiology
  - For known cardiovascular disease
  - For decreased LV function for monitoring and treatment with carvedilol and/or ACE inhibitors
- Lifestyle behaviors (see recommendations in Figure 15-3)
- Lipid management
  - LDL < 100 mg/dl (< 70 mg/dl for high-risk patients)
  - Total cholesterol < 200 mg/dl
  - HDL ≥ 40 mg/dl for men, ≥ 50 mg/dl for women
  - Triglycerides ≤ 150 mg/dl (hs-CRP) ≤ 1 mg/dl
- Blood pressure management
  - Maintain BP ≤ 130/85 mm Hg
  - Ideal ≤ 120/80 mm Hg
- Waist circumference
  - ≤ 35 inches for women
  - ≤ 40 inches for men
- Maintain glucose ≤ 100 mg/dl
- Insulin ≤ 15 mg/dl

Long-Term Surveillance Following Cardiotoxic Cancer Treatment
- Annual cardiology assessment to determine LV function either by echocardiography or multigated blood pool scan* (MUGA)
- Lipid profile
- Glucose
- Insulin
- Waist circumference
- Weight
- BP
- Assessment of lifestyle behaviors

---

* Additional testing may be required for those who have received left chest radiation alone or in combination with cardiotoxic chemotherapy in order to evaluate for coronary and/or valvular fibrosis.

ACE—angiotensin-converting enzyme; BP—blood pressure; ECG—electrocardiogram; HDL—high-density lipoprotein; hs-CRP—high-sensitivity cardiac C-reactive protein; LDL—low-density lipoprotein; Lp(a)—lipoprotein-a; LV—left ventricular

Note. Based on information from Lenihan & Esteva, 2008; Levine et al., 2010; Redig & Munshi, 2010; Shenoy et al., 2011.

(less than 1,500 mg/day), refined carbohydrates, whole-fat dairy products, and sweetened beverages, and one that does not include trans-fatty acids. Moderate-intensity physical activity of 30 minutes most days of the week is recommended for adults to reduce cardiovascular risk (AHA, 2010; Artinian et al., 2010). Exercise has been shown to improve cardiovascular fitness (Dunn et al., 2005; Manson et al., 2002; Stampfer, Hu, Manson, Rimm, & Willett, 2000), reduce blood pressure (Pescatello et al., 2004; Whelton, Chin, Xin, & He, 2002), and improve lipid levels (Kelley, Kelley, & Tran, 2004a, 2004b). Exercise as a risk reduction and health promotion strategy in cancer survivors has a strong evidence base (deBacker, Schep, Backs, Vreugdenhil, & Kulpers, 2009; Kim, Kang, & Park, 2009; Schmitz et al., 2010; Speck, Courneya Mâsse, Duval, & Schmitz, 2010). Exercise in cancer survivors has been shown to improve overall cardiovascular fitness, aerobic capacity, quality of life, psychosocial functioning, muscle strength, and body composition and reduce depression, anxiety, fatigue, and sleep alterations (deBacker et al., 2009; Duijts, Faber, Oldenburg, van Beurden, & Aaronson, 2011; Ferrer, Huedo-Medina, Johnson, Ryan, & Pescatello, 2011; Jones et al., 2011; Kim et al., 2009; Schmitz et al., 2010; Speck et al., 2010). It also has been shown to decrease risk of recurrence and improve survival (Holick et al., 2008; Holmes, Chen, Feskanich, Kroenke, & Colditz, 2004). For cancer survivors who are overweight or obese, weight loss is indicated. To achieve an energy balance that results in weight loss, more time engaged in moderate-intensity exercise per day is required (e.g., 60 minutes), and healthy diet plus increased energy expenditure will enhance outcomes (Chaput et al., 2011; Goodpaster et al., 2010; Slentz et al., 2004). Dietary intervention alone can improve the quality of a survivor's diet, indicating adoption of the recommended healthy risk reduction diet (Demark-Wahnefried et al., 2007; Pekmezi & Demark-Wahnefried, 2011; Pierce et al., 2007). However, although a few studies have suggested that diet combined with cognitive-behavioral therapy or counseling can result in weight loss and improved lipid levels (Thomson et al., 2009), dietary modification alone appears to be an insufficient stimulus as a weight loss intervention, especially in overweight and obese survivors (Demark-Wahnefried et al., 2007; Demark-Wahnefried & Jones, 2008; Loprinzi et al.,1996; Saquib et al., 2009). Combined diet and exercise interventions that include components of cognitive-behavioral therapy (e.g., motivation, feedback) are indicated to effect behavior changes and achieve goals of weight loss for overweight and obese cancer survivors.

Lifestyle behaviors, specifically physical activity, should be recommended to all survivors to maintain a healthy lipid profile or reduce elevated lipids (Kelley et al., 2004a, 2004b). Pharmacologic therapy is the cornerstone of management for patients with elevated lipids. Statins (3-hydroxyl 3-methyl glutaryl coenzyme A reductase [HMG COA] inhibitors) have an established benefit in primary and secondary prevention of acute coronary syndromes, cerebrovascular accidents (Amarenco et al., 2006), and venous thromboembolism (Glynn et al., 2009). Statins target lipid metabolism, have significant anti-inflammatory properties, and also reduce cardiovascular morbidity and mortality in patients with cancer (Katz, 2005; Katz et al., 2005). Also, a substantial body of literature from observational studies reports an association between statin use and a decrease in cancer incidence (Blais, Desgagné, & LeLorier, 2000; Cauley et al., 2003; Farwell et al., 2008; Fortuny et al., 2006; Karp, Behlouli, Lelorier, & Pilote, 2008; Khurana, Bejjanki, Caldito, & Owens, 2007; Poynter et al., 2005; Shannon et al., 2005). A lower incidence of venous thromboembolism has also been reported in patients with cancer who are taking statins (Khemasuwan, DiVietro, Tangdhanakanond, Pomerantz, & Eiger, 2010). Statins have been shown to induce apoptosis and inhibit tumor growth, angiogenesis, and metastases along multiple cell lines and may act synergistically with chemotherapy to improve cancer outcomes (Li, Park, Ye, Kim, & Kim, 2006; Nowakowski et al., 2010; Vaklavas, Chatzizisis, & Tsimberidou, 2011). The addition of pravastatin to induction chemotherapy for acute myeloid leukemia appeared to enhance the antitumor effect (Kornblau et al., 2007). Statins may have a role in reducing the risk of recurrence. A prospective, randomized, placebo-controlled phase III trial of rosuvastatin (Crestor®) in patients with stage I or stage II colon cancer is ongoing (see http://clinicaltrials .gov, Identifier: NCT01011478). A similar trial with atorvastatin (Lipitor®) in colorectal cancer was recently completed with results pending (see http://clinicaltrials.gov, Identifier: NCT00335504).

Conclusion

Susceptibility to CVD in cancer survivors is multifactorial and requires the scientific and clinical knowledge of cardiology and oncology specialists (Giordano & Hortobagyi, 2007; Lenihan & Esteva, 2008). It is a critical time for cardiology and oncology to collaborate in risk identification and develop risk reduction interventions to enhance the quality of life for cancer survivors and decrease all-cause mortality (Albini et al., 2010; Giordano & Hortobagyi, 2007; Lenihan & Esteva, 2008; Zambelli et al., 2011). Early identification of CVD risk factors, along with early referral to cardiology, provides the opportunity to target interventions to reduce risk and improve quality of life and survival outcomes. Survivors are interested in what they can do to improve their health and reduce their risks of comorbid illness (Knobf, 2002), yet health promotion information is not routinely provided by oncologists (Arora, Reeve, Hays, Clauser, & Oakley-Girvan, 2011). Nursing practice is based upon a health and wellness continuum that lends itself to a comprehensive focus of care (Pender, Murdaugh, & Parsons, 2011). Nurses are uniquely situated to address this gap in care. Promotion of healthy lifestyle behaviors (physical activity, healthy diet, smoking cessation, and stress management) is an important therapeutic strategy to the long-term survival of this vulnerable population (Knobf & Coviello, 2011).

Interdisciplinary collaboration in the follow-up care and for health promotion is essential to coordination and continuity of care. Providers with expertise from oncology, cardiology, exercise physiology, nutrition science, psychology, and primary care need to develop and maintain a coordinated effort to support the care of cancer survivors who are at risk for chronic illness. Research is needed to validate the cardiovascular risk interventions to improve outcomes in cancer treatment.

References

Abu-Khalaf, M.M., & Harris, L. (2009). Anthracycline-induced cardiotoxicity: Risk assessment and management. *Oncology, 23,* 239, 244, 252.

Albert, C.M., Chae, C.U., Rexrode, K.M., Manson, J.E., & Kawachi, I. (2010). Phobic anxiety and risk of coronary heart disease and sudden death among women. *Circulation, 111,* 480–487. doi:10.1161/01 .CIR.0000153813.64165.5D

Albini, A., Pennesi, G., Donatelli, F., Cammarota, R., De Flora, S., & Noonan, D.M. (2010). Cardiotoxicity of anticancer drugs: The need for cardio-oncology and cardio-oncological prevention. *Journal of the National Cancer Institute, 102,* 14–25. doi:10.1093/jnci/djp440

Amarenco, P., Bogousslavsky, J., Callahan, A., 3rd, Goldstein, L.B., Hennerici, M., Rudolph, A.E., ... Zivin, J.A. (2006). High-dose atorvastatin after stroke or transient ischemic attack. *New England Journal of Medicine, 355,* 549–559. doi:10.1056/NEJMoa061894

American Cancer Society. (2012). Cancer facts and figures 2012. Retrieved from http://www.cancer. org/Research/CancerFactsFigures/index

American Heart Association. (2010). Heart disease and stroke statistics. Retrieved from http://www. americanheart.org/downloadable/heart/1265665152970DS-3241%20HeartStrokeUpdate_2010.pdf

Arora, N.K., Reeve, B.B., Hays, R.D., Clauser, S.B., & Oakley-Girvan, I. (2011). Assessment of quality of cancer-related follow-up from the cancer survivor's perspective. *Journal of Clinical Oncology, 29,* 1280–1289. doi:10.1200/JCO.2010.32.1554

Artinian, N.T., Fletcher, G.F., Mozaffarian, D., Kris-Etherton, P., VanHorn, L., & Lichetenstein, A.H. (2010). Interventions to promote physical activity and dietary lifestyle changes for cardiovascular risk factor reduction in adults: A scientific statement from the American Heart Association. *Circulation, 122,* 406–441. doi:10.1161/CIR.0b013e3181e8edf1

Auner, H.W., Tinchon, C., Linkesh, W., Tiran, A., Quehenberger, F., Link, H., & Still, H. (2003). Prolonged monitoring of troponin T in the detection of anthracycline cardiotoxicity in adults with hematologic malignancies. *Annals of Hematology, 82,* 218–222.

Babio, N., Bulló, M., & Salas-Salvadó, J. (2009). Mediterranean diet and metabolic syndrome: The evidence. *Public Health Nutrition, 12,* 1607–1617. doi:10.1017/S1368980009990449

Bambs, C., Kip, K.E., Dinga, A., Mulukutla, S.R., Aiyer, A.N., & Reis, S.E. (2011). Low prevalence of "ideal cardiovascular health" in a community-based population: The Heart Strategies Concentrating on Risk Evaluation (Heart SCORE) Study. *Circulation, 123,* 850–857. doi:10.1161/CIRCULATIONAHA.110.980151

Beckie, T.M., Fletcher, G.F., Beckstead, J.W., Schocken, D.D., & Evans, M.E. (2008). Adverse baseline physiological and psychosocial profiles of women enrolled in a cardiac rehabilitation clinical trial. *Journal of Cardiopulmonary Rehabilitation and Prevention, 28,* 52–60. doi:10.1097/01.HCR.0000311510.16226.6e

Bender, C.M., Ergÿn, F.S., Rosenzweig, M.Q., Cohen, S.M., & Sereika, S.M. (2005). Symptom clusters in breast cancer across 3 phases of the disease. *Cancer Nursing, 28,* 219–225. doi:10.1097/00002820-200505000-00011

Bennet, A., Di Angelantonio, E., Erquo, S., Eiriksdottir, G., Sigurdsson, G., Woodward, M., ... Gudnason, V. (2008). Lipoprotein(a) levels and risk of future coronary heart disease: Large-scale prospective data. *Archives of Internal Medicine, 168,* 598–608. doi:10.1001/archinte.168.6.598

Berger, J.S., Jordan, C.O., Lloyd-Jones, D., & Blumenthal, R.S. (2010). Screening for cardiovascular risk in asymptomatic patients. *Journal of the American College of Cardiology, 53,* 1169–1177. doi:10.1016/j.jacc.2009.09.066

Bittner, V. (2009). Menopause, age and cardiovascular risk. *Journal of American College of Cardiology, 54,* 2374–2375. doi:10.1016/j.jacc.2009.10.008

Blais, L., Desgagné, A., & LeLorier, J. (2000). 3-Hydroxy-3-methylglutaryl coenzyme A reductase inhibitors and the risk of cancer: A nested case-control study. *Archives of Internal Medicine, 160,* 2363–2368. doi:10.1001/archinte.160.15.2363

Bouchard, C., Després, J.P., & Mauriège, P. (1993). Genetic and nongenetic determinants of regional fat distribution. *Endocrine Reviews, 14,* 72–93. doi:10.1210/edrv-14-1-72

Boyd, D.B. (2003). Insulin and cancer. *Integrative Cancer Therapies, 2,* 315–329. doi:10.1177/1534735403259152

Braga-Basaria, M., Dobs, A.S., Muller, D.C., Carducci, M.A., John, M., Egan, J., & Basaria, S. (2006). Metabolic syndrome in men with prostate cancer undergoing long-term androgen-deprivation therapy. *Journal of Clinical Oncology, 24,* 3979–3983. doi:10.1200/JCO.2006.05.9741

Braithwaite, D., Tammemagi, C.M., Moore, D.H., Ozanne, E.M., Hiatt, R.A., Belkora J., ... Esserman, L. (2009). Hypertension is an independent predictor of survival disparity between African-American and white breast cancer patients. *International Journal of Cancer, 124,* 1213–1219. doi:10.1002/ijc.24054

Cabana, M.D., & Kim, C.K. (2003). Physician adherence to preventive cardiology guidelines for women. *Women's Health Issues, 13,* 142–149. doi:10.1016/S1049-3867(03)00034-3

Cardinale, D., Colombo, A., Torrisi, R., Sandri, M.T., Civelli, M., Salvatici, M., ... Cipolla, C.M. (2010). Trastuzumab-induced cardiotoxicity: Clinical and prognostic implications of troponin I evaluation. *Journal of Clinical Oncology, 28,* 3910–3916. doi:10.1200/JCO.2009.27.3615

Cardinale, D., Sandri, M.T., Colombo, A., Colombo, N., Boeri, M., Lamantia, G., ... Cipolla, C.M. (2004). Prognostic value of troponin I in cardiac risk stratification of cancer patients undergoing high-dose chemotherapy. *Circulation, 109,* 2749–2754. doi:10.1161/01.CIR.0000130926.51766.CC

Cardinale, D., Sandri, M.T. , Martinoni, A., Borghini, E., Civelli, M., Lamantia, G., ... Cipolla, C.M. (2002). Myocardial injury revealed by plasma troponin I in breast cancer patients treated with high-dose chemotherapy. *Annals of Oncology, 13,* 710–715. doi:10.1093/annonc/mdf170

Cardinale, D., Sandri, M.T., Martinoni, A., Tricca, A., Civelli, M., Lamantia, G., ... Fiorentini, C. (2000). Left ventricular dysfunction predicted by early troponin I release after high-dose chemotherapy. *Journal of the American College of Cardiology, 36,* 517–522. doi:10.1016/S0735-1097(00)00748-8

Cauley, J.A., Zmuda, J.M., Lui, L.Y., Hillier, T.A., Ness, R.B., Stone, K.L., ... Bauer, D.C. (2003). Lipid-lowering drug use and breast cancer in older women: A prospective study. *Journal of Women's Health, 12,* 749–756. doi:10.1089/154099903322447710

Chapman, J.W., Meng, D., Shepherd, L., Parulekar, W., Inge, J.N., & Muss, H. (2008). Competing causes of death from a randomized trial of extended adjuvant endocrine therapy for breast cancer. *Journal of the National Cancer Institute, 100,* 252–260. doi:10.1093/jnci/djn014

Chaput, J.P., Klingenberg, L., Rosenkilde, M., Gilbert, J.A., Tremblay, A., & Sjödin, A. (2011). Physical activity plays an important role in body weight regulation. *Journal of Obesity.* doi:10.1155/2011/360257

Chen, T.H., Gona, P., Sutherland, P.A., Benjamin, E.S., Wilson, P.W., Larson, M.G., ... Robins, S.J. (2009). Long-term c-reactive protein variability and prediction of metabolic risk. *American Journal of Medicine, 122,* 53–61. doi:10.1016/j.amjmed.2008.08.023

Chen, X., Lu, W., Zheng, Y., Gu, K., Chen, Z., Zheng, W., & Shu, X. (2010). Exercise, tea consumption, and depression among breast cancer survivors. *Journal of Clinical Oncology, 28,* 991–998. doi:10.1200/JCO.2009.23.0565

Chobanian, A.V., Bakris, G.L., Black, H.R., Cushman, W.C., Green, L.A., Izzo, J.L., Jr., ... Roccella, E.J. (2003). The seventh report of the Joint National Committee on Prevention, Detection, Evaluation, and Treatment of High Blood Pressure: The JNC 7 report. *JAMA, 289,* 2560–2572. doi:10.1001/jama.289.19.2560

Christian, A.H., Mills, T., Simpson, S.L., & Mosca, L. (2006). Quality of cardiovascular disease preventative care and physician/practice characteristics. *Journal of General Internal Medicine, 21,* 231–237. doi:10.1111/j.1525-1497.2006.00331.x

Clarke, R., Peden, J.F., Hopewell, J.C., Kyriakou, T., Goel, A., Heath, S., ... Farrall, M. (2009). Genetic variants associated with Lp(a) lipoprotein level and coronary disease. *New England Journal of Medicine, 361,* 2518–2528. doi:10.1056/NEJMoa0902604

Collins, P., Rosano, G., Casey, C., Daly, C., Gambacciani, M., Hadji, P., ... Stramba-Badiale, M. (2007). Management of cardiovascular risk in the perimenopausal women: A consensus statement of European cardiologists and gynecologists. *Climacteric, 10,* 508–526. doi:10.1080/13697130701755213

Coviello, J., LeClerque, S., & Knobf, M.T. (in press). Assessing and managing metabolic syndrome and cardiovascular risk in mid-life women. *Journal of Cardiovascular Nursing.*

D'Agostino, R.B., Sr., Vasan, R.S., Pencina, M.J., Wolf, P.A., Cobain, M., Massaro, J.M., & Kannel, W.B. (2008). General cardiovascular risk profile for use in primary care: The Framingham Heart Study. *Circulation, 117,* 743–753. doi:10.1161/CIRCULATIONAHA.107.699579

Daher, I.N., & Yeh, E.T.H. (2008). Vascular complications of selected cancer therapies. *Nature Clinical Practice: Cardiovascular Medicine, 5,* 797–805. doi:10.1038/ncpcardio1375

deBacker, I.C., Schep, G., Backs, F.J., Vreugdenhil, G., & Kulpers, H. (2009). Resistance training in cancer survivors: A systematic review. *International Journal of Sports Medicine, 30,* 703–712. doi:10.1055/s-0029-1225330

Demark-Wahnefried, W., Clipp, E.C., Lipkus, I.M., Lobach, D., Snyder, D.C., Sloane, R., ... Kraus, W.E. (2007). Main outcomes of the FRESH START trial: A sequentially tailored, diet and exercise mailed print intervention among breast and prostate cancer survivors. *Journal of Clinical Oncology, 25,* 2709–2718. doi:10.1200/JCO.2007.10.7094

Demark-Wahnefried, W., & Jones, L.W. (2008). Promoting a healthy lifestyle among cancer survivors. *Hematology/Oncology Clinics of North America, 22,* 319–342. doi:10.1016/j.hoc.2008.01.012

Demark-Wahnefried, W., Peterson, B., McBride, C., Lipkus, I., & Clipp, E. (2000). Current health behaviors and readiness to pursue life-style changes among men and women diagnosed with early stage prostate and breast carcinomas. *Cancer, 88,* 674–684.

Derweesh, I.H., Diblasio, C.J., Kincade, M.C., Malcolm, J.B., Lamar, K.D., Patterson, A.L., ... Wake, R.W. (2007). Risk of new-onset diabetes mellitus and worsening glycaemic variables for established diabetes in men undergoing androgen-deprivation therapy for prostate cancer. *BJU International, 100,* 1060–1065.

Duijts, S.F., Faber, M.M., Oldenburg, H.S., van Beurden, M., & Aaronson, N.K. (2011). Effectiveness of behavioral techniques and physical exercise on psychosocial functioning and health-related quality of life in breast cancer patients and survivors—A meta-analysis. *Psycho-Oncology, 20,* 115–126. doi:10.1002/pon.1728

Dunn, A.L., Marcus, B.H., Kampert, J.B., Garcia, M.E., Kohl, H.W., & Blair, S.N. (2005). Comparison of lifestyle and structured interventions to increase physical activity and cardiorespiratory fitness. *JAMA, 281,* 327–334. doi:10.1001/jama.281.4.327

Erickson, K., Patterson, R.E., Flatt, S.W., Natarajan, L., Parker, B.A., Heath, D.D., ... Pierce, J.P., (2011). Clinically defined type 2 diabetes mellitus and prognosis in early-stage breast cancer. *Journal of Clinical Oncology, 29,* 54–60. doi:10.1200/JCO.2010.29.3183

Erqou, S., Kaptoge, S., Perry, P.L., Di Angelantonio, E., Thompson, A., White, I.R., ... Danesh, J. (2009). Lipoprotein(a) concentration and the risk of coronary heart disease, stroke, and nonvascular mortality. *JAMA, 302,* 412–423. doi:10.1001/jama.2009.1063

Eshtiaghi, R., Esteghamati, A., & Nakhjavani, M. (2010). Menopause is an independent predictor of metabolic syndrome in Iranian women. *Maturitas, 65,* 262–266. doi:10.1016/j.maturitas.2009.11.004

Esteva, F.J., & Hortobagyi, G.N. (2006). Comparative assessment of lipid effects of endocrine therapy for breast cancer: Implications for cardiovascular disease prevention in postmenopausal women. *Breast, 15,* 301–312. doi:10.1016/j.breast.2005.08.033

Ewer, M.S., & Ewer, S.M. (2010). Cardiotoxicity of anticancer treatments: What the cardiologist needs to know. *Nature Review Cardiology, 7,* 564–575. doi:10.1038/nrcardio.2010.121

Ewer, M.S., & Gluck, S. (2009). A woman's heart. The impact of adjuvant endocrine therapy on cardiovascular health. *Cancer, 115,* 1813–1826. doi:10.1002/cncr.24219

Ewer, M.S., Swain, S.M., Cardinale, D., Fadol, A., & Suter, T.M. (2011). Cardiac dysfunction after cancer treatment. *Texas Heart Institute Journal, 38,* 248–252.

Eyre, H., Kahn R., & Robertson R. (2004). Preventing cancer, cardiovascular disease and diabetes. A common agenda for the American Cancer Society, the American Diabetes Association and the American Heart Association. *Circulation, 109,* 3244–3255. doi:10.1161/01.CIR.0000133321.00456.00

Farwell, W.R., Scranton, R.E., Lawler, E.V., Lew, R.A., Brophy, M.T., Fiore, L.D., & Gaziano, J.M. (2008). The association between statins and cancer incidence in a veterans population. *Journal of the National Cancer Institute, 100,* 134–139. doi:10.1093/jnci/djm286

Ferdinand, K.C. (2006). Ethnic, gender, and age-related differences in treatment of dyslipidemia. *American Journal of Managed Care, 12*(Suppl. 15), s400–s404.

Ferketich, A.K., Schwartzbaum, J.A., Frid, D.J., & Moeschberger, M.L. (2000). Depression as an antecedent to heart disease among women and men in the NHANES I Study. *Archives of Internal Medicine, 160,* 1261–1268. doi:10.1001/archinte.160.9.1261

Ferrer, R.A., Huedo-Medina, T.B., Johnson, B.T., Ryan, S., & Pescatello, L.S. (2011). Exercise interventions for cancer survivors: A meta-analysis of quality of life outcomes. *Annals of Behavioral Medicine, 41,* 32–47. doi:10.1007/s12160-010-9225-1

Fortuny, J., de Sanjosé, S., Becker, N., Maynadié, M., Cocco, P.L., Staines, A., ... Boffetta, P. (2006). Statin use and risk of lymphoid neoplasms: Results from the European Case-control study EPILYMPH. *Cancer Epidemiology, Biomarkers and Prevention, 15,* 921–925. doi:10.1158/1055-9965.EPI-05-0866

Gallo, W.T., Bradley, E.H., Falba, T.A., Dubin, J.A., Cramer, L.D., Bogardus, S.T., Jr., & Kasl, S.V. (2004). Involuntary job loss as a risk factor for subsequent myocardial infarction and stroke: Findings from the Health and Retirement Survey. *American Journal of Industrial Medicine, 45,* 408–416. doi:10.1002/ajim.20004

Gaspard, U. (2009). Hyperinsulinaemia, a key factor of the metabolic syndrome in postmenopausal women. *Maturitas, 62,* 362–365. doi:10.1016/j.maturitas.2008.11.026

Gaziano, J.M. (2008). Global burden of cardiovascular disease. In P. Libby, R. Bonow, D. Mann, & D. Zipes (Eds.), *Braunwald's heart disease: A textbook of cardiovascular medicine* (8th ed., pp. 1–22). Philadelphia, PA: Elsevier Saunders.

Germanakis, I., Kalmanti, M., Parthenakis, F., Nikitovic, D., Stiakaki, E., Patrianakos, A., & Vardas, P.E. (2006). Correlation of plasma N-terminal pro-brain natriuretic peptide levels with left ventricle mass in children treated with anthracyclines. *International Journal of Cardiology, 108,* 212–215. doi:10.1016/j.ijcard.2005.05.006

Gidding, S.S. (2010). Assembling evidence to justify prevention of atherosclerosis beginning in youth. *Circulation, 122,* 2493–2494. doi:10.1161/CIRCULATIONAHA.110.992123

Giordano, S.H., & Hortobagyi, G. (2007). Local recurrence or cardiovascular disease: Pay now or later [Editorial]. *Journal of the National Cancer Institute, 99,* 340–341. doi:10.1093/jnci/djk085

Glynn, R.J., Danielson, E., Fonseca, F.A.H., Genest, J., Gotto, A.M., Jr., Kastelein, J.J., ... Ridker, P.M. (2009). A randomized trial of rosuvastatin in the prevention of venous thromboembolism. *New England Journal of Medicine, 360,* 1851–1861. doi:10.1056/NEJMoa0900241

Goodpaster, B.H., DeLany, J.P., Otto, A.D., Kuller, L., Vockley, J., South-Paul, J.E., ... Jakicic, J.M. (2010). Effects of diet and physical activity interventions on weight loss and cardiometabolic risk factors in severely obese adults. *JAMA, 304,* 1795–1802. doi:10.1001/jama.2010.1505

Goodwin, P.J., Ennis, M., Pritchard, K.I., Trudeau, M.E., Koo, J., Maddamas, Y., ... Hood, N. (2002). Fasting insulin and outcome in early-stage breast cancer: Results of a prospective cohort study. *Journal of Clinical Oncology, 20,* 42–51. doi:10.1200/JCO.20.1.42

Goodwin, P.J., Ligibel, J.A., & Stambolic, V. (2009). Metformin in breast cancer: Time for action [Editorial]. *Journal of Clinical Oncology, 27,* 3271–3273. doi:10.1200/JCO.2009.22.1630

Granger, C.B. (2006). Prediction and prevention of chemotherapy-induced cardiomyopathy. Can it be done? *Circulation, 114,* 2432–2433. doi:10.1161/CIRCULATIONAHA.106.666248

Grundy, S.M., Cleeman, J.I., Merz, C.N., Brewer, H.B., Clark, L.T., Hunninghake, D.B., ... Stone, N.S. (2004). Implications of recent clinical trials for the National Cholesterol Education Program Adult Treatment Panel III guidelines. *Circulation, 110,* 227–239. doi:10.1161/01.CIR.0000133317.49796.0E

Hamer, M., Chida, Y., & Stamatakis, E. (2010). Association of very highly elevated C-reactive protein concentration with cardiovascular events and all-cause mortality. *Clinical Chemistry, 56,* 132–135. doi:10.1373/clinchem.2009.130740

Hamer, M., Molloy, G.J., & Stamatakis, E. (2008). Psychological distress as a risk factor for cardiovascular events: Pathophysiological and behavioral mechanisms. *Journal of the American College of Cardiology, 52,* 2156–2162. doi:10.1016/j.jacc.2008.08.057

Hanrahan, E.D., Gonzalez-Argulo, A.M., Giordano, S.H., Rouzier, R., Broglio, K.R., Hortobagyi, G.N., & Valero, V. (2007). Overall survival and cause-specific mortality of patients with stage T1a, bNOMO breast carcinoma. *Journal of Clinical Oncology, 25,* 4952–4960. doi:10.1200/JCO.2006.08.0499

Harbeck, N., & Thomssen, C. (2011). A new look at node-negative breast cancer. *Oncologist, 16*(Suppl. 1), 51–60. doi:10.1634/theoncologist.2011-S1-51

Harlan, L.C., Klabunde, C.N., Ambs, A.H., Gibson, T., Bernstein, L., McTiernan, A., … Ballard-Barbash, R. (2009). Comorbidities, therapy and newly diagnosed conditions for women with early stage breast cancer. *Journal of Cancer Survivorship, 23,* 89–98. doi:10.1007/s11764-009-0084-3

Hayakawa, H., Komada, Y., Hirayama, M., Hori, H., Ito, M., & Sakurai, M. (2001). Plasma levels of natriuretic peptides in relation to doxorubicin-induced cardiotoxicity and cardiac function in children with cancer. *Medical and Pediatric Oncology, 37,* 4–9. doi:10.1002/mpo.1155

Healthy People 2020. (2012). 2020 topics and objectives: Heart disease and stroke. Retrieved from http://www.healthypeople.gov/2020/topicsobjectives2020/objectiveslist.aspx?topicId=21

Hegel, M.T., Collins, E.D., Kearing, S., Gillock, K.L., Moore, C.P., & Ahles, T.A. (2008). Sensitivity and specificity of the Distress Thermometer for depression in newly diagnosed breast cancer patients. *Psycho-Oncology, 17,* 556–560. doi:10.1002/pon.1289

Holick, C.N., Newcomb, P.A., Trentham-Dietz, A., Titus-Ernstoff, L., Bersch, A.J., Stampfer, M.J., … Willett, W.C. (2008). Physical activity and survival after diagnosis invasive breast cancer. *Cancer Epidemiology, Biomarkers and Prevention, 17,* 379–386. doi:10.1158/1055-9965.EPI-07-0771

Holmes, M.D., Chen, W.Y., Feskanich, D., Kroenke, C.H., & Colditz, G.A. (2005). Physical activity and survival after breast cancer diagnosis. *JAMA, 293,* 2479–2486. doi:10.1001/jama.293.20.2479

Hunt, S.A. (2005). ACC/AHA 2005 guideline update for the diagnosis and management of chronic heart failure in the adult: A report of the American College of Cardiology/American Heart Association Task Force on Practice Guidelines (writing committee to update the 2001 guidelines for the evaluation and management of heart failure). *Journal of the American College of Cardiology, 46*(6), e1–e82. doi:10.1016/j.jacc.2005.08.022

Hunt, S.A., Abraham, W.T., Chin, M.H., Feldman, A.M., Francis, G.S., Ganiats, T.G., … Yancy, C.W. (2009). 2009 focused update incorporated into the ACC/AHA 2005 guidelines for the diagnosis and management of heart failure in adults: A report of the American College of Cardiology Foundation/America Heart Association Task Force on Practice Guidelines: Developed in collaboration with the International Society for Heart and Lung Transplantation. *Circulation, 119,* e391–e479. doi:10.1161/CIRCULATIONAHA.109.192065

Ingram, C., & Brown, J. (2004). Patterns of weight and body composition change in premenopausal women with early stage breast cancer. *Cancer Nursing, 27,* 483–490. doi:10.1097/00002820-200411000-00008

Institute of Medicine. (2004). *Meeting the psychological needs of women with breast cancer.* Washington, DC: National Academies Press.

Inzucchi, S.E., Bergenstal, R.M., Buse, J.B., Diamant, M., Ferrannini, E., Nauck, M., … Matthews, D.R. (2012). Management of hyperglycemia in type 2 diabetes: A patient-centered approach: Position statement of the American Diabetes Association (ADA) and the European Association for the Study of Diabetes (EASD). *Diabetes Care, 35,* 1364–1379. doi:10.2337/dc12-0413

Iribarren, C., Karter, A.J., Go, A.S., Ferrara, A., Liu, J.Y., Sidney, S., & Selby, J.V. (2001). Glycemic control and heart failure among adult patients with diabetes. *Circulation, 103,* 2668–2673. doi:10.1161/01.CIR.103.22.2668

Irwin, M.L., McTiernan, A., Baumgartner, R.N., Baumgartner, K.B., Bernstein, L., Gilliland, F.D., & Ballard-Barbash, R. (2005). Changes in body fat and weight after a breast cancer diagnosis: Influence of demographic, prognostic, and lifestyle factors. *Journal of Clinical Oncology, 23,* 774–782. doi:10.1200/JCO.2005.04.036

Jones, L.W., Haykowsky, M.J., Swartz, J.J., Douglas, P.S., & Mackey, J.R. (2007). Early breast cancer therapy and cardiovascular injury. *Journal of the American College of Cardiology, 50,* 1435–1441. doi:10.1016/j.jacc.2007.06.037

Jones, L.W., Liang, Y., Pituskin, E.N., Battaglini, C.L., Scott, J.M., Hornsby, W.E., & Haykowsky, M. (2011). Effects of exercise training on peak oxygen consumption in patients with cancer: A meta-analysis. *Oncologist, 16,* 112–120. doi:10.1634/theoncologist.2010-0197

Jurcut, R., Wildiers, H., Ganame, J., D'hooge, J., Paridaems, R., & Voight, J. (2008). Detection and monitoring of cardiotoxicity—What does modern cardiology offer? *Supportive Care in Cancer, 16,* 437–445. doi:10.1007/s00520-007-0397-6

Kalinowski, A., Plowes, N.J.R., Huang, Q., Berdejo-Izquierdo, C., Russell, R.R., & Russell, K.S. (2010). Metalloproteinase-dependent cleavage of neuregulin and autocrine stimulation of vascular endothelial cells. *FASEB Journal, 24,* 2567–2575. doi:10.1096/fj.08-129072

Karp, I., Behlouli, H., Lelorier, J., & Pilote, L. (2008). Statins and cancer. *American Journal of Medicine, 121,* 302–309. doi:10.1016/j.amjmed.2007.12.011

Katz, M.S. (2005) Therapy insight: Potential of statins for cancer chemoprevention and therapy. *Nature Clinical Practice Oncology, 2*, 82–89. doi:10.1038/ncponc0097

Katz, M.S., Minsky, B.D., Saltz, L.B., Riedel, E., Chessin, D.B., & Guillem, J.G. (2005). Association of statin use with a pathologic complete response to neoadjuvant chemoradiation for rectal cancer. *International Journal of Radiation Oncology, Biology, Physics, 62*, 1363–1370. doi:10.1016/j.ijrobp.2004.12.033

Keating, N.L., O'Malley, A.J., & Smith, M.R. (2006). Diabetes and cardiovascular disease during androgen deprivation therapy for prostate cancer. *Journal of Clinical Oncology, 24*, 4448–4456. doi:10.1200/JCO.2006.06.2497

Kelley, G.A., Kelley, K.S., & Tran, Z.V. (2004a). Aerobic exercise and lipids and lipoproteins in women: A meta-analysis of randomized controlled trials. *Journal of Women's Health, 13*, 1148–1164. doi:10.1089/jwh.2004.13.1148

Kelley, G.A., Kelley, K.S., & Tran, Z.V. (2004b). Walking, lipids, and lipoproteins: A meta-analysis of randomized controlled trials. *Preventive Medicine, 38*, 651–661. doi:10.1016/j.ypmed.2003.12.012

Kenchaiah, S., Gaziano, J.M., & Vasan, R.S. (2004). Impact of obesity on the risk of heart failure and survival after the onset of heart failure. *Medical Clinics of North America, 88*, 1273–1294. doi:10.1016/j.mcna.2004.04.011

Kenchaiah, S., Narula, J., & Vasan, R.S. (2004). Risk factors for heart failure. *Medical Clinics of North America, 88*, 1145–1172. doi:10.1016/j.mcna.2004.04.016

Khakoo, A.Y., & Yeh, E.T. (2008). Therapy insight: Management of cardiovascular disease in patients with cancer and cardiac complications of cancer therapy. *Nature Clinical Practice Oncology, 5*, 655–667. doi:10.1038/ncponc1225

Khemasuwan, D., DiVietro, M.L., Tangdhanakanond, K., Pomerantz, S.C., & Eiger, G. (2010). Statins decrease the occurrence of venous thromboembolism in patients with cancer. *American Journal of Medicine, 123*, 60–65. doi:10.1016/j.amjmed.2009.05.025

Khurana, V., Bejjanki, H.R., Caldito, G., & Owens, M.W. (2007). Statins reduce the incidence of lung cancer in humans: A large case-control study of US Veterans. *Chest, 131*, 1282–1288. doi:10.1378/chest.06-0931

Kim, C.-J., Kang, D.-H., & Park, J.-W. (2009). A meta-analysis of aerobic exercise interventions for women with breast cancer. *Western Journal of Nursing Research, 31*, 437–461. doi:10.1177/0193945908328473

Knobf, M.T. (2002). Carrying on the experience of premature menopause in women with early stage breast cancer. *Nursing Research, 51*, 9–17. doi:10.1097/00006199-200201000-00003

Knobf, M.T. (2007). Psychosocial responses in breast cancer survivors. *Seminars in Oncology Nursing, 23*, 71–83. doi:10.1016/j.soncn.2006.11.009

Knobf, M.K., & Coviello, J.S. (2011). Lifestyle interventions for cardiovascular risk reduction in women with breast cancer. *Current Cardiology Reviews, 7*, 250–257.

Knobloch, K., Tepe, J., Lichtinghagen, R., Luck, H.J., & Vogt, P.M. (2008). Simultaneous hemodynamic and serological cardiotoxicity monitoring during immunotherapy with trastuzumab. *International Journal of Cardiology, 125*, 113–115. doi:10.1016/j.ijcard.2007.01.010

Kornblau, S.M., Banker, D.E., Stirewalt, D., Shen, D., Lemker, E., Verstovsek, S., ... Appelbaum, F.R. (2007). Blockade of adaptive defensive changes in cholesterol uptake and synthesis in AML by the addition of pravastatin to idarubicin + high dose Ara-C: A phase 1 study. *Blood, 109*, 2999–3006. doi:10.1182/blood-2006-08-044446

Kriegbaum, M., Christensen, U., Lund, R., Prescott, E., & Osler, M. (2008). Job loss and broken partnerships: Do the number of stressful life events influence the risk of ischemic heart disease in men? *Annals of Epidemiology, 18*, 743–745. doi:10.1016/j.annepidem.2008.04.010

Kroenke, C.H., Chen, W.Y., Rosner, B., & Holmes, M.D. (2005). Weight, weight gain and survival after breast cancer diagnosis. *Journal of Clinical Oncology, 23*, 1370–1378. doi:10.1200/JCO.2005.01.079

Ky, B., Kimmel, S.E., Safa, R.N., Putt, M.E., Sweitzer, M.K., Fang, J.C., ... Cappola, T.P. (2009). Neuregulin-1β is associated with disease severity and adverse outcomes in chronic heart failure. *Circulation, 120*, 310–317. doi:10.1161/CIRCULATIONAHA.109.856310

Lemmens, K., Doggen, K., & De Keulenaer, G.W. (2007). Role of neuregulin-1/ErbB signaling in cardiovascular physiology and disease. *Circulation, 116*, 954–960. doi:10.1161/CIRCULATIONAHA.107.690487

Lenihan, D.J., & Esteva, F.J. (2008). Multidisciplinary strategy for managing cardiovascular risk when treating patients with early stage breast cancer. *Oncologist, 13*, 1224–1234. doi:10.1634/theoncologist.2008-0112

Lethborg, C.E., Kissane, D., Burns, W.I., & Snyder, R. (2000). "Cast adrift": The experience of completing treatment among women with early stage breast cancer. *Journal of Psychosocial Oncology, 18*(4), 73–90. doi:10.1300/J077v18n04_05

Levine, G.N., D'Amico, A.V., Berger, P., Clark, P.E., Eckel, R.H., Keating, N.L., ... Zakai, N. (2010). Androgen-deprivation therapy in prostate cancer and cardiovascular risk: A science advisory from the American Heart Association, American Cancer Society, and American Urological Association: Endorsed by the American Society for Radiation Oncology. *Circulation, 121*, 833–840. doi:10.1161/CICULATIONAHA.109.192695

Lewis, S. (2007). Do endocrine treatments for breast cancer have a negative impact on lipid profiles and cardiovascular risk in postmenopausal women? *American Heart Journal, 153*, 182–188. doi:10.1016/j.ahj.2006.10.034

Li, Y.C., Park, M.J., Ye, S.K., Kim, C.W., & Kim, Y.N. (2006). Elevated levels of cholesterol-rich lipid rafts in cancer cells are correlated with apoptosis sensitivity induced by cholesterol depleting agents. *American Journal of Pathology, 168*, 1107–1118. doi:10.2353/ajpath.2006.050959

Ligibel, J.A., O'Malley, A., Fisher, M., Daniel, G., Winer, E.P., & Keating, N.L. (2010, December). *Aromatase inhibitors and risk of myocardial infarction, stroke, and fracture.* Paper presented at San Antonio Breast Cancer Symposium, San Antonio, TX.

Lipscombe, L.L., Goodwin, P.J., Zinman, B., McLaughlin, J.R., & Hux, J.E. (2008). The impact of diabetes on survival following breast cancer. *Breast Cancer Research and Treatment, 109*, 389–395. doi:10.1007/s10549-007-9654-0

Lloyd-Jones, D.M., Leip, E.P., Larson, M.G., D'Agostino, R.B., Beiser, A., Wilson, P.W., ... Levy, D. (2006). Prediction of lifetime risk for CVD risk factor burden at 50 years of age. *Circulation, 113*, 791–798. doi:10.1161/CIRCULATIONAHA.105.548206

Loprinzi, C.L., Athmann, L.M., Kardinal, C.G., O'Fallon, J.R., See, J.A., Bruce, B.K., ... Rayson, S. (1996). Randomized trial of dietician counseling to try to prevent weight gain associated with breast cancer adjuvant chemotherapy. *Oncology, 53*, 228–232. doi:10.1159/000227565

Lorenzo, C., Williams, K., Hunt, K.S., & Haffner, J. (2007). National Cholesterol Education Program-Adult Treatment Panel III, International Diabetes Foundation, and the World Health Organization definition of the metabolic syndrome as prediction of incident cardiovascular disease and diabetes. *Diabetes Care, 30*(8), 8–13. doi:10.2337/dc06-1414

Maitland, M.L., Bakris, G.L., Black, H.R., Chen, H.X., Durand, J.-B., Elliott, W.J., ... Tang, W.H.W. (2010). Initial assessment, surveillance, and management of blood pressure in patients receiving vascular endothelial growth factor signaling pathway inhibitors. *Journal of the National Cancer Institute, 102*, 596–604. doi:10.1093/jnci/djq091

Manson, J.E., Greenland, P., LaCroix, A.Z., Stefanik, M.L., Mouton, C.P., & Oberman, A. (2002). Walking compared with vigorous exercise for the prevention of cardiovascular events in women. *New England Journal of Medicine, 347*, 716–725. doi:10.1056/NEJMoa021067

Martin, M., Esteva, F.J., Alba, E., Khandheria, B., Pérez-Isla, L., García-Sáenz, J.A., ... Zamorano, J. (2009). Minimizing cardiotoxicity while optimizing treatment efficacy with trastuzumab: Review and expert recommendations. *Oncologist, 14*, 1–11. doi:10.1634/theoncologist.2008-0137

Matthews, K.A., Crawford, S.L., Chae, C.U., Everson-Rose, S.A., Sowers, M.F., Sternfeld, B., & Sutton-Tyrell, K. (2009). Are changes in cardiovascular disease risk factors in midlife women due to chronological aging or to the menopause transition? *Journal of the American College of Cardiology, 54*, 2366–2373. doi:10.1016/j.jacc.2009.10.009

Maurea, N., Coppola, C., Ragone, G., Frasci, G., Bonelli, A., Romano, C., & Iaffaioli, R.V. (2010). Women survive breast cancer but fall victim to heart failure: The shadows and lights of targeted therapy. *Journal of Cardiovascular Medicine, 11*, 861–868. doi:10.2459/JCM.0b013e328336b4c1

May, H.T., Horne, B.D., Carlquist, J.F., Sheng, X., Joy, E., & Catinella, A.P. (2009). Depression after coronary artery disease is associated with heart failure. *Journal of the American College of Cardiology, 53*, 1440–1447. doi:10.1016/j.jacc.2009.01.036

McInnes, J., & Knobf, M.T. (2001). Weight gain and quality of life in women with breast cancer on adjuvant chemotherapy for early stage breast cancer. *Oncology Nursing Forum, 28*, 675–684.

McNicholas, W.T. (2009). Chronic obstructive pulmonary disease and obstructive sleep apnea: Overlaps in pathophysiology, systemic inflammation, and cardiovascular disease. *American Journal of Respiratory and Critical Care Medicine, 180*, 692–700. doi:10.1164/rccm.200903-0347PP

Mosca, L., Banka, C.L., Benjamin, E.J., Berra, K., Bushnell, C., Dolor, R.J., ... Wenger, N.K. (2007). Evidence-based guidelines for cardiovascular disease prevention in women: 2007 update. *Circulation, 115*, 1481–1501. doi:10.1161/CIRCULATIONAHA.107.181546

Mosca, L., Barrett-Connor, E., & Wenger, N.K. (2011). Sex/gender differences in cardiovascular disease prevention: What a difference a decade makes. *Circulation, 124*, 2145–2154. doi:10.1161/CIRCULATIONAHA.110.968792

Mosca, L., Benjamin, E.J., Berra, K., Bezanson, J.L., Dolor, R.J., Lloyd-Jones, D.M., ... Wenger, N.K. (2011). Effectiveness-based guidelines for the prevention of cardiovascular disease in women—2011 update: A guideline from the American Heart Association. *Circulation, 123,* 1243–1262. doi:10.1161/ CIR.0b013e31820faaf8

Mosca, L., Linfante, A.H., Benjamin, E.J., Berra, K., Hayes, S.N., Walsh, B.W., ... Simpson, S.L. (2005). National study of physician awareness and adherence to cardiovascular prevention guidelines. *Circulation, 111,* 499–510.

Mouhayar, E., & Salahudeen, A. (2011). Hypertension in cancer patients. *Texas Heart Institute Journal, 38,* 263–265.

Murray, L.J., Ramakrishnan, S., O'Toole, L., Manifold, I.H., Purohit, O.P., & Coleman, R.E. (2010). Adjuvant trastuzumab in routine clinical practice and the impact of cardiac monitoring guidelines on treatment delivery. *Breast, 19,* 339–344. doi:10.1016/j.breast.2010.02.001

National Cholesterol Education Program Expert Panel on Detection, Evaluation, and Treatment of High Blood Cholesterol in Adults. (2001). Executive summary of the third report of the National Cholesterol Education Program (NCEP) Expert Panel on Detection, Evaluation, and Treatment of High Blood Cholesterol in Adults (Adult Treatment Panel III). *JAMA, 285,* 2486–2497. doi:10.1001/ jama.285.19.2486

Ng, R., Better, N., & Green, M.D. (2006). Anticancer agents and cardiotoxicity. *Seminars in Oncology, 33,* 2–14. doi:10.1053/j.seminoncol.2005.11.001

Nguyen, A.B., Rohatgi, A., Garcia, C.K., Ayers, C.R., Das, S.R., Lakoski, S.G., ... de Lemos, J.A. (2011). Interactions between smoking, pulmonary surfactant protein B, and atherosclerosis in the general population: The Dallas Heart Study. *Atherosclerosis, Thrombosis, and Vascular Biology, 31,* 2136–2143. doi:10.1161/ATVBAHA.111.228692

Nichols, H.B., Trentham-Dietz, A., Egan, K.M., Titus-Ernstoff, L., Holmes, M.D., Bersch, A.J., ... Newcomb, P.A. (2009). Body mass index before and after breast cancer diagnosis: Associations with all-cause, breast cancer and cardiovascular disease mortality. *Cancer Epidemiology, Biomarkers and Prevention, 18,* 1403–1409. doi:10.1158/1055-9965.EPI-08-1094

Nicolucci, A. (2010). Epidemiological aspects of neoplasms in diabetes. *Acta Diabetologica, 47,* 87–95. doi:10.1007/s00592-010-0187-3

Norgren, L., Hiatt, W.R., Dormandy, J.A., Nehler, M.R., Harris, K.A., & Fowkes, F.G.R (2007). Inter-Society Consensus for the Management of Peripheral Arterial Disease (TASC II). *Journal of Vascular Surgery, 45*(Suppl. 1), S5–S67. doi:10.1016/j.jvs.2006.12.037

Norris, C.M., Ljubsa, A., & Hegadoren, K.M. (2009). Gender as a determinant of responses to a self-screening questionnaire on anxiety and depression by patients with coronary artery disease. *Gender Medicine, 6,* 479–487. doi:10.1016/j.genm.2009.09.001

Nowakowski, G.S., Maurer, M.J., Habermann, T.M., Ansell, S.M., Macon, W.R., Ristow, K.M., ... Cerhan, J.R. (2010). Statin use and prognosis in patients with diffuse large B-cell lymphoma and follicular lymphoma in the rituximab era. *Journal of Clinical Oncology, 28,* 412–417. doi:10.1200/JCO.2009.23.4245

Pan, A., Okereke, O.I., Sun, Q., Logroscino, G., Manson, J.E., Willett, W.C., ... Rexrode, K.M. (2011). Depression and incident stroke in women. *Stroke, 42,* 2770–2775. doi:10.1161/STROKEAHA.111.617043

Patnaik, J.L., Byers, T., DiGuiseppi, C., Dabelea, D., & Denberg, T.D. (2011). Cardiovascular disease competes with breast cancer as the leading cause of death for older females diagnosed with breast cancer: A retrospective cohort study. *Breast Cancer Research, 13,* R64. doi:10.1186/bcr2901

Peairs, K.S., Barone, B.B., Snyder, C.F., Yeh, C.-H., Stein, K.B., Derr, R.L., ... Wolff, A.C. (2011). Diabetes mellitus and breast cancer outcomes: A systematic review and meta-analysis. *Journal of Clinical Oncology, 29,* 40–46. doi:10.1200/JCO.2009.27.3011

Pekmezi, D.W., & Demark-Wahnefried, W. (2011). Updated evidence in support of diet and exercise interventions in cancer survivors. *Acta Oncologica, 50,* 167–178. doi:10.3109/0284186X.2010.529822

Pelletier, P., Lapointe, A., Laflamme, N., Piche, M.E., Weisnagel, A., Lemeiux, S., ... Bergeon, J. (2009). Discordances among different tools used to estimate cardiovascular risk in postmenopausal women. *Canadian Journal of Cardiology, 25,* e413–e416. doi:10.1016/S0828-282X(09)70535-5

Pender, N.J., Murdaugh, C.L., & Parsons, M.A. (2011). *Health promotion in nursing practice* (6th ed.). Upper Saddle River, NJ: Pearson Education.

Peng, X., Pentassuglia, L., & Sawyer, D.B. (2010). Emerging anticancer therapeutic targets and the cardiovascular system: Is there cause for concern? *Circulation Research, 106,* 35–46. doi:10.1161/ CIRCRESAHA.109.211276

Pescatello, L.S., Franklin, B.A., Fagard, R., Farquhar, W.B., Kelley, G.A., & Ray, C.A. (2004). American College of Sports Medicine position stand. Exercise and hypertension. *Medicine and Science in Sports and Exercise, 36,* 533–553. doi:10.1249/01.MSS.0000115224.88514.3A

Picard, C., Plu-Bureau, G., Neves-e Castro, M., & Gompel, A. (2008). Insulin resistance, obesity and breast cancer risk. *Maturitas, 60,* 19–30. doi:10.1016/j.maturitas.2008.03.002

Pichon, M.F., Cvitkovic, F., Hacene, K., Delaunay, J., Lokiec, F., Collignon, M.A., & Pecking, A.P. (2005). Drug-induced cardiotoxicity studied by longitudinal B-type natriuretic peptide assays and radionuclide ventriculography. *In Vivo, 19,* 567–576.

Pierce, J.P., Natarajan, L., Caan, B.J., Parker, B.A., Greenberg, E.R., Flatt, S.W., ... Stefanick, M.L. (2007). Influence of a diet very high in vegetables, fruit, and fiber and low in fat on prognosis following treatment for breast cancer: The Women's Healthy Eating and Living (WHEL) randomized trial. *JAMA, 298,* 289–298. doi:10.1001/jama.298.3.289

Poynter, J.N., Gruber, S.B., Higgins, P.D., Almog, R., Bonner, J.D., Rennert, H.S., ... Rennert, G. (2005). Statins and the risk of colorectal cancer. *New England Journal of Medicine, 352,* 2184–2192. doi:10.1056/NEJMoa043792

Redig, A.J., & Munshi, H.G. (2010). Care of the cancer survivor: Metabolic syndrome after hormone-modifying therapy. *American Journal of Medicine, 123,* 87.e1–87.e6. doi:10.1016/j.amjmed.2009.06.022

Ridker, P.M., Buring, J.E., Rifai, N., & Cook, N.R. (2007). Development and validation of improved algorithms for the assessment of global cardiovascular risk in women: The Reynolds Risk Score. *JAMA, 297,* 611–619. doi:10.1001/jama.297.6.611

Roger, V.L., Go, A.S., Lloyd-Jones, D.M., Benjamin, E.J., Berry, J.D., Borden, W.B., ... Turner, M.B. (2012). Heart disease and stroke statistics—2012 update: A report from the American Heart Association. *Circulation, 125,* e2–e220. doi:10.1161/CIR.0b013e31823ac046

Rose, D.P., Komninou, D., & Stephenson, G.D. (2004). Obesity, adipocytokines and insulin resistance in breast cancer. *Obesity Reviews, 5,* 153–165. doi:10.1111/j.1467-789X.2004.00142.x

Saarto, T., Blomqvist, C., Ehnholm, C., Taskinen, M., & Elomaa, I. (1996). Effects of chemotherapy-induced castration on serum lipids and apoproteins in premenopausal women with node-positive breast cancer. *Journal of Clinical Endocrinology and Metabolism, 81,* 4453–4457. doi:10.1210/jc.81.12.4453

Saigal, C.S., Gore, J.L., Krupski, T.L., Hanley, J., Schonlau, M., & Litwin, M. (2007). Androgen deprivation therapy increases cardiovascular morbidity in men with prostate cancer. *Cancer, 110,* 1493–1500. doi:10.1002/cncr.22933

Saquib, N., Rock, C.L., Natarajan, L., Flatt, S.W., Newman, V.A., Thomson, C.A., ... Pierce, J.P. (2009). Does a healthy diet help weight management among overweight and obese people? *Health Education and Behavior, 36,* 518–531. doi:10.1177/1090198108314617

Schmitz, K.H., Courneya, K.S., Matthews, C., Demark-Wahnefried, W., Galvão, D.A., Pinto, B.M., ... Schwartz, A.L. (2010). American College of Sports Medicine Roundtable on exercise guidelines for cancer survivors. *Medicine and Science in Sports and Exercise, 42,* 1409–1426. doi:10.1249/MSS.0b013e3181e0c112

Shannon, J., Tewoderos, S., Garzotto, M., Beer, T.M., Derenick, R., Palma, A., & Farris, P.E. (2005). Statins and prostate cancer risk: A case-control study. *American Journal of Epidemiology, 162,* 318–325. doi:10.1093/aje/kwi203

Shenoy, C., Klem, I., Crowley, A.L., Patel, M.R., Winchester, M.A., Owusu, C., & Kimmick, G.G. (2011). Cardiovascular complications of breast cancer therapy in older adults. *Oncologist, 16,* 1138–1143. doi:10.1634/theoncologist.2010-0348

Siegel, R., Desantis, C., Virgo, K., Stein, K., Mariotto, A., Smith, T., ... Ward, E. (2012). Cancer treatment and survivorship statistics, 2012. *CA: A Cancer Journal for Clinicians, 62,* 220–241. doi:10.3322/caac.21149

Slentz, C.A., Duscha, B.D., Johnson, J.L., Ketchum, K., Aiken, L.B., Samsa, G.P., ... Kraus, W.E. (2004). Effects of the amount of exercise on body weight, body composition and measures of central obesity. *Archives of Internal Medicine, 164,* 31–39. doi:10.1001/archinte.164.1.31

Speck, R.M., Courneya, K.S., Mâsse, L., Duval, S., & Schmitz, K.H. (2010). An update of controlled physical activity trials in cancer survivors: A systematic review and meta-analysis. *Journal of Cancer Survivorship, 4,* 87–100. doi:10.1007/s11764-009-0110-5

Stampfer, M.J., Hu, F.B., Manson, J.E., Rimm, E.B., & Willett, W.C. (2000). Primary prevention of coronary heart disease in women through diet and lifestyle. *New England Journal of Medicine, 343,* 16–22. doi:10.1056/NEJM200007063430103

Stangl, V., Baumann, G., & Stangl, K. (2002). Coronary artherogenic risk factors in women. *European Heart Journal, 23,* 1738–1752.

Székely, A., Balog, P., Benkö, E., Breuer, T., Székely, J., Kertai, M.D., ... Thayer, J.F. (2007). Anxiety predicts mortality and morbidity after coronary artery surgery—A 4-year follow-up study. *Psychosomatic Medicine, 69,* 625–631. doi:10.1097/PSY.0b013e31814b8c0f

Taylor, J.Y., Sun, Y.V., Hunt, S.C., & Kardia, S.L. (2010). Gene-environment interaction for hypertension among African American women across generations. *Biological Research for Nursing, 12,* 149–155. doi:10.1177/1099800410371225

Thomson, C.A., Stopeck, A.T., Bea, J.W., Cussler, E., Nardi, E., Frey, G., & Thompson, P.A. (2010). Changes in body weight and metabolic indexes in overweight breast cancer survivors enrolled in a randomized trial of low-fat vs. reduced carbohydrate diets. *Nutrition and Cancer, 62,* 1142–1152. doi:10.1080/01635581.2010.513803

Thomson, C.A., Thompson, P.A., Wright-Bea, J., Nardi, E., Frey, G.R., & Stopeck, A. (2009). Metabolic syndrome and elevated C-reactive protein in breast cancer survivors on adjuvant hormone therapy. *Journal of Women's Health, 18,* 2041–2047. doi:10.1089/jwh.2009.1365

Todaro, J.F., Shen, B.-J., Niaura, R., & Tilkemeier, P.L. (2005). Prevalence of depressive disorders in men and women enrolled in a cardiac rehabilitation. *Journal of Cardiopulmonary Rehabilitation and Prevention, 25,* 71–75. doi:10.1097/00008483-200503000-00003

Traish, A.M., Saad, F., & Guay, A. (2009). The dark side of testosterone deficiency: II. Type 2 diabetes and insulin resistance. *Journal of Andrology, 30,* 23–32. doi:10.2164/jandrol.108.005751

Tsai, H.K., D'Amico, A.V., Sedetsky, N., Chen, M.H., & Carroll, P.R. (2007). Androgen deprivation therapy for localized prostate cancer and the risk of cardiovascular mortality. *Journal of the National Cancer Institute, 99,* 1516–1524. doi:10.1093/jnci/djm168

Tsimberidou, A.M., Minotti, G., & Cardinale, D. (2011). Managing cardiac risk factors in oncology clinical trials. *Texas Heart Institute Journal, 38,* 266–267.

Vaklavas, C., Chatzizisis, Y.S., & Tsimberidou, A.M. (2011). Common cardiovascular medications in cancer therapeutics. *Pharmacology and Therapeutics, 130,* 177–190. doi:10.1016/j.pharmthera.2011.01.009

van den Belt-Dusebout, A.W., Nuver, J., de Wit, R., Gietema, J.A., ten Bokkel Huinink, W.W., Rodrigus, P.T.R., … van Leeuwen, F.E. (2006). Long-term risk of cardiovascular disease in 5-year survivors of testicular cancer. *Journal of Clinical Oncology, 24,* 467–475. doi:10.1200/JCO.2005.02.7193

Verma, S., & Ewer, M.S. (2011). Is cardiotoxicity being adequately assessed in current trials of cytotoxic and targeted agents in breast cancer? *Annals of Oncology, 22,* 1011–1018. doi:10.1093/annonc/mdq607

Warren, T.Y., Wilcox, S., Dowda, M., & Baruth, M. (2012). Independent association of waist circumference with hypertension and diabetes in African American women, South Carolina, 2007–2009. *Preventing Chronic Disease, 9,* 110170. doi:10.5888/pcd9.110170

Whelton, S.P., Chin, A., Xin, X., & He, J. (2002). Effects of aerobic exercise on blood pressure: A meta-analysis randomized controlled trials. *Annals of Internal Medicine, 136,* 493–503.

Wulsin, S.R., & Singal, B.M. (2003). Do depressive symptoms increase the risk for the onset of coronary disease? A systematic quantitative review. *Psychosomatic Medicine, 65,* 201–210. doi:10.1097/01.PSY.0000058371.50240.E3

Yancy, C.W. (2011). Is ideal cardiovascular health attainable? *Circulation, 123,* 850–857. doi:10.1161/CIRCULATIONAHA.110.016378

Zambelli, A., Della Porta, M.G., Eleuteri, E., De Giuli, L., Catalano, O., Tondini, C., & Riccardi, A. (2011). Predicting and preventing cardiotoxicity in the era of breast cancer targeted therapies. Novel molecular tools for clinical issues. *Breast, 20,* 176–183. doi:10.1016/j.breast.2010.11.002

Index

The letter f after a page number indicates that relevant content appears in a figure; the letter t, in a table.

A

abciximab, 68–69, 70t
Abl protein, 35
acute coronary syndrome (ACS), 55. *See also* coronary artery disease; myocardial ischemia/infarction
classification of, 65f, 65–67
diagnosis of, 58–64, 59t, 62f, 63t–64t
differential diagnosis, 62–64, 64t, 142
nursing management, 70–71, 72f
pharmacologic therapy, 67–70, 70t
prevention of, 71–73
risk factors for, 270
signs/symptoms of, 58, 59t
acute decompensated heart failure (ADHF), 163–164, 173–176, 174f–175f, 176t. *See also* heart failure
acute GVHD (aGVHD), 140–141
acute lymphoblastic leukemia (ALL), 35–36
acute myeloid leukemia, 132t
adenosine, for SVT, 208–209
ADHERE (Acute Decompensated Heart Failure National Registry), 174
advanced cardiac life support (ACLS), 227
AFFIRM trial (Atrial Fibrillation Follow-Up

Investigation of Rhythm Management), 199–200
aflibercept, 97t
African American women, CVD risk in, 16, 272
age
and CVD risk, 269–270, 276
and HSCT eligibility, 135
alcohol intake, 185
aldosterone receptor antagonists, 179t, 183
alemtuzumab, for aGVHD, 141
allogeneic HSCT, 133
alteplase, 68
amiodarone, 70, 183, 200, 202t–203t, 212, 232–234
analgesia. *See also specific agents*
for chest pain, 69, 70t
QT prolongation with, 222t
androgen suppression therapy, 277
anemia, 58
angioedema, 180
angiography, 9–10, 15f, 61–62, 62f, 63t, 114
angiosarcoma, 6, 8, 8f
angiotensin-converting enzyme (ACE) inhibitors, 22–23
for ACS, 69, 70t
for heart failure, 178–180, 179t
for hypertension, 101, 102t
nursing implications, 180
angiotensin receptor blockers
for heart failure, 179t, 180
for hypertension, 101, 102t
anthracycline-induced cardiotoxicity, 13–14, 31, 78, 79t
differential diagnoses for, 18f

dose effects, 16, 17f
heart failure from, 151t, 159, 162, 168
management of, 22–24, 25f
pathophysiology of, 14
reversibility of, 23
risk factors for, 14–16
anthracyclines, 13, 79t
antiarrhythmic agents, 70, 200
avoided with heart failure, 183
QT prolongation with, 222t, 233
for V-fib, 235
anticoagulant therapy, 67–69, 70t. *See also specific agents*
in A-fib, 259–260
and bleeding risk, 204–205, 206t
bridge protocol, 258–259, 259t, 261
with mechanical prosthetic heart valves, 260–261, 261t
preoperative, 257–259
for thromboembolism, 118t, 118–121, 120t–122t, 124
antidepressants, QT prolongation with, 222t
antiembolic stockings, 123t, 125, 126f
antiemetics, 222t
antifungals/antimicrobials, 222t
antiplatelet agents, 67–69, 70t
antipsychotics, 222t
antithymocyte globulin (ATG), 139

anxiety, as CVD risk, 270–271, 278
aortic stenosis, 144
apical ballooning syndrome, 141–142
apixaban, 121
aromatase inhibitors (AIs), 275
arrhythmias. *See also specific conditions*
  from HSCT conditioning, 139, 148–149
  from RT, 42–43, 44*t*, 50*t*
  from surgery, 253
arsenic, 221*t*
ARTEMIS study (ARixtra for Thromboembolism Prevention in Medical Indications), 124
aspirin, 67, 70*t*, 257–258, 259*t*, 262
asystole, 149, 150*t*, 160
atenolol, 230
atherosclerosis, 55–56
  in diabetes, 273
  from RT, 43
atorvastatin, 286
atrial fibrillation (A-fib), 195, 197, 198*f*
  after HSCT, 139, 148–149, 150*t*
  anticoagulation therapy and, 259–260
  management of, 199–200, 201*t*–203*t*
  pathophysiology/classification of, 197–198
  risk factors for, 198–199
atrial flutter (AFL)
  management of, 201*t*–203*t*, 207
  pathophysiology/classification, 205–206
  risk factors for, 207
  "sawtooth" ECG pattern, 205, 206*f*
atrioventricular blocks (AVBs)
  classification of, 210, 210*f*–211*f*
  management of, 212–213
  pathophysiology of, 210–212
  risk factors for, 212
atrioventricular (AV) node, 6, 197
atropine, 212–213
autologous HSCT, 131–133
autonomic dysfunction, from RT, 45*t*
autonomic neuropathy, 253*t*
autotransplantation, cardiac, 5
AV node reentrant tachycardia, 208
AV reentrant tachycardia, 208
axitinib, 97*t*

B

bare metal stents, 262, 263*f*
basic cardiac life support (BCLS), 227
Bazett formula, for QTc, 219
beta-blockers, 22–23
  for ACS, 69, 70*t*, 71
  for A-fib, 201*t*–202*t*
  for AVBs, 212
  for heart failure, 179*t*, 180–181
  for hypertension, 101, 102*t*
  nursing implications, 181
  for PVCs, 229–230
bevacizumab
  cardiotoxicity of, 32*f*, 34–35, 57, 57*t*, 161*t*, 162
  hypertension from, 97*t*
  thrombosis risk with, 110
biomarkers, cardiac, 19–20, 22*t*, 59*t*, 59–60, 171*t*, 172–173, 283–284
biopsy, cardiac, 84, 171*t*, 171–172
bisoprolol, 23, 179*t*, 181
bivalirudin, 70*t*
bleeding risk assessment, 204–205, 206*t*
bleomycin, pericarditis from, 79*t*
blood pressure monitoring
  with coronary artery disease, 71–72
  with hypertension, 101–103, 103*t*
BNP (biomarker), 19–20, 22*t*, 143, 171*t*, 172–173, 283
bone marrow aspiration, 134*t*
bone marrow registries, 131, 133, 135
bortezomib, cardiotoxicity of, 161*t*
brachytherapy, 41
bradycardia, 197, 209, 253*t*
brain natriuretic peptide (BNP) (biomarker), 19–20, 22*t*, 143, 171*t*, 172–173, 283
breast cancer
  CVD risk with, 271–276, 276*f*
  radiation therapy for, 40, 40*t*, 46–47, 48*t*
  targeted therapy for, 13, 33
bridge anticoagulation therapy, 258–259, 259*t*, 261
broken-heart syndrome, 141–142
Brugada syndrome, 235
bumetanide, 181–182
busulfan, for HSCT conditioning, 138–139

C

calcific pericardium, 81, 82*f*
calcineurin inhibitors, 95, 98–99
calcium channel blockers
  for A-fib, 201*t*–202*t*
  for AVBs, 212
  avoided with heart failure, 183
  for hypertension, 101, 102*t*
candesartan, 69, 179*t*
captopril, 70*t*, 179*t*
cardiac assessment, 24, 26*f*, 268
  before chemotherapy, 252
  for heart failure, 167–170, 168*f*, 170*f*
  before HSCT, 135, 136*t*, 136–137
  preoperative, 252–257, 254*t*–255*t*, 256*f*
  stepwise approach, 255, 256*f*
cardiac autotransplantation, 5
cardiac biomarkers, 19–20, 22*t*, 59*t*, 59–60, 171*t*, 172–173, 283–284
cardiac biopsy, 84, 171*t*, 171–172
cardiac catheterization, 61–62, 62*f*, 63*t*, 71, 84
cardiac diagnostic tests, 19–20, 21*t*–22*t*. *See also specific tests*
cardiac magnetic resonance imaging (C-MRI), 9–10, 19–20, 21*t*
  for heart failure, 171*t*, 172
  for myocarditis, 84, 84*t*
  for pericarditis, 81*t*
  preoperative, 257
cardiac resynchronization therapy (CRT) device, 227, 236, 239
cardiac stents, 72*t*, 261–262
cardiac tamponade, 86. *See also* pericardial effusion
  after HSCT, 146, 150*t*
  chemotherapeutic agents causing, 253*t*
  diagnostic studies of, 89–91, 90*f*, 91*t*
  management of, 91, 147
  pathophysiology of, 86–89, 88*f*–90*f*
  signs/symptoms of, 89, 146
cardiac thrombosis, 200, 262
cardiac tumors. *See also* left atrial tumors; left ventricular tumors; right atrial tumors; right ventricular tumors

diagnosis of, 9–10. *See also* diagnostic tests
incidence of, 1
cardiomyopathy, 160
    clinical presentation of, 16–19, 18*f*
    follow-up testing for, 24
    from HSCT, 141–142, 149*t*
    HSCT with, 151
    management of, 22–26, 25*f*
    mechanisms of, 18*f*
    nonischemic, 152
    from RT, 45*t*, 49*t*
cardioprotective agents, 23
cardiotoxicity, 160. *See also* specific conditions
    from chemotherapy, 57, 57*t*, 253*t*
    definition of, 31
    from HSCT conditioning, 138
    risk factors for, 14–16, 15*f*
    type I/type II, 31
cardiovascular disease (CVD)
    with breast cancer, 271–276, 276*f*
    epidemiology of, 251–252, 267–268
    in general population, 268–271
    in men, 276–277
    prevention of, 284–286
    risk factors for, 268–271, 279*t*, 281*f*–282*f*
    screening/surveillance for, 277–284, 279*t*–280*t*, 281*f*–282*f*, 285*f*
    in survivorship, 277
cardiovascular implantable electronic devices (CIEDs), 227
    and central venous access, 241–242
    components of, 235–236, 236*f*–237*f*
    electromagnetic interference, 240–241
    electrosurgery and, 240
    "magnet mode," 239–240
    perioperative considerations, 240
    programming of, 236–238, 237*f*
    radiation therapy and, 242–245, 244*t*, 247*t*
cardioversion, 148, 200, 232
Carney syndrome, 2
carotid sinus massage, 208
carvedilol, 23, 179*t*, 181, 230
catheter ablation
    for SVT, 209
    for VT, 232

catheterization, cardiac, 61–62, 62*f*, 63*t*, 71, 84
cediranib, 97*t*
CHADS$_2$ scoring system, 204, 205*t*, 260, 260*f*
chemotherapy. *See also* specific agents
    CAD from, 57
    cardiac assessment before, 252
    cardiotoxicity of, 57, 57*t*, 253*t*
    heart failure from, 161*t*, 162
    pericarditis from, 78, 79*t*
    postoperative, 5
chest pain
    with acute coronary syndrome, 58, 60, 63
    differential diagnosis of, 64*t*
    management of, 69, 71, 80–81
    with pericarditis, 79–81, 145–146
    with SICM, 142
chest x-ray
    for heart failure, 171*t*
    for myocarditis, 84*t*
    for pericarditis, 81*t*, 146
    for pulmonary embolism, 115*f*
Chiari network, 6
chronic GVHD (cGVHD), 153
chronic heart failure, 164, 176–177, 178*t*. *See also* heart failure
chronic lymphocytic leukemia, 132*t*
chronic myeloid leukemia (CML), 35–36, 132*t*
cigarette smoking, 24–25, 185, 270
cisplatin, 91, 199
clofarabine, cardiotoxicity of, 161*t*
clonidine, 212
clopidogrel, 67–68, 70*t*, 257–258, 262
CLOT trial (Comparison of LMWH vs. Oral Anticoagulation Therapy), 120
colchicine, 147
colorectal cancer, postoperative A-fib and, 199
Common Terminology Criteria for Adverse Events (CTCAE), 18–19, 96, 96*t*
computed tomography (CT), 40, 81*t*, 114–115, 115*f*–116*f*

computed tomography angiography (CTA), 9, 61, 63*t*
conditioning, for HSCT, 135, 137–139
conduction system dysfunction, from RT, 42–43, 44*t*, 50*t*
congestive heart failure (CHF), 143, 160, 200, 253, 253*t*. *See also* heart failure
constrictive pericarditis, 81
contrast venography, for DVT diagnosis, 115*f*
COPE trial (Colchicine for Acute Pericarditis), 147
core performance measures, 176, 177*t*
coronary angiography, 61–62, 62*f*
coronary arteriography, 171*t*
coronary artery calcium score, 61
coronary artery disease (CAD), 160. *See also* acute coronary syndrome
    HSCT with, 151
    pathophysiology/mechanisms of, 55–56
    prevention of, 71–73
    risk factors for, 56*f*, 56–58, 57*t*, 71–72
    from RT, 43, 44*t*, 45, 49*t*
coronary artery plaques, 56
cor pulmonale, 6
corticosteroids
    for aGVHD, 140
    hypertension from, 99
    for pericarditis pain, 147
coughing, from ACE inhibitors, 180
couplets, 228
creatine kinase-MB (CK-MB) (biomarker), 59, 59*t*, 60
crista terminalis, 6
CURE trial (Clopidogrel in Unstable Angina to Prevent Recurrent Events), 67
cyclophosphamide
    cardiotoxicity of, 159, 161*t*, 168
    for HSCT conditioning, 138–139, 143
    pericarditis from, 79*t*
    QT prolongation from, 233
cyclosporine
    for aGVHD, 140–141
    dyslipidemia from, 153
    hypertension from, 95, 98–99
cytarabine, pericarditis from, 79*t*
cytokine-release syndrome, 141

D

dabigatran, 121, 121*t*, 259
dacarbazine, for sarcoma, 5
dalteparin, 118*t*, 120, 120*t*, 123*t*
dasatinib, 36–37, 161*t*, 221*t*
daunorubicin, 57, 79*t*
D-dimer assays, 113
deep vein thrombosis (DVT),
    109. *See also* venous
    thromboembolism
  diagnostic tests for, 113–115,
    114*f*–115*f*
  differential diagnosis of, 112,
    113*f*
  signs/symptoms of, 110,
    113*f*, 125–126
  treatment of, 117–121, 118*t*
defibrillation, 224*t*, 235, 238–
    239
demand ischemia, 58
depression, as CVD risk, 270–
    271, 278
device interrogation reports, 239
dexrazoxane, 23–24
diabetes, 56, 72–73, 273–274
diagnostic tests, 19–20, 21*t*–22*t*.
    See also specific tests
diastolic dysfunction, 165–166,
    166*f*
  after HSCT, 144–145
  from RT, 42, 49*t*
dietary modification, 26, 184,
    284–286
diffuse nonspecific myocardial
    fibrosis, 42
digitalis, 179*t*, 182–183
Digitalis Investigation Group
    trial, 182
digoxin, 148, 182–183, 201*t*–
    202*t*, 212
diltiazem, 201*t*–202*t*
dimethylbusulfan, for HSCT
    conditioning, 138
direct current cardioversion
    (DCCV), 200
disseminated intravascular co-
    agulation (DIC), 113
diuretics
  for heart failure, 176*t*, 181–
    182
  for hypertension, 101, 102*t*
  nursing implications, 182
dobutamine
  for heart failure, 176*t*
  for pulmonary embolism,
    117
docetaxel
  A-fib with, 199
  cardiotoxicity of, 57, 57*t*, 161*t*
  for sarcoma, 5

dofetilide, 183, 200, 203*t*, 233
dopamine, 176*t*
dose
  of anthracyclines, 16, 17*f*
  of radiation therapy, 41,
    48*t*, 58
doxorubicin
  A-fib with, 199
  cardiotoxicity of, 57, 161*t*
  dose effects, 17*f*
  for leukemia, 9
  pericarditis from, 79*t*
  for sarcoma, 5
  VT with, 231
drug-eluting stents, 261–262
dual-chamber implant, 236
duplex ultrasonography, for
    DVT diagnosis, 115*f*
dyslipidemia
  with breast cancer, 275
  with GVHD, 153
  from steroid therapy, 140
dyspnea, 17

E

Eastern Cooperative
    Oncology Group
    (ECOG) performance
    score, 134–135
echocardiography, 9, 19–20,
    21*t*, 36
  for ACS, 60, 63*t*
  during A-fib, 200
  for heart failure, 171*t*, 172
  before HSCT, 135, 136*t*, 137
  for myocarditis, 84*t*
  for pericarditis, 81*t*, 146–
    147
  preoperative, 256–257
  for pulmonary embolism,
    115*f*–116*f*
  of SICM, 142
EINSTEIN-DVD study (Oral
    Rivaroxaban Versus
    Standard Therapy), 121
electrical alternans, 80
electrocardiogram (ECG), 19–
    20, 21*t*, 278
  for ACS, 60, 63*t*, 66*f*
  for A-fib, 148
  for atrial flutter, 205, 206*f*
  for heart failure, 171*t*
  before HSCT, 135, 136*t*
  interpretation of, 195–197,
    196*f*–197*f*, 219*f*
  for myocarditis, 84*t*
  for pericarditis, 80, 80*f*, 81*t*,
    146, 146*f*
  preoperative, 255–256

for pulmonary embolism,
    115, 117*f*
  of SICM, 142
  for ventricular tachycar-
    dia, 149
  for V-fib, 234*f*
electrolytes, monitoring of,
    26, 231
electromagnetic radiation, 40.
    See also radiation therapy
enalapril, 23, 179*t*
endocarditis, 85*f*, 85–86, 87*f*–
    88*f*
endomyocardial biopsy (EMB),
    171*t*, 171–172
endoplasmic reticulum (ER)
    homeostasis, 35
engraftment, following HSCT,
    139–141
enoxaparin, 69, 70*t*, 118*t*, 120*t*,
    123*t*, 124
epirubicin, 161*t*
eplerenone, 179*t*, 183
eptifibatide, 68–69, 70*t*
ErbB2 receptor, 13–14, 32–34,
    283–284
erlotinib, 57, 57*t*
esmolol, 70*t*, 201*t*
esophageal cancer
  postoperative A-fib and, 199
  RT for, 40*t*, 47, 48*t*
ESSENCE trial (Efficacy and
    Safety of Subcutaneous
    Enoxaparin in Unstable
    Angina and Non-Q-Wave
    MI), 69
etoposide, for HSCT condition-
    ing, 138
exercise, 26, 184, 272–273,
    285–286
external beam radiation, 41. *See
    also* radiation therapy

F

fever, 58
fibromas, 6
fibrosis, from RT, 42, 44*t*
first-degree AVB, 210, 210*f*, 211
first heart sound (S$_1$), 5
5-fluorouracil (5-FU), 57, 57*t*,
    228, 233
5-HT$_3$ antagonists, 222*t*
flecainide, 203*t*
fludarabine, for HSCT condi-
    tioning, 139
fluid restriction/management,
    144, 184
fluoroquinolones, 222*t*
fluvastatin, 153

follow-up testing, 24
fondaparinux, for thromboembolism, 118, 118t, 119, 123t, 124
fosinopril, 179t
fractionation, of radiation therapy, 41, 138
Framingham Risk Assessment for Coronary Heart Disease (FRACHD), 73, 278–279, 281f–282f
Fridericia formula, for QTc, 219
furosemide, 176t, 181–182

G

gemcitabine, 5, 199
glucocorticoids
    for aGVHD, 140
    dyslipidemia from, 153
glycoprotein IIb/IIIa inhibitors, 68–69
glycoside. *See* digoxin
Gorlin syndrome, 6
graduated compression stockings, 123t, 125, 126f
graft-versus-host disease (GVHD), 133, 152
    acute, 140–141
    chronic, 153

H

harvesting, of stem cells, 133, 134t. *See also* hematopoietic stem cell transplantation
HAS-BLED assessment, 205, 206t
head and neck surgery, hypertension from, 99
heart, anatomy of, 2f
heart failure (HF), 31, 159–160
    causes of, 160, 161t, 162f
    classification of, 163–167
    diagnostic tests for, 170–173, 171t
    drugs to avoid with, 183–184
    evaluation for, 167–170, 168f, 170f
    from HSCT, 143–145, 150t
    management of, 173–185, 176t, 179t
    pathophysiology of, 160–162, 239
    risk factors for, 161f
    signs/symptoms of, 169f, 169–170

stages of, 162–163, 163t
symptom management, 185
heart sounds, 5
helical CT scan, 114, 115f–116f
hematopoietic stem cell transplantation (HSCT), 95, 98, 131
    A-fib following, 199
    cardiac evaluation before, 135, 136t, 136–137
    cardiovascular complications from, 141–150, 149t–150t, 151–153
    conditioning for, 135, 137–139
    diseases treated with, 131–132, 132t
    engraftment following, 139–141
    long-term effects, 151–153
    patient selection for, 133–135
    with preexisting cardiac disease, 151
    stem cell harvesting for, 133, 134t
    types of, 132–133
hemorrhagic myocarditis, 253t
heparin. *See* low-molecular-weight heparin; unfractionated heparin
heparin-induced thrombocytopenia (HIT), 119, 122, 122t
hepatojugular reflux, 168, 169f
HER2 receptor, 13–14, 32–34, 283–284
high-sensitivity cardiac C-reactive protein (hs-CRP), 269, 281
Hodgkin lymphoma, 40t, 48t, 132, 132t
    RT for, 40t, 43–46, 48t
Hounsfield, Godfrey, 40
human leukocyte antigen (HLA) matching, 131, 133
hydralazine, 179t
hypertension (HTN), 14–15, 95
    with breast cancer, 272
    chemotherapeutic agents causing, 253t
    definitions/classifications, 96, 96t
    diagnostic tests for, 100–101
    management of, 101–105, 102t, 105
    nursing implications, 105
    pathophysiology of, 97t, 97–99, 98f
    resistant/refractory, 103, 104t

risk factors for, 99, 100f
    from steroid therapy, 140
hypertrophic cardiomyopathy, 235
hypotension, 142, 144, 148
hypothyroidism, 36
    post-HSCT, 152–153

I

ibutilide, 200, 204
idarubicin, 161t
ifosfamide, 5, 161t
image-guided radiation therapy, 40
imatinib, 32f, 35, 37, 79t, 161t, 162
impedance plethysmography, for DVT diagnosis, 115f
implantable cardioverter defibrillator (ICD), 227, 238–239, 244t–245t
IMPROVE survey, 124
indomethacin, 80
infection
    after HSCT, 140
    endocarditis from, 85, 85f
    myocardial ischemia from, 58
    pericarditis from, 78, 78f
inferior vena cava (IVC) filter, 123
inflammation, role in CVD, 269
inotropic agents, for pulmonary embolism, 117
intensity-modulated radiation therapy (IMRT), 40
interdisciplinary team approach, 24, 25f
interleukin, 231
intermittent pneumatic compression, 123t, 125
international normalized ratio (INR), 258, 259t
interrogation reports, for implantable devices, 239
intracardial mapping, 232
ionizing radiation, 40. *See also* radiation therapy
isoproterenol, 223–224, 224t
isosorbide dinitrate, 179t

K

Karnofsky performance score, 134
kidney function tests, before HSCT, 135

L

labetalol, 230
Lambl excrescences, 2
lapatinib, 32*f*, 33, 37, 161*t*, 221*t*
left atrial appendage, 198
left atrial tumors, 1–5, 3*f*
  clinical manifestations of, 3–4
  diagnostic evaluation of, 4–5
  incidence of, 1
  postoperative management, 5
  treatment/prognosis of, 5
left atrium, 1
left-sided heart failure, 164
left ventricle, 6
left ventricular dysfunction (LVD), 31. *See also* targeted therapies
  after HSCT, 145
  incidence of, 32, 32*f*
  mechanisms for, 36
  monitoring of, 36–37
left ventricular ejection fraction (LVEF), 19–20, 33, 36–37, 137, 165–166, 257
left ventricular failure, 164
left ventricular tumors, 6
lenalidomide, 83–84
leukemia, 8–9, 35, 131–132, 132*t*
levosimendan, 176*t*
lidocaine, 70, 224*t*, 234
lifestyle modifications, 24–26, 71–73, 184–185, 270, 284–286
lipid-lowering therapy, 69, 72, 153, 286
lipomas, 2
lipomatous hypertrophy of interatrial septum, 8
lisinopril, 70*t*, 179*t*
liver function tests, 135, 153
loop diuretics, 181–182. *See also* diuretics
low-density lipoprotein (LDL), 56, 69, 72, 140, 153, 275
low-molecular-weight heparin (LMWH), 69, 259*t*, 261
  for thromboembolism, 118–120, 122, 124
Lp(a) (genetic marker), 280–281
L-thyroxine, 153
lung cancer
  postoperative A-fib and, 199
  RT for, 40, 40*t*, 47, 48*t*
lung function tests, for HSCT, 135
lymphomas, 3, 132, 132*t*

M

macroangiopathy, 271
macrolides, 222*t*
magnesium sulfate, 223, 224*t*, 234
magnetic resonance imaging (MRI), 40, 115
  cardiac, 9–10, 19–20, 21*t*, 81*t*, 84, 84*t*, 171*t*, 172
  preoperative, 257
  for venous thromboembolism diagnosis, 115*f*
magnets, CIED response to, 239–240
malignant pericardial effusion, 91
MD Anderson Symptom Inventory-Heart Failure (MDASI-HF), 17, 185, 186*f*–187*f*
mechanical foot pumps, 125
mechanical prosthetic heart valves, 260–261, 261*t*
MEDENOX study (Medical Patients with Enoxaparin), 124
melphalan, 138–139, 199
menopause, CVD risk with, 275–276
mesothelioma, 9
metabolic syndrome, 73, 273–274, 274*t*, 280*t*
metastatic tumors, to heart, 9
methotrexate, pericarditis from, 79*t*
metoprolol, 23, 70*t*, 179*t*, 181, 201*t*–202*t*, 230
milrinone, 176*t*
mitomycin, cardiotoxicity of, 161*t*
mitoxantrone, cardiotoxicity of, 161*t*
modifiable risk factors
  for CAD, 56, 56*f*, 71–72
  for hypertension, 99, 100*f*
morphine, 69, 70*t*
motesanib, 97*t*
mucositis, 145
multigated acquisition (MUGA) scan, 19–20, 21*t*, 36
  for heart failure diagnosis, 172
  before HSCT, 135, 136*t*, 137
  preoperative, 257
multiple-hit hypothesis, 271–272, 284
multiple myeloma, 132*t*
myeloablation, 137
myeloablative conditioning, for HSCT, 137–138

myelodysplastic syndrome, 132*t*
myocardial damage, from RT, 42, 44*t*
myocardial infarction, 160, 252–253
myocardial ischemia, 47, 56–58, 160
  chemotherapeutic agents causing, 253*t*
  definition/diagnosis of, 58–64, 59*t*, 62*f*, 63*t*–64*t*
  VT caused by, 231
myocardial perfusion imaging, 36*t*, 60–61, 171*t*
myocardial "stunning," 141. *See also* myocarditis
myocarditis, 82–83, 83*f*
  from cytokine release, 141
  diagnostic studies of, 84, 84*t*
  medical management of, 84–85
  pathophysiology of, 83
  signs/symptoms of, 83–84, 84*f*
myoglobin (biomarker), 59*t*
myopericarditis, 91
myxomas, 2

N

narcotics, BP monitoring with, 103
National Health and Nutrition Examination Survey (NHANES), 271
National Marrow Donor Program, 131, 133, 135
NBG pacemaker code, 237*f*
nebivolol, 230
nesiritide, 176*t*
neuregulin, 283–284
neutropenia, 145
New York Heart Association (NYHA), functional classification of heart failure, 159, 167, 167*t*
nilotinib, 221*t*
nitrates, 69, 70*t*, 71
nitric oxide (NO), 97
nitroglycerin, 69, 70*t*, 71, 176*t*
non-Hodgkin lymphoma, 132, 132*t*
  A-fib with, 199
  RT for, 40*t*, 48*t*
nonischemic cardiomyopathy, 152, 160
nonmodifiable risk factors
  for CAD, 56, 56*f*
  for hypertension, 99, 100*f*

nonmyeloablative (NMA) conditioning, 138–139
nonsteroidal anti-inflammatory drugs (NSAIDs)
 avoided with heart failure, 184
 BP monitoring with, 102
 for pericarditis pain, 80, 147
nonsustained ventricular tachycardia, 228, 229*f*
norepinephrine, for pulmonary embolism, 117
normal sinus rhythm (NSR), 197, 197*f*, 199–200, 203*t*.
 See also electrocardiogram
NSTEMI (non-ST-elevation MI), 59, 65, 66*f*, 66–67
nuclear stress test, 60–61, 63*t*, 171*t*
Nurses' Health Study, 270

O

omeprazole, 68
opioids, 103, 222*t*
orthopnea, 164
outpatient clinic checklist, for chronic heart failure, 177, 178*t*
overweight/obesity, 274–275, 286

P

pacemakers, 209, 212, 227, 235, 236*f*. *See also* cardiac implantable electronic devices
 code system, 236, 237*f*
 in ICDs, 238–239
 programming of, 236–238, 237*f*
 radiation therapy and, 244*t*–245*t*
paclitaxel, cardiotoxicity of, 57, 57*t*, 162
pancytopenia, 138, 147
papillary fibroelastomas, 2
paradoxical hemodynamic instability (PHI), 147–148
paragangliomas, 3, 4*f*
parietal pericardium, 78, 145
paroxysmal A-fib, 198
paroxysmal nocturnal dyspnea, 164
particulate radiation, 40. *See also* radiation therapy
patient/family education. *See also* lifestyle modifications
 on ACS, 71

on heart failure, 184
on hypertension, 105
pazopanib, 97*t*, 221*t*
percutaneous coronary intervention (PCI), 262, 263*f*
performance status, for HSCT, 134–135
pericardial cavity, 78
pericardial constriction, 81
pericardial effusion, 78, 89*f*–90*f*, 91. *See also* cardiac tamponade; pericarditis
 diagnostic tests for, 91*t*, 146, 146*f*
 with pericarditis, 81, 146–148, 150*t*
 from radiation therapy, 42, 47
pericardial fluid, 90–91
pericardial friction rub, 79–80, 146
pericardial sac, 42, 78
pericardial window, 90–91, 147
pericardiocentesis, 81, 89–91, 147
pericarditis
 after HSCT, 145–148, 150*t*
 anatomy/pathophysiology of, 78, 78*f*, 79*t*
 diagnostic studies for, 79–80, 80*f*, 81*t*, 146, 146*f*
 medical management of, 80–81, 147–148
 from RT, 42, 44*t*, 49*t*
 signs/symptoms of, 79, 79*f*, 145–146
pericardium, 9, 78. *See also* pericarditis
peripheral stem cell collection, 134*t*
permanent A-fib, 198
persistent A-fib, 198
physical activity, 26, 184, 272–273, 285–286
platelet-derived growth factor receptor (PDGFR), 35
platelet transfusions, 144
positron-emission tomography (PET), 40, 61, 63*t*
potassium chloride, 224*t*
prasugrel, 68
pravastatin, 153, 286
predicted lifetime risk, for CVD, 278
prednisone, for leukemia, 9
pre–heart failure, 272
premature ventricular contractions (PVCs), 227–230, 228*f*
PREVENT study (Prevention of Recurrent Venous Thromboembolism), 124

primary cardiac tumors. *See* cardiac tumors
PR interval, 196, 219*f*. *See also* electrocardiogram
propafenone, 203*t*
propranolol, 201*t*–202*t*, 230
prostate cancer, CVD risk with, 276–277
proton pump inhibitors (PPIs), 68
proton therapy, 41. *See also* radiation therapy
PROVE-IT-TIMI 22 study, 69
pulmonary angiography, 114, 115*f*
pulmonary embolectomy, 123
pulmonary embolism (PE), 109. *See also* venous thromboembolism
 diagnostic tests for, 113–115, 114*f*–115*f*
 differential diagnosis of, 112, 113*f*
 with right atrial tumors, 6
 signs/symptoms of, 111, 113*f*
 treatment for, 117–121, 118*t*, 123
pulmonary hypertension, 7
P-wave deflection, 195, 196*f*. *See also* electrocardiogram

Q

QRS complex, 195–196, 196*f*, 219*f*. *See also* electrocardiogram
QT interval, 196, 218–219, 219*f*. *See also* electrocardiogram
 formulas for correcting (QTc), 219
QT prolongation, 217, 233. *See also* torsades de pointes
 diagnosis of, 218–220, 220*t*
 incidence of, 217–218
 medications causing, 220–221, 221*t*–222*t*, 253*t*
 pathophysiology of, 220
 prevention of, 221*f*
 risk factors for, 218*f*
quinapril, 179*t*

R

radiation-induced heart disease (RIHD), 39
 nursing implications, 47–48, 49*t*–50*t*, 50*f*
 pathophysiology of, 42–43

risk factors for, 50*f*, 57–58
types of, 44*t*–45*t*, 49*t*–50*t*, 81,
  86, 87*f*–88*f*, 99
radiation therapy, 39, 40*t*, 40–41
  effect on CIEDs, 242–243,
    244*t*, 247*t*
  endocarditis from, 86, 87*f*–
    88*f*
  heart failure from, 168
  as HSCT conditioning, 137–
    138
  hypertension from, 99
  pericarditis from, 81
  planning/delivery of, 41,
    41*f*, 48*t*, 58
radionuclide scanning, 81*t*
radiosensitivity, 41
ramipril, 70*t*, 179*t*
rate control strategy
  for A-fib, 199–200, 201*t*–202*t*
  for atrial flutter, 207
rate response, in pacemaker, 238
reduced-intensity conditioning (RIC), for HSCT,
  135, 139
remodeling, of left ventricle, 272
resistant hypertension, 103, 104*t*
respiration synchronized radiation therapy, 40
respiratory-gated radiation
  therapy, 40
reteplase, 68
rhabdomyomas, 6
rhythm control strategy
  for A-fib, 199–204, 203*t*
  for atrial flutter, 207
ribosomal S6 kinase (RSK), 36
right atrial tumors, 6–7, 7*f*, 7–8
right atrium, 6
right-sided heart failure, 164
right ventricle, 8
right ventricular tumors, 8–9
rituximab, 231
rivaroxaban, 120–121, 121*t*
romidepsin, 221*t*
rosuvastatin, 153, 286
RR interval, 218–219

S

sarcoma, 5–8, 8*f*
Sarcoma Meta-Analysis
  Collaboration, 5
"sawtooth" ECG pattern, with
  atrial flutter, 205, 206*f*
screening, cardiac, 24, 26*f*
second-degree AVB, type I
  (Wenckebach), 210–211,
  211*f*

second-degree AVB, type II,
  210–211, 211*f*, 212
second heart sound (S_2), 5
selective estrogen receptor
  modulators, 275
selective serotonin reuptake inhibitors, 222*t*
sequential compression devices
  (SCDs), 123*t*, 125
serum glutamic-oxaloacetic
  transaminase (SGOT),
  135
serum glutamic pyruvic transaminase (SGPT), 135
sick sinus syndrome, 209–210
single-photon emission computed tomography
  (SPECT), 36*t*, 60–61, 171*t*
sinoatrial node (SAN), 197
sinus node, 209
smoking, 24–25, 185, 270
sorafenib, 57, 57*t*, 97*t*, 101, 161*t*
sotalol, 200, 203*t*, 233
spiral CT scan, 114, 115*f*–116*f*
spironolactone, 179*t*, 183
statin therapy, 69, 153, 286
stem cells, 133. *See also* hematopoietic stem cell transplantation
STEMI (ST-elevation MI), 59,
  65–66, 66*f*, 68, 68*f*
stent placement, 72*t*, 258, 261–
  262
steroid therapy
  dyslipidemia from, 153
  hypertension from, 99
  for pericarditis pain, 80–
    81, 147
streptokinase, 117–118
stress echocardiography, 60,
  63*t*. *See also* cardiography
stress-induced cardiomyopathy
  (SICM), 141–142
stress testing, before HSCT,
  136*t*
stroke risk, 204, 205*t*, 260
sunitinib, 32*f*, 35–37, 97*t*, 101,
  161*t*, 221*t*
supraventricular tachycardia
  (SVT), 148, 207*f*, 207–
  209
survivorship, 267–268, 277
syncope, 231
systolic dysfunction, 145, 164–
  165, 165*f*

T

tachycardia, 58, 148–149, 197,
  209

tacrolimus, hypertension from,
  95, 98–99
takotsubo cardiomyopathy,
  141–142
tamoxifen, 233, 275
targeted therapies, 31. *See also*
  specific agents
  cardiac monitoring during,
    36–37
  cardiotoxicity of, 34–36
  mechanism of action, 32–36
temporary ventricular pacing,
  for TdP, 223, 224*t*
testicular cancer, CVD risk
  with, 276–277
thalidomide, 231
thiazide-type diuretics, for hypertension, 101, 102*t*
thiotepa, 81*t*, 138–139
third-degree AVB, 210–212,
  212*f*
three-dimensional (3-D) echocardiography, 20, 21*t*
thrombocytopenia, 62, 67
  with atrial flutter, 207
  heparin-induced, 119, 124
  with pericardial effusion,
    148
thrombolytic agents, 68, 117
thyroid function, 152–153, 171*t*
tinzaparin, 118*t*, 120*t*, 123*t*
tirofiban, 68–69
tissue plasminogen activators
  (TPAs), 117–118
tobacco use, 24–25, 185, 270
torsades de pointes (TdP), 149,
  217–218, 223*f*, 223–224,
  224*t*, 227, 232–234, 233*f*,
  253*t*
torsemide, 176*t*
total body irradiation (TBI),
  for HSCT conditioning,
  137–139. *See also* radiation therapy
trandolapril, 179*t*
transesophageal echocardiography (TEE), 9, 200. *See
  also* echocardiography
transthoracic echocardiography, 9, 21*t*, 116*f*. *See also*
  echocardiography
trastuzumab, 13–14, 32*f*, 32–34
trastuzumab-induced cardiotoxicity, 32*f*, 32–33, 159,
  161*t*, 162, 168. *See also*
  heart failure
  cardiac monitoring dur-
    ing, 37
  differential diagnoses for,
    18*f*
  management of, 22–24, 25*f*

pathophysiology of, 14
reversibility of, 23
risk factors for, 14–16
tricyclic antidepressants, 222*t*
troponin I (biomarker), 19–20, 22*t*, 59–60, 59*t*, 171*t*, 172–173, 283
Trousseau, Armand, 109
Trousseau sign of malignancy, 109, 122, 122*t*
T wave/U wave, 195, 196*f*. *See also* electrocardiogram
type 2 MI, 58
tyrosine kinase inhibitors, for leukemia, 9

U

umbilical cord, stem cells harvested from, 134*t*
unfractionated heparin (UFH), 69, 70*t*, 71
for thromboembolism, 118*t*, 118–119, 122, 123*t*, 124
unstable angina, 65, 67
urokinase, 117–118

V

vagal maneuver, 208

Valsalva maneuver, 208
valsartan, 179*t*
valvular disease, from RT, 43, 44*t*, 50*t*
vandetanib, 97*t*, 221*t*
vascular changes, from RT, 45*t*
vascular endothelial growth factor (VEGF), 34–36, 97
VEGF receptor-2 (VEGFR2), 97
venous thromboembolism (VTE), 109. *See also* deep vein thrombosis; pulmonary embolism
with A-fib, 204
chemotherapeutic agents causing, 253*t*
diagnostic tests for, 113–115, 114*f*–115*f*
differential diagnosis of, 112, 113*f*
nursing implications, 125–126
pathogenesis of, 110, 110*t*, 111*f*
prevention of, 123*t*, 123–125, 124*f*, 126*f*
recurrence management, 122*t*, 122–123
signs/symptoms of, 110–111, 113*f*
treatment of, 117–121, 118*t*

ventilation/perfusion (V/Q) scan, 114, 115*f*
ventricular fibrillation (V-fib), 227, 234*f*, 234–235
after HSCT, 149, 150*t*
management of, 232
ventricular tachycardia (VT), 148–149, 150*t*, 227, 230*f*, 230–232
verapamil, 201*t*–202*t*
vincristine, for leukemia, 9
viral titers, 84*t*, 171*t*
Virchow triad, 110
visceral pericardium, 78, 145
vitamin K antagonists (VKAs), 119–120. *See also* warfarin
volume overload, 140, 143–145
vorinostat, 221*t*
VSP inhibitors, hypertension with, 95, 97, 97*t*, 101

W

warfarin, 120, 120*t*, 257–259, 259*t*, 261
weight management, 184–185, 272, 274–275, 286
white-coat hypertension, 105
Wolff-Parkinson-White syndrome, 208, 235